Inflammatory bowel disease nursing

Note

Health and social care practice and knowledge are constantly changing and developing as new research and treatments, changes in procedures, drugs and equipment become available.

The authors, editor and publishers have, as far as is possible, taken care to confirm that the information complies with the latest standards of practice and legislation.

Inflammatory bowel disease nursing

edited by

Kathy Whayman, Julie Duncan and Marian O'Connor

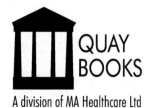

QUAY
BOOKS

A division of MA Healthcare Ltd

Quay Books Division, MA Healthcare Ltd, St Jude's Church, Dulwich Road, London
SE24 0PB

British Library Cataloguing-in-Publication Data
A catalogue record is available for this book

© MA Healthcare Limited 2011

ISBN-10: 1 85642 404 9
ISBN-13: 978 1 85642 404 2

Printed by CLE, Huntingdon, Cambridgeshire

Contents

Foreword   vii
Preface   ix
About the editors   xi
Contributors   xiii

Part 1
The nature of inflammatory bowel disease

Chapter 1
Pathophysiology   3
Louise Langmead

Chapter 2
Epidemiology   29
Clive Onnie

Chapter 3
Clinical features   47
Ailsa L. Hart

Part 2
Clinical management

Chapter 4
Investigating inflammatory bowel disease   61
Siew C. Ng and Nisha Patel

Contents

Chapter 5
Nursing assessment   81
Julie Duncan

Chapter 6
**Medical management of inflammatory bowel disease in the
adult general setting**   95
Kirstin M. Taylor and Peter M. Irving

Chapter 7
Management of the patient with more complex IBD   117
Jeremy Sanderson and Melissa Smith

Chapter 8
Dietary considerations in IBD   139
Miranda Lomer

Chapter 9
Surgical management   159
Sue Clark

Chapter 10
Ileoanal pouch care   179
Zarah L. Perry-Woodford and Simon D. McLaughlin

Chapter 11
Caring for stomas and fistulae   201
Jennie Burch

Chapter 12
Intestinal failure   223
Jeremy Nightingale and Hannah Middleton

Chapter 13
Fertility, pregnancy and IBD   241
Julie Duncan and Lisa Younge

Chapter 14
Care of children and adolescents with IBD   **259**
John M. E. Fell

Chapter 15
Managing the transition from paediatric to adult care   **281**
Kay Greveson and Vikki Garrick

Chapter 16
Psychosocial aspects of inflammatory bowel disease   **295**
Sonya Chelvanayagam and Anton Emmanuel

Chapter 17
**Living with inflammatory bowel disease – a patient's
experience**   **315**
Sneha Wadhwani and Marian O'Connor

Chapter 18
Living with IBD – the role of patient support organisations **325**
Helen Terry

Chapter 19
Supporting and educating patients   **333**
Kathy Whayman

Part 3
Advancing practice

Chapter 20
Organisation of IBD care   **359**
Richard Driscoll

Chapter 21
Developing the role of the Clinical Nurse Specialist in IBD **375**
Cath Stansfield, Julie Duncan, Marian O'Connor and Kathy Whayman

Contents

Chapter 22
Setting up specialist nursing services   **397**
Marian O'Connor

Chapter 23
Getting research into practice   **415**
Christine Norton

Chapter 24
**A vision of the future: celebrating the increasing sphere of
influence**   **425**
Isobel Mason

Index   **437**

Foreword

Rozlynn Prescott

I was diagnosed with ulcerative colitis back in March 2008. Unfortunately, I became so ill I had to take six months off work. My weight plummeted from ten stone to six and a half. Before I got UC, I was confident, ambitious, energetic and sociable, and I loved sport. Within weeks of getting IBD, this all changed. Months later, and thankfully in remission, I discovered I was pregnant. After being so ill, it was a miracle it happened and I soon forgot about the past and looked to the future. Pregnancy was bliss and I felt good again until the eighth month, when I felt the symptoms return. Our beautiful, healthy daughter, Ava Grace Prescott, was born on 26 May 2009. When I returned home with my little girl I became extremely ill within days. I tried breastfeeding but found this impossible, as I spent most of my time, both day and night, on the toilet. My husband finally convinced me to return to hospital. I was admitted immediately and put under the care of my consultant gastroenterologist and his team. I was told that if my bowel was not removed, I would die. This was just two weeks after giving birth. I couldn't get my head around it all, and when I was informed that I would have to have a stoma bag my heart sank. Despite having a wonderful baby girl, I cried and told them I would rather die. The gastroenterologists were very caring and took time to explain to me that if I had my large colon removed, it would mean no more colitis, that a bag was not for life, and that I could have it reversed. It took a while, but they convinced me and I did, for the first time, see light at the end of the tunnel.

Once the decision had been taken, I was booked in for emergency surgery. This was a success, and for two months I was honoured to have a brilliant team help me recover. Since then I've had my ileoanal pouch formed and reversal. It was a really tough time and I ask myself how I got through it all. But I did and it was thanks to the amazing, dedicated medical team I was lucky enough to have care for me. These included the stoma care and IBD specialist nurses, the anaesthetist, surgeons, gastroenterologists, pain team, physiotherapists and dietitians. The ward nurses' care and attention kept me going and they did everything to help so that

I could spend as much time as possible with my beautiful baby when I began to recover. It was all hands on deck and I never had a moment's peace – and that of course was a good thing! Importantly, my family formed their own team and rallied together to help in any way they could. They all were equally fantastic and I couldn't have got through any of this without them. I realised then how important, supportive and loving a family can be, and that I was one of the lucky ones. They dropped everything and were there for me, my husband and my little girl 24/7.

My experience highlights the importance of the multidisciplinary team in caring for patients with IBD and their loved ones. The role that nurses play in providing holistic, high quality care is so valuable. Nurses need to have access to educational material which can then be translated directly into patient care. This is where a book such as *Inflammatory Bowel Disease Nursing* comes in: to help future nurses and members of the team develop their understanding of IBD and, most importantly, communicate that knowledge to their patients.

Kathy, Julie and Marian have brought together an impressive group of professionals and patients – all experts in their field – to create a comprehensive, practical and relevant text. Any nurse working in IBD practice will find this book an invaluable asset to support their clinical care and learning ventures.

Preface

One of the motivations behind the development of this book was the surprising discovery by one of the editors (Julie), that there was no existing inflammatory bowel disease nursing textbook to support and inform her in her new role as an IBD nurse. At the same time it had been identified by Kathy and Marian that the academic IBD modules they were running at the Burdett Institute of GI Nursing would benefit from a dedicated supporting text.

There are many excellent tomes written by doctors for doctors. These texts form an important part of the education of nurses caring for people with IBD. They can, however, lack the practical applicability that nurses need to help them provide high quality, holistic, evidence-based care. Hence, *Inflammatory Bowel Disease Nursing* has been written around real-life (anonymised) case studies with the role of the nurse in mind. We have been privileged to have expert authors contribute to this book, who have shared their extensive experience, and without whom this book would have not been possible.

The book has been divided into three parts. The first is entitled The Nature of IBD. This part includes chapters on the pathophysiology, epidemiology and clinical features of IBD, providing a sound basis for the rest of the book.

The second part is entitled Clinical Management, a comprehensive part which draws on both evidence-based practice and the extensive clinical expertise of the authors. There is a unique patient translation summary at the end of each clinical chapter to aid the nurse explain the key points of the chapter to their patients in easily understood language. Within this section, there is an important chapter outlining one contributor's personal experience of being diagnosed with IBD and their subsequent adaptation to living with the condition. This gives insight into the patient's perspective and the effects of the disease and its treatment on lifestyle, as well as highlighting the importance of a multidisciplinary approach to care.

Finally, the third section is entitled Advancing Practice. This section is aimed predominantly at established IBD nurses and those who are interested in working in a specialist role. Chapters are written with the purpose of providing practical and strategic support for nurses and other professionals in setting up and developing services and specialist skills.

This is not a text by nurses for nurses, but rather reflects the multidisciplinary nature of IBD teams and of IBD care. This is achieved with excellent contributions from gastroenterologists, surgeons, nurses, dietitians, support groups and, very importantly, patients who are at the centre of IBD management. Although specifically aimed at nurses we strongly feel that the book will be useful to all healthcare professionals caring for people with IBD.

Kathy Whayman, Julie Duncan, Marian O'Connor
December 2010

Acknowledgements

We'd like to thank all the contributors for sharing their expertise so willingly, and Quay Books for their guidance. Our colleagues have been a huge source of support, advice and encouragement; Claire Taylor and Marlene Sastrillo deserve particular mention. Special thanks to our families for their enthusiasm for the project and belief in us, particularly Ian Gray, and Kate and Andrew Duncan. Finally, big thanks and love to Matt, Jimi and James for their patience, ongoing support, encouragement, and tolerance of all the disrupted evenings, weekends and holidays!

Kathy, Julie and Marian
December 2010

About the editors

Kathy Whayman MSc PGDip (Healthcare Ed) DipN RN qualified in 1991 and moved to St Mark's Hospital to specialise in gastrointestinal care. She took up post as a Macmillan Colorectal Nurse specialist in 2001, whilst completing her MSc in 2003. Kathy then became a Lecturer for The Burdett Institute of Gastrointestinal Nursing, in partnership with King's College London and St Mark's Hospital, helping to set up and deliver education programmes for GI nursing. This work involved developing clinical modules on IBD care, and included the first Masters-level module in IBD Advanced Nursing Practice. Research interests include gastrointestinal patient information and education, most specifically in inflammatory bowel disease (IBD) and colorectal cancer nursing service development. Kathy coedited *The Oxford Handbook of Gastrointestinal Nursing* and has presented to UK and European nursing forums on education for nurses, self-management, informational care in IBD and colorectal cancer nursing practice. Kathy has now taken a career break following the birth of her second child, and looks forward to contributing to gastrointestinal nursing care again in the near future.

Julie Duncan MSc RGN currently works as a Clinical Nurse Specialist in Inflammatory Bowel Disease at Guy's and St Thomas' NHS Foundation Trust, London. She developed her interest in GI/colorectal nursing during her training at Edinburgh Royal Infirmary. She worked at St Mark's Hospital from 1995 and in 2000 joined the internationally renowned team of Biofeedback Specialist Nurses, becoming the Lead Nurse for the service in 2002. She was active in the teaching and research commitments of both the clinical service and The Burdett Institute of Gastrointestinal Nursing, including being clinical lead for the bowel continence and biofeedback modules. She has extensive experience in developing and leading specialist nursing services at St Mark's Hospital, Royal Marsden Hospital, London and now Guy's and St Thomas'. Julie has presented widely nationally and internationally. She retains part-time lecturing responsibilities as clinical lead for the MSc IBD module with the Burdett Institute.

Marian O'Connor RGN joined the team at St. Mark's Hospital in 2005 as an IBD Clinical Nurse Specialist, and took over as the Lead Nurse for this service in 2008. Marian is currently the clinical lead for the IBD Degree (BSc) module at the Burdett Institute of Gastrointestinal Nursing, providing lectures and tutorial support. On a European Nursing level, Marian is currently the Networking Officer for NECCO (Nurses European Colitis & Crohn's Organisation) and the chair in waiting for NECCO, due to commence from February 2011.

Marian has presented at various meetings and conferences at national, European and international level on IBD Nursing. She also peer reviews articles for publication for the *British Journal of Nursing* and *Gastrointestinal Nursing* (GIN), and her recent publications include two chapters for the *Oxford Handbook of Gastrointestinal Nursing*. Marian has completed the BSc and MSc IBD Nursing Modules, and is planning to commence her Masters in GI Nursing in January 2011.

Contributors

Jennie Burch MSc, BSc, RN is an enhanced recovery nurse facilitator at St Mark's Hospital, Harrow, UK. Jennie has varied experience in colorectal nursing including almost eight years as a stoma specialist nurse, working with people with inflammatory bowel disease, high-output stomas, enterocutaneous fistulae and colorectal cancer. She has written several articles and a edited a book entitled *Stoma Care*.

Sonya Chelvanayagam MSc, RN, PgDip (Learning & Teaching) is a Senior Lecturer in Mental Health at the University of Hertfordshire. She is a registered mental health nurse and adult nurse who has worked in a variety of settings with people who experience either physical or mental illnesses or a combination of physical symptoms and mental health problems. Sonya works currently on a part-time basis, both as a Nursing Research Fellow at the Burdett Institute for Gastrointestinal Nursing and as a Senior Lecturer in Mental Health at the University of Hertfordshire.

Sue Clark MD FRCS (Gen Surg) is Consultant Colorectal Surgeon at St Mark's Hospital, Harrow, and Honorary Senior Lecturer in Surgery at Imperial College, London. She has a clinical and research interests in inherited colorectal cancers and inflammatory bowel disease. In particular, she performs high volumes of ileoanal pouch surgery, and is active in studying and managing pouch dysfunction.

Richard Driscoll worked as a Social Worker in London before becoming Administrator and Patients' Advocate to the Home Dialysis Programme of St Bartholomew's Hospital. He then worked with Vicky Clement-Jones in establishing CancerBACKUP as a leading provider of cancer information before moving to his current role as Chief Executive for Crohn's and Colitis UK. During his 19 years in post he has developed the charity to be the leading provider of information and support to patients as well as campaigning for better services and raising funds for research. He also chaired the working group that produced the UK IBD Service Standards in 2009.

Anton Emmanuel BSc, MD, FRCP obtained his medical degree from London University. He is a Senior Lecturer in Neuro-Gastroenterology at University College London and Consultant Gastroenterologist at University College Hospital, the National Hospital for Neurology and Neurosurgery (Queen Square) and the Royal National Orthopaedic Hospital (Stanmore). He currently supervises eight postgraduate research fellows undertaking higher degrees. He is the Chairman of the Neurogastroenterology section of the British Society of Gastroenterology and Medical Director of Core, the largest UK gastrointestinal charity.

John Fell is head of Paediatric Gastroenterology at Chelsea and Westminster Hospital London, running the paediatric inflammatory bowel disease clinical services for West London, and an Honorary Senior Lecturer with Imperial College. His research has focused on mucosal inflammation in paediatric gastrointestinal disorders, and in particular the effects of nutritional therapy in Crohn's disease.

Vikki Garrick BSc RGN RSCN qualified as RGN in 1991 then as RSCN in 1993. Vikki worked in the Royal Hospital for Sick Children in Glasgow as a staff nurse in the burns unit for seven years in total as a junior then senior staff nurse. Vikki became a Paediatric Tissue Viability Nurse Specialist in 2000, which is where the crossover with Inflammatory Bowel Disease (IBD) occurred. She has set up and rolled out the Paediatric IBD Nursing service in Glasgow over the course of the last four years and managed a caseload of approximately 300 children and families, successfully implementing the first programme in the UK for the home administration of methotrexate for paediatric patients with IBD. She is also a founder member and now chair of the first national paediatric IBD nurse forum as part of the RCN special interest group. This group has been instrumental in raising awareness of paediatric issues and the need for family-centred care in paediatric IBD.

Kay Greveson qualified as a nurse in 2001 and has a background working on a medical Gastroenterology ward and endoscopy. She has been working as an IBD specialist nurse for the past four years, initially at Sheffield Teaching hospitals, and for the past two years at the Royal Free Hospital, London. She is a qualified independent nurse prescriber and is currently working towards her Masters degree. She has particular research interests in transitional care in IBD and screening for latent tuberculosis prior to anti-TNF therapy. She has published on these topics in a variety of medical and nursing journals and has presented both nationally and internationally. She has been involved in various national projects, including the NICE appraisals for anti-tnf in Crohn's and ulcerative colitis, and more recently a RCN nurse advisor for the Biologics registry.

Ailsa Hart BA (Hons) BMBCh, MRCP, PhD is Honorary Consultant Gastroenterologist at St Mark's Hospital and Senior Clinical Lecturer for Imperial College.

Peter Irving is a Consultant Gastroenterologist at Guy's and St Thomas' Hospitals in London specialising in inflammatory bowel disease. He is widely published in the field and is regularly invited to talk on the management of IBD. He has edited two IBD textbooks and co-authored an information book for patients. He is on the editorial boards of Crohn's and Colitis UK and the journal *Inflammatory Bowel Diseases*.

Louise Langmead MBBS MD FRCP is a Consultant Gastroenterologist at The Royal London Hospital, specialising in Inflammatory Bowel Disease with a research interest in complementary therapy for IBD.

Miranda Lomer qualified as a dietitian in 1990. In 2002 she completed a PhD on diet and Crohn's disease. In 2007, Dr Lomer was appointed as a Consultant Dietitian in Gastroenterology at Guy's and St Thomas' Hospitals, London with a joint academic position at King's College London. Her research interests are diet and the nutritional management of inflammatory bowel disease and functional gut disorders. She has been the chair of the Gastroenterology Specialist Group of the British Dietetic Association (BDA) from 2006–2010.

Isobel Mason RGN, MSc, MCGI is currently employed at the Royal Free Hospital as a Nurse Consultant in Gastroenterology, leading and developing other nurses within the speciality and making strategic decisions about improving and advancing nursing practice. Her clinical role includes a busy inflammatory bowel disease nursing service alongside two other clinical nurse specialists, and clinics for patients with dyspepsia, coeliac disease, iron deficiency anaemia and family history of colorectal cancer. Isobel chaired the Royal College of Nursing Gastroenterology & Stoma Care Forum until January 2009, representing the group in the development of the Quality Care Standards for IBD care.

Simon McLaughlin is a Consultant Gastroenterologist at the Royal Bournemouth Hospital and Visiting Research Fellow in the Nutritional Sciences Division, King's College London. Simon's area of clinical interest is inflammatory bowel disease. His MD thesis was on the pathogenesis and management of pouchitis and he has published widely in this area.

Hannah Middleton completed the Diploma HE in Nursing Studies at King's College London. Following this training, she was appointed as a staff nurse within the neurology department of King's College Hospital. She occupied this post for just over five years, at which point she was successful in application for a fixed term nutrition nurse position at University College London Hospitals. Due to the temporary nature of this role she progressed to Inflammatory Bowel Disease nurse and has been in this specialty since 2008. Hannah has been fortunate to have gained experience in the nursing of the patient with both intestinal failure and inflammatory bowel disease. She has had the opportunity to work within specialist teams which have offered tremendous support and knowledge. Recently, Hannah has thoroughly enjoyed completing her first Master's module in inflammatory bowel disease advanced practice, and hopes to continue with her Master's programme at King's College London.

Siew C. Ng MBBS PhD MRCP is a Gastroenterologist at the Prince of Wales Hospital, Chinese University of Hong Kong. She qualified from St Bartholomew's and the Royal London School of Medicine and Dentistry in 2000, trained in gastroenterology in London from 2000 to 2004, and was awarded a PhD in the modulation of immune cells with bacteria therapy in intestinal inflammation by Imperial College London in 2009. She has published extensively and received several research prizes. Her research interests include inflammatory bowel disease and intestinal infections.

Jeremy Nightingale MD FRCP has been a Consultant Gastroenterologist at St Mark's Hospital specialising in intestinal failure and inflammatory bowel disease since April 2006. For 10 years previously he was a Consultant Gastroenterologist and General Physician at Leicester Royal Infirmary, where he set up and established a nutrition support team. He originally trained at St Mark's Hospital under the guidance of Professor J. E. Lennard-Jones. He was awarded the Sir David Cuthbertson Medal by the Nutrition Society in 1993 for his work on the problems of a short bowel. He has edited a bestselling textbook entitled *Intestinal Failure*. He is the chairman of the BAPEN (British Association of Parenteral and Enteral Nutrition) Regional Representatives and chairman of the independent charity The Nightingale Trust for Nutritional Support (1109586). He is the vice chairman of the Royal College of Physicians Nutrition Committee and is a member of the British Society of Gastroenterology Small Bowel and Nutrition Committee. Jeremy has published and lectured widely, and has represented the BSG on NICE clinical guideline development on Nutritional Support for Adults. He is currently the editor of the *British Journal of Home Healthcare*. He became the treasurer to the Coloproctology Section of the RSM in 2009. Jeremy is also Co-chair of the Intestinal Failure Unit in St Mark's Hospital and an Honorary Senior Lecturer with Imperial College.

Christine Norton RN MA PhD is Nurse Consultant (Bowel Control) St Mark's Hospital Harrow and Professor of Clinical Nursing and Innovation at Bucks New University and Imperial College Healthcare NHS Trust London. Christine combines clinical practice with research and teaching, leading a team of nurses and physiotherapists who treat patients with functional bowel disorders. She chaired the 2007 NICE guideline on faecal incontinence and publishes and lectures widely.

Clive Onnie BSc(Hons) MSc PhD MRCP is a Consultant Gastroenterologist at the Whittington Hospital, London, and Honorary Senior Lecturer, Royal Free and University College Medical School. He undertook his research in the Genetics of Inflammatory Bowel Disease, and acts as the Medical Adviser to the North London Chapter of Crohn's and Colitis UK.

Nisha Patel qualified from the Royal Free and University College Hospital Medical School in 2004. She underwent postgraduate training at Hammersmith, St Mary's and Charing Cross Hospitals. She was appointed to the North West Thames Gastroenterology and Internal Medicine registrar rotation in 2008 and is currently at the West Middlesex Hospital. She has published and presented widely at international and national gastroenterology conferences and has an interest in inflammatory bowel disease.

Zarah Perry-Woodford RN DipN is currently pursuing her MSc in gastrointestinal nursing. Zarah has served in the Royal Air Force as a military nurse on a general/ colorectal ward. In 2002, she joined St Mark's Hospital and worked as a Senior Staff nurse on Frederick Salmon ward and then as a Clinical Nurse Specialist in stoma care, where she managed patients with stomas, ileoanal pouches, enterocutaneous fistulae and those with intestinal failure. Since 2005 Zarah has worked as the Clinical Nurse Specialist in Pouch Care providing expert care to patients with ileoanal pouches both pre- and post-operation. She also runs an outpatient nurse-led clinic and email and telephone helpline. She has researched and published in a variety of medical and nursing journals and enjoys contributing to undergraduate and postgraduate education.

Jeremy Sanderson is a Consultant Gastroenterologist at Guy's and St. Thomas' Hospital and Senior Clinical Research Fellow in the Nutritional Sciences Division, King's College London. He qualified in 1984 at Charing Cross Hospital and undertook his Post-Graduate training in London and Australia. He was appointed Consultant at Guy's and St. Thomas' Hospital in 1995. His major clinical interest is in the optimal management of Crohn's disease and ulcerative colitis but other specialist areas include colonoscopy, oral manifestations of IBD and irritable bowel syndrome. His research interests include the genetics, microbiology and immunology of Crohn's disease and individualised medicine through pharmacogenetics. He is a regular lecturer on IBD and has published widely in this field. He was secretary of the British Society of Gastroenterology from 2001 to 2005.

Melissa Smith BSc (Hons), MB, ChB, MA (Medical Ethics), PGCert Med Ed, MRCP is a Gastroenterology Specialist Registrar at Guy's and St Thomas' NHS Foundation Trust, completing research into the optimisation of immunomodulation in IBD.

Cath Stansfield is a IBD Nurse Specialist at Salford Royal Hospitals NHS Trust, and the current chair of the RCN IBD Nurses Network. She has a wide experience of IBD and IBD nursing spanning over 12 years as a specialist nurse, and additional experience in medical gastroenterology and intestinal failure. Her current interests include service redesign for patients with complex Crohn's disease. Cath has a number of publications in national and international nursing journals, along with presentations at both national and international level.

Kirstin Taylor MBBS MRCP is a research registrar in IBD genetics at Guy's and St Thomas' Hospitals NHS Foundation Trust & King's College London.

Helen Terry BA (Hons), CQSW is Director of Information and Support at Crohn's and Colitis UK. She is a member of the Association's Senior Management Team. and her responsibilities include managing the Association's information and support services, including the production of Crohn's and Colitis UK's publications. She is editor-in-chief of *NACC News*, the Association's quarterly newsletter, and she takes the staff lead in Crohn's and Colitis UK's programmes of research and campaigning on issues related to living with IBD. Helen is also a member of the Information Standard Executive Council (Crohn's and Colitis UK is the working title for the National Association for Colitis and Crohn's Disease.)

Sneha Wadhwani was diagnosed with IBD aged 14 years while at secondary school. With the care she received and her determination she managed to progress through education and schooling as normal with no loss of time due to the illness. She studied at University of Leicester Medical School and qualified as a doctor in 2002. Sneha went on to train in General Practice under the esteemed Riverside Vocational Training Scheme in Chelsea, London, and qualified as a GP in 2006, attaining diplomas in paediatrics, obstetrics, and gynaecology and family planning along the way. She ended the year on a high by marrying her husband. In 2007 she became a partner in a large practice in Harpenden, Hertfordshire, and in

2010 completed the Postgraduate Certificate in Medical Education and became a GP trainer. This was shortly followed in 2010 by the birth of her daughter. Her treatment has continued throughout and is ongoing. IBD has been a huge part of her life, and has helped to define who she is both as a person and also as a doctor. Though times have often been hard and some things have been a struggle, it has given her more than it has taken away.

Lisa Younge RGN, BSc (Hons) works as the IBD nurse specialist at Bart's and the London NHS Trust, having previously worked at the Whittington Hospital and St Mark's Hospital in similar roles. Her focus is on patient support, and her service includes nurse-led clinics and running the telephone helpline service for IBD patients in the trust, working in close collaboration with the MDT to ensure continuity and accessibility for patients. She is the current chair of the European Nursing Network for IBD – NECCO – and has published on various aspects of both therapies and the nursing role within IBD.

The nature of inflammatory bowel disease

The nature of inflammatory bowel disease

CHAPTER I

Pathophysiology

Louise Langmead

Introduction

Inflammatory bowel disease (IBD) is exactly what it sounds like: a disease of the bowel in which it becomes inflamed. Specifically, IBD describes an idiopathic, chronic, relapsing and remitting inflammatory disorder of the gastrointestinal tract.

Two main conditions are included under the heading of IBD. These are ulcerative colitis and Crohn's disease. There are also a number of other rarer conditions which may be classified as IBD (Figure 1.1). There is much overlap between the different conditions both in the way they affect people, the bowel pathology, and their association with other conditions. There is also overlap among possible factors which probably contribute to the development of the different types of IBD, such as genes.

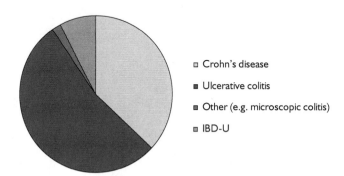

□ Crohn's disease

■ Ulcerative colitis

▨ Other (e.g. microscopic colitis)

▨ IBD-U

Figure 1.1 Classifications of IBD.

The normal gut

In order to understand the pathophysiology of IBD, it is worth revising the anatomy and physiology of the healthy gut. For patients, terminology in the human gut can be confusing because there is often more than one word used for the same part. A simple explanation can make it is easier to appreciate how disease of different parts can cause quite different problems and symptoms.

Anatomy

The human gut (Figure 1.2) is a long hollow tube which starts at the mouth. Next is the oesophagus, then the stomach, the small intestine, the large intestine and finally the anus. The small intestine is made up of the duodenum, jejunum and ileum. The large intestine is made up of the colon and rectum which attaches to the anus. The gut is attached to various other organs along its course, including the liver and pancreas, which are important in its digestive function.

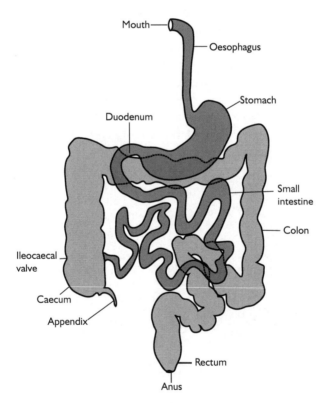

Figure 1.2 The human gut.

Physiology

The overall functions of the gut are to get food into the body, to convert it into useful fuel to be delivered to the organs, and to dispose of the waste products.

Digestion

The gut, the salivary glands, pancreas, liver and gall bladder are all organs of digestion. Food is processed in the stomach by a combination of chemical hydrolysis by gastric acid, digestion by proteolytic enzymes and salivary amylase, and mechanical breakdown due to gastric motility. Further digestion occurs in the upper small bowel, where pancreatic juices containing proteases, lipase and amylase are released into the duodenum under the influence of the hormones cholecystokinin and secretin, among others. Fat is emulsified in the presence of bile which is also released through the common bile duct into the duodenum. The combined fluid volume from gastric, pancreatic, biliary and small bowel secretion, in response to eating a meal, is up to 7 litres. The major function of the small intestine is to absorb fluid, ions and nutrients as the products of digestion (sugars, amino acids and fats) back across the gut mucosa into the capillaries. In order to achieve this, the small intestinal lumen has an enormous surface area, thanks to the presence of crypts and villi along its length as well as microvilli on each epithelial cell (Figure 1.3). Nutrients are carried in the blood to the liver, to be stored or utilised as energy. What remains in the small intestine at the end of this process passes into the colon through the ileocaecal valve. At this point, the bowel content is liquid. However, as it passes along the colon, most of the water is reabsorbed through the colonic wall into the mesenteric vessels. By the time the stool reaches the rectum it is therefore solid, not liquid. Passage of fluid and food along the GI tract is facilitated by peristalsis, which is a coordinated contraction of the muscle layers of the gut to cause propulsion of a bolus along the tube. The act of defecation is controlled by a complex process including sensation of rectal distension and conscious and subconscious control of the anal sphincters.

Malfunction

When any part of the gut becomes diseased, processes can go wrong in a variety of ways, causing illness. This may result in symptoms in the affected organ (for example a stomach ulcer causing pain) or it may cause failure of energy production (for example weight loss due to malabsorption). Symptoms of IBD will be discussed in more detail in Chapter 3.

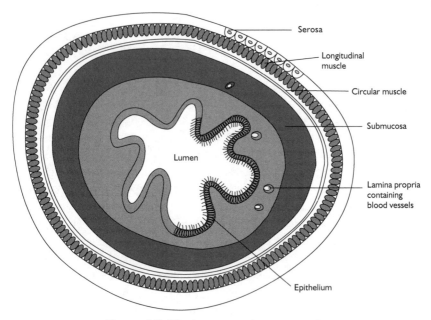

Serosa

Longitudinal
muscle

Circular muscle

Submucosa

Lumen

Lamina propria
containing
blood vessels

Epithelium

Figure 1.3 The human gut in cross-section.

The mucosal immune system

The lamina propria of the gut mucosa houses a large number of immune cells which form the mucosal immune system. This is in constant flux with the systemic immune system, with recruitment of cells to the gut from the blood under complex control mechanisms. The intestinal mucosa is continuously exposed to a wide variety of luminal antigens originating from the diet and resident micro-organisms. To avoid an acute inflammatory response to such antigen exposure, mucosal immune cells behave differently from their systemic counterparts. There is a so-called immunological tolerance which results from down regulation of lymphocyte and macrophage activation by antigen exposure. Regulation of the mucosal response to antigens is determined in part by a balance of pro-inflammatory and anti-inflammatory molecules, particularly cytokines which are in turn, regulated by nuclear transcription factors.

CD 4 T lymphocytes play an important role in initiating immune responses. They provide help in activating other immune cells among a variety of other effector functions. When naïve CD4 cells are activated by antigenic stimulation, they expand and differentiate into different subsets with individual characteristics. These are Th1 and Th2 and more recently recognised Th17 subsets (Bettelli *et*

Table 1.1 Th1/Th2 and Th17 cytokine profiles in inflammation.

Th1 cytokines	Th2 cytokines	Th17 cytokines
IFN-γ	IL-4	IL-17
TNF-β	IL-5	IL-23
IL-12	IL-6	IL-6
IL-2	IL-10	TGF beta

al., 2007). The cytokine profiles of these subsets can be seen in Table 1.1 Th1 and Th2 cells are the two principal subtypes of T-cells and have been identified according to their primary role and profile of cytokine release. Cytokines are low molecular weight peptides secreted by many different cell types, including macrophages, lymphocytes, polymorphs and epithelial cells in the gut mucosa. They have important regulatory effects on both the cells which secrete them, and the adjacent cells, in inflammation.

Th1 cells are important in cell-mediated immunity and release predominantly IL-2, interferon γ, TNF-β and IL-12. Th2 cells are important in the humoral immune response and secrete mainly IL-4, IL-5 and IL-10. Th 17 cells may play a role in defence against extracellular pathogens not adequately cleared by Th1 cells. They require a specific set of cytokines and transcription factors for their differentiation. They produce a family of IL 17 cytokines which appear to have pro-inflammatory functions (Kolls and Linden, 2004).

A breakdown in balance leads to dysregulated activity of mucosal immune cells in response to non-pathogenic organisms, or dietary antigens, and a state of chronic inflammation (Duchmann *et al.*, 1995).

Patient translation summary: the role of bacteria in our guts

There are more bacteria in our gastrointestinal tract than there are cells in our body. The 10^{13} bacteria that live in our bowels are made up of several hundred different species. They reside mostly in the colon and perform a variety of important functions including aiding digestion and helping to prevent infections by pathogenic (disease-causing) bacteria. There is increasing understanding that bacterial flora are also important in the development of IBD. In particular, the way they interact with the immune system in the gut seems to play a vital role in control of inflammation.

Inflammatory bowel disease

Ulcerative colitis

Ulcerative colitis (UC) is a condition in which part or all of the lining of the rectum and colon becomes inflamed and ulcerated. Although inflammation and ulceration of the bowel can occur for a variety of reasons, such as dysentery or as a side-effect of radiotherapy, by definition the cause in UC is not known.

The disease can affect anyone at any time. It is a chronic condition, but the inflammation may wax and wane either with or without treatment, so that a typical pattern of flare-up or relapse occurs between periods of remission.

The pattern of UC in the bowel is very typical. It (nearly) always affects the rectum and then extends up the colon to a differing degree in each individual. In clinical practice it is the macroscopic extent of disease which is used to predict response to treatment and long-term prognosis. For most patients, if the diagnosis is left-sided colitis at the beginning it is not very likely to become more extensive

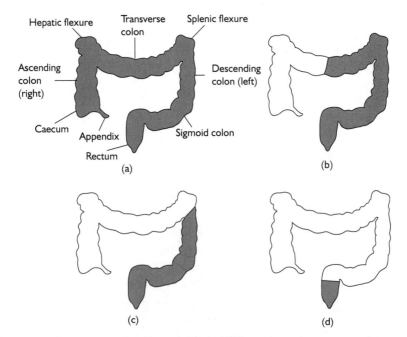

Figure 1.4 The extent of ulcerative colitis. (a) Extensive colitis = pan colitis, total colitis: entire colon and rectum inflamed; (b) subtotal colitis = rectum, sigmoid, descending and transverse colon inflamed; (c) distal colitis = left-sided colitis: rectum, sigmoid and descending colon inflamed; (d) proctitis = rectum only inflamed.

with time or subsequent flare-ups. Similarly, extensive disease does not tend to regress to limited with time. In severe total ulcerative colitis, the distal ileum is occasionally involved ('backwash ileitis'), but this is not clinically important. The extent of UC be seen in Figure 1.4.

Crohn's disease

Crohn's disease is less easy to classify than UC because its effects are more variable in both nature and locality. It was first described by and named after Burrill Crohn, an American gastroenterologist, in 1932. The disease is now recognised to cover a wide variety of presentations and patterns of gut inflammation. The typical features of Crohn's disease may occur separately or together.

Crohn's disease can cause problems in any part of the gut, from ulcers in the mouth to abscesses around the anus. It is classically patchy so that there are areas of inflammation interspersed with normal gut. However, in about half of people with Crohn's disease, the area affected is limited to the terminal ileum and some, or all, of the large bowel. When Crohn's disease affects the large bowel only, it can sometimes be difficult to distinguish it from ulcerative colitis. The sites affected by CD can be seen in Figure 1.5.

Crohn's disease may affect only the mucosa of the gut (like UC) or the inflammation can go deeper into the bowel wall, causing a perforation or fistula to form. This allows bowel contents to leak causing abscess formation. A fistula (Figure 1.6) is an abnormal channel causing a connection between two surfaces that are not normally linked, e.g. between the gut lumen and the skin. These occur in approximately one third of patients with Crohn's disease at some point in their lives. The commonest place to develop fistulae is around the anus.

Another complication of Crohn's disease occurs when the bowel lumen becomes narrowed as a result of healing and scarring after inflammation resolves. This causes strictures which can cause obstruction of the bowel.

Some people are more prone to inflammatory type Crohn's causing ulceration and bleeding of the gut mucosa, whereas some are more prone to 'penetrating' disease which causes abscesses, perforations and fistula formation. Others seem to be more likely to have stricturing disease. Some people have more than one type of Crohn's disease at the same time and some will change from one type to another over time. Different criteria have been developed to help unify the way phenotypes of Crohn's disease are described (see Chapter 3).

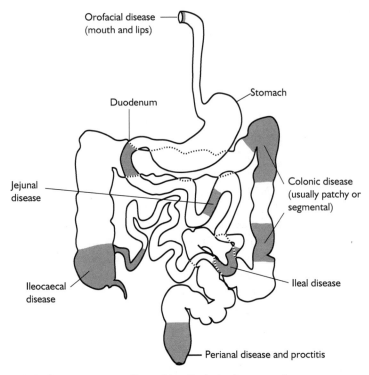

Figure 1.5 Common sites affected by Crohn's disease, where one or more sites may be involved in any individual.

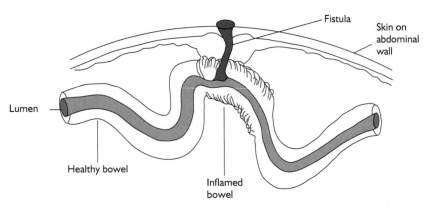

Figure 1.6 Fistula.

Pathology

The macroscopic and microscopic appearances of the bowel play a key role in the diagnosis of ulcerative colitis and Crohn's disease.

Ulcerative colitis

The hallmark of UC is diffuse mucosal inflammation (Figure 1.7(a)). There is hyperaemia, granularity, surface pus and blood. In more severe cases there may be extensive ulceration. Healing is by granulation and can lead to formation of multiple pseudopolyps.

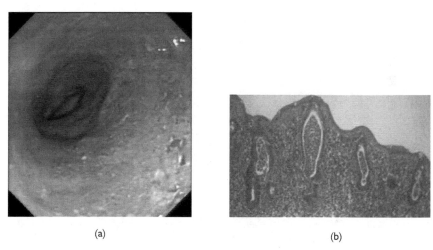

(a)   (b)

Figure 1.7 (a) Colonoscopic appearance of ulcerative colitis; (b) microscopic appearance of ulcerative colitis – intense inflammatory cell infiltration of the lamina propria, goblet cell depletion and crypt abscesses.

Histopathology

Microscopically, acute and chronic inflammatory cells infiltrate the lamina propria and crypts producing crypt abscesses (Figure 1.7(b)). Crypt architecture is distorted with shortened and bifid crypts. Goblet cells appear depleted due to loss of mucin. The mucosa is oedematous with epithelial ulceration.

In long-standing ulcerative colitis chronic inflammation may lead to dysplasia, in which epithelial cell nuclei are enlarged, crowded and lose their polarity. Colonic carcinoma may also occur.

Crohn's disease

Typically Crohn's disease causes inflammation in segments with normal gut in between (skip lesions). Initially there is enlargement of lymphoid follicles with surrounding erythema, visible as red ring or small aphthous ulcer. Superficial ulceration progresses to deep fissuring ulcers with the normal mucosa between appearing like cobblestones (cobblestoning) as shown in Figure 1.8(a).

Inflammation and fibrosis predispose to intestinal strictures, presenting with obstructing symptoms, and to local perforation of the gut wall, leading to abscess formation or fistulation.

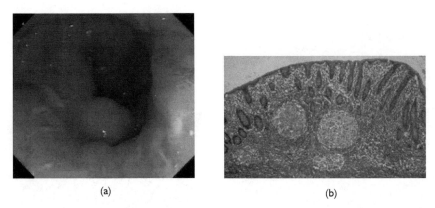

(a)   (b)

Figure 1.8 (a) Endoscopic view of Crohn's colitis; (b) histopathology slide of Crohn's colitis. Three large epithelioid granulomas with multinucleate giant cells are visible.

Histopathology

In Crohn's disease the hallmark is transmural chronic inflammation with inflammatory cell infiltration, with ulceration and formation of microabscesses throughout all layers of the gut wall (Figure 1.8(b)). Noncaseating granulomas are found in about 25% of patients investigated with colonoscopic biopsies, and in 60% of those examined after surgical resection of the bowel. This does not appear to be an important independent factor in prognosis.

There is an increased risk of cancer in chronically inflamed areas of small intestinal, anorectal, and, particularly, colorectal mucosa.

IBD (unclassified)

In some patients with chronic colitis, the pathological features are not typical of either ulcerative colitis or Crohn's disease. The term IBD (unclassified) (IBD-U) or 'colitis of uncertain type or etiology' (CUTE) is preferable to the term 'indeterminate' colitis.

Aetiology

The cause of IBD is unknown, but a widely accepted hypothesis is that in genetically predisposed individuals, luminal bacteria (or their products) gain access to the gut mucosa through an abnormally permeable epithelial layer, triggering an inappropriately prolonged and/or severe mucosal inflammatory response (Figures 1.9 and 1.10).

Different mechanisms may account for subsets of disease. For example, various genetic polymorphisms of proteins which sense, or otherwise interact with, the microbial environment in the gut have been shown to predispose to Crohn's disease. This seems to be consistent with the proposal that the disease results, at least in some individuals, from an inappropriate immunologic response to the normal commensal microbiota. However, molecular analysis of the gut microbiota has raised the possibility that a subset of patients with Crohn's disease or ulcerative colitis have an abnormal or altered microbial composition in the gut.

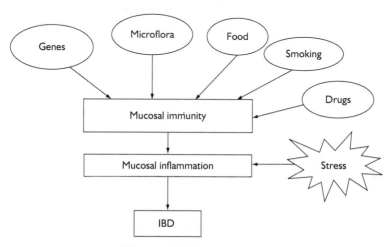

Figure 1.9 Triggers in IBD.

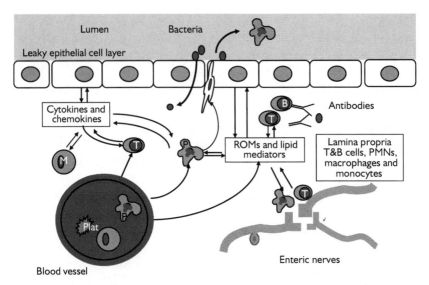

Figure 1.10 Diagrammatic representation of luminal and mucosal events leading to chronic inflammation in IBD. PMN = polymorphonucleocyte; M = macrophage; T = T lymphocyte; P = PMN; Plat = platelet; ROM = reactive oxygen metabolite.

Genetic factors

The importance of genes in IBD first became apparent when studies showed that relatives of people with IBD were more likely to develop the condition themselves. The risk of IBD is increased 10-fold in the first-degree relatives of patients and there is a high concordance rate for identical twins, particularly in Crohn's disease.

Extensive research over the last few years has helped to unravel the genetics of IBD. Ulcerative colitis and Crohn's disease are likely to be related, heterogeneous polygenic disorders. Genetic studies show that the two diseases are distinct, sharing some, but not all susceptibility genes. Genome scanning techniques using microsatellite markers have been employed to highlight areas of chromosomes linked to disease such as those on chromosomes 12 (IBD2) and 16 (IBD1) (Cavanaugh, 2001). Some of the pathophysiological abnormalities in IBD, such as abnormal immune regulation, increased gut permeability and defective colonic mucus, are probably genetically determined, while the clinical variability of IBD may also reflect genetic heterogeneity.

The contribution of genes to the development of IBD is, however, relatively small. For example, someone with two copies of the high-risk version of the IBD1

Patient translation summary
If I have IBD, will my children get it?

- Crohn's disease runs in families more than UC.
- The chance of developing IBD is higher for closer relatives than distant ones.
- Certain racial groups, such as Jews, have a higher incidence of IBD.
- Siblings > parents > children are at the highest risk of getting IBD.
- A sibling of someone with Crohn's disease is 20–40 times more likely to develop IBD than a member of the general population.
- Overall risk for a first degree relative is about 1 in 15.
- 90–95% of brothers or sisters of someone with IBD will not develop it.
- For UC, the risk is less.
- When both parents have IBD, their children have about a 1 in 3 chance of also developing IBD.

Identical twins are exact genetic copies of each other. If one twin develops Crohn's disease, the other has about a 50% chance of getting it too. If the development of IBD was entirely due to genes, you would expect that if one twin has IBD then the other would always get it too. The fact that they don't tells us something – other factors must be involved too.

gene (one from each parent) is between 20 and 40 times more likely to develop Crohn's disease than somebody with two low-risk copies. However, they still only have about a 1 in 30 chance of developing Crohn's. Put another way, over 95% of people with two copies of the high-risk version do not develop Crohn's disease.

To understand some of the recent advances in IBD genetics it might be worth revising some of the basics!

Humans have about 30,000 genes. These genes, combined with other factors, are responsible for determining what we look like and what illnesses we get. Human genetic material is stored in the nucleus of cells in 23 pairs of chromosomes which contain our DNA (deoxyribonucleic acid). We inherit one of each pair of chromosomes from each of our parents. Therefore we all have two copies of every gene. Genes are a code for every aspect of humans as individuals.

In the simplest form there may only be two possible variables for a gene. Each variable is called an allele. An individual may therefore carry two of one allele (homozygote) or one of each allele (heterozygote) (see Figure 1.11). For some genes there is very little variation and the majority of the population have a single common allele (often called wild-type). A gene mutation occurs when an unusual

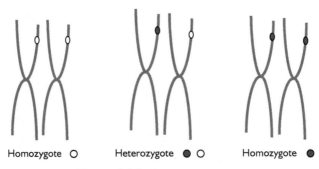

Homozygote ○   Heterozygote ● ○   Homozygote ●

Figure 1.11 Genetic variation.

change is seen in the allele which may effect the way the gene product functions. A person with one copy of a mutated allele is termed a heterozygote and someone with two copies is a homozygote.

NOD2

The most significant advance in the genetics of IBD relates to a gene location on chromosome 16, IBD1, which contributes to susceptibility to Crohn's disease. The NOD2 gene, renamed capsase-activating recruitment domain (CARD 15) gene, is located in the peak region of linkage on chromosome 16. It has been established that three mutations are associated with Crohn's disease. There is a greater than forty-fold increased risk of Crohn's disease for individuals who are homozygous for all three. About 40% of European patients with familial Crohn's disease carry one of the three NOD2 mutations. NOD2 mutations predispose in particular to fibrostenosing small-bowel and right-sided colonic Crohn's disease. The protein encoded by wild-type (normal) NOD2 is an intracellular pattern recognition receptor that can be activated by a component of bacterial peptidoglycan. NOD2 is therefore implicated in susceptibility to Crohn's disease through a disruption of the innate immune response to bacterial components (Ogura *et al.*, 2001).

However, because NOD2 mutations account for only 20–30% of cases and are not linked with Crohn's disease in Japanese and others of Oriental descent, this genetic risk factor, like others, is neither necessary nor sufficient for the development of Crohn's disease.

Autophagy-related gene defects

Autophagy (self-eating) is a normal cellular event in the homeostatic control of growth and development by which cellular components are degraded or recycled. It is also central to the processing of intracellular pathogens. Variants in the autophagy-related 16-like 1 gene (ATLG 16L1) (Hampe *et al.*, 2007) and the IRGM gene (immunity related GTPase family, M) have been confirmed as genetic susceptibility factors for Crohn's disease but not ulcerative colitis (Massey and Parkes, 2007). The resulting increased intracellular bacterial load may lead to the secondary TH1 activity within the mucosa that characterizes Crohn's disease.

Interleukin-23 receptor (IL-23 R)
Several polymorphisms of the gene encoding IL-23 R have been linked with Crohn's disease (conferring protection or risk), and also contribute to the risk of ulcerative colitis (Dubinsky *et al.*, 2007). IL-23 is a pivotal cytokine in the generation of TH17 effector cells and interleukin-17 (IL-17), which contribute to chronic mucosal inflammatory disease, particularly Crohn's disease (see below).

The ECM locus (extracellular matrix protein I)
This has recently been identified as a susceptibility locus for ulcerative colitis (Consortium UIG, 2009). The extracellular matrix protein 1 encoded here is a glycoprotein expressed in the small and large bowel that interacts with the basement membrane, inhibits matrix metalloproteinase 9, and can activate NF-κB.

Recently much work has been focused on genes that may determine aspects of clinical phenotype such as disease extent or severity, or response to treatment. Identification of these genes in the future may lead to better prognostication and targeting of therapy.

Environmental factors
Epidemiological evidence has identified a number of environmental factors which appear to play a causative role in IBD (Table 1.2). Refer to Chapter 2 for further detail.

Factors which have been implicated in aetiology include cow's milk products in UC, and microparticles and increased consumption of refined sugar in Crohn's disease.

Breastfeeding and cows' milk
Several studies have suggested that breastfeeding may protect against developing IBD. The length of time for which breastfeeding occurs may also be important (benefits up to 1 year have been suggested). It may be related to delaying exposure to cow's milk. Up to 5% of patients with ulcerative colitis improve by avoiding cow's milk (Wright and Truelove, 1965), but no definite causative role or individual component has ever been established.

Table 1.2 Possible environmental disease-modifying factors in IBD.

Crohn's disease	Ulcerative colitis
Smoking	Non-smoking
Mycobacterium paratuberculosis	Milk (rarely)
Measles	Enteric infection
MMR vaccine	
NSAIDs	NSAIDs
Antibiotics	Antibiotics
Oral contraceptives	Oral contraceptives
Stress	Stress
Dietary factors	

Sugar and refined carbohydrate
Epidemiological studies have suggested that patients with Crohn's disease eat more sugar and sweets than control individuals (Mayberry *et al.*, 1981). However, restriction of dietary sugar has not been shown to produce clinical benefit. It is possible that a higher intake of sugar and refined carbohydrate may be a result of IBD rather than a cause. In addition, diets high in these substances are found chiefly in the developed world, and may simply be confounding factors.

Fibre
The role of dietary fibre is not clear. Some studies have shown that fibre intake is lower in patients with IBD. However, this may be because fibre could exacerbate symptoms in people with active disease (Galvez *et al.*, 2005).

Margarine
The role of fat, particularly chemically processed hydrogenated fats such as margarine was in part prompted by the geographical distribution of Crohn's and UC, and the fact that IBD was first recognised around the time that margarine was introduced into Western diets. Studies examining an association between IBD and margarine have produced conflicting results, as have those examining the relative contributions of saturated and unsaturated fats (Maclean *et al.*, 2005).

In support of a role for dietary factors in its aetiology, the use of elemental diets in Crohn's disease produces symptomatic and objective remission in up to

90% of compliant patients; however, on return to normal eating most patients soon relapse (Hunter, 1998).

Smoking

The explanation for the relationship between cigarette smoking and inflammatory bowel disease remains an enigma. Many case control studies confirm the negative association of smoking with ulcerative colitis and conversely a positive association with Crohn's disease (Calkins, 1989). Only 1 in 8 people with UC smoke, compared with about 1 in 4 of the general population in the UK. In contrast, Crohn's is a disease of smokers, with some studies showing that more than half of people with Crohn's disease smoke.

It is also evident that smoking among patients with Crohn's disease predisposes to relapse (Duffy *et al.*, 1990) and recurrence after surgery (Sutherland *et al.*, 1990). Smoking also decreases the effectiveness of some treatments.

Most importantly, stopping smoking is an effective treatment for active Crohn's and decreases the chance of having a disease flare by more than 50%. The beneficial effects on relapse rate and on the need for corticosteroid and immunosuppressive therapy have been shown clearly (Cosnes, 2001). The beneficial effects of giving up smoking occur fairly rapidly and are long lasting, with ex-smokers having similar risks of relapse as those who have never smoked.

The reason why Crohn's is associated with smoking, but UC with non-smoking, is not clear, although many theories have been suggested. These include that smoking alters the quality of mucus produced by the bowel (mucus protects the lining of the bowel); that it alters the way the bowel contracts; that it alters blood supply to the gut; that it has effects on the immune system; and that it has a direct effect on inflammation within the bowel itself.

Hygiene theory

The fact that IBD is more common in the West prompted the theory that an increase in standards of hygiene might somehow predispose people to IBD. The thinking behind this relates to the development of the immune system. As sanitation standards increase, children are exposed to fewer infections and encounter them later in life. Why infections should protect against IBD is unclear, but similar associations have been seen with asthma and multiple sclerosis.

Infective agents

The resemblance of ulcerative colitis to infective diarrhoea and Crohn's disease to intestinal tuberculosis has led to a wide search for infective agents to which IBD

> ## Patient translation summary
>
> ### Smoking in Crohn's disease
> - Increases the risk of developing Crohn's disease
> - Makes Crohn's disease more active
> - Makes medications used to treat Crohn's disease less effective
> - Makes recurrence of Crohn's disease after surgery worse
>
> ### Stopping smoking
> - Is an effective treatment for active Crohn's
> - Decreases the chance of having a disease flare by more than 50%
> - Works quickly; ex-smokers have similar risk of relapse as those who have never smoked
> - It's never too late!

could be attributed. As yet no single agent has been confirmed in a causal role, but a number have been implicated as either initiating or perpetuating the mucosal inflammation.

Escherichia coli (E. coli)
Several groups have identified a virulent form of enteroadherent *E. coli* in patients with Crohn's disease (Rhodes, 2007). Whether this is causal or consequential to defective innate immunity is unclear.

Measles virus
Earlier claims that measles virus and measles vaccination may predispose to Crohn's disease have been discounted.

Mycobacterium paratuberculosis
The observation that pathological processes in Crohn's disease closely resemble those of intestinal tuberculosis, and particularly Johne's disease in cattle, which is caused by *Mycobacterium paratuberculosis*, has led to investigation of the role of this agent in human IBD. The initial isolation of *M. paratuberculosis* (MAP) from tissue from patients with Crohn's disease (McFadden *et al.*, 1987; Sanderson *et al.*, 1992) provoked the hypothesis of a causative role for this agent. However, these results have not been consistently reproducible (Clarkston *et al.*, 1998; Chiba *et al.*, 1998; Kanazawa *et al.*, 1999). Furthermore, a placebo-controlled trial

of an antibiotic regime which is bactericidal against MAP gave negative results (Selby, 2007).

Drugs

The oral contraceptive pill has been associated epidemiologically with prevalence of Crohn's disease in particular (Cornish *et al.*, 2008). Relapse of IBD may be precipitated by non-steroidal anti-inflammatory drugs (NSAIDs), perhaps as a result of inhibition of the synthesis of cytoprotective prostaglandins (Kefalakes *et al.*, 2009), and by antibiotics, probably secondary to changes in enteric flora.

Pathogenesis

The initiating factor or factors in IBD are unknown, but there is good understanding of the amplification phase and final common pathway of tissue injury in both forms of the disease.

Upregulation of the expression of nuclear transcription factors, such as NF-κB, leads to excessive mucosal release of cytokines, growth factors, reactive oxygen metabolites, nitric oxide, eicosanoids (leukotrienes, thromboxanes and prostaglandins), platelet-activating factor, proteases, neuropeptides and other inflammatory mediators (Figure 1.10).

The immunologic disturbances in ulcerative colitis include prominent autoimmune responsiveness e.g. antinuclear cytoplasmic antibodies (ANCA), whereas those in Crohn's disease appear to be primarily directed against components of the gut microbiota, e.g. antisaccharomyces c antibody (ASCA). In both disorders, this might suggest an underlying defect in immune regulation, but evidence for a primary immunoregulatory defect in humans with either disorder remains to be shown.

Host factors

Intestinal barrier function

Disruption of mucosal barrier function, measured using absorption of 600 kD polymers of polyethylene glycol, has been demonstrated in patients with IBD (Almer *et al.*, 1993). Increased permeability, measured using the lactulose/mannitol test, precedes the onset of relapse in Crohn's disease (D'Inca, 1999). Increased mucosal permeability is also demonstrable in relatives of patients with IBD in response to insult with aspirin (Hilsden, 1996), lending support to the theory that disturbed barrier function may be a primary defect in the development of chronic inflammation in IBD. The observation that permeability abnormalities are also seen in spouses of patients with Crohn's disease, however, disputes the hypothesis of a primary defect and suggests an environmental effect causing barrier dysfunction (Soderholm, 1999). Disruption of epithelial cell barrier function can occur in response to cytokines such as TNFα, which might be released from lamina propria cells in response to a primary environmental insult such as microbial infection. Whether it be a primary or secondary defect, it is likely that once disturbance of barrier function occurs, allowing penetration of luminal bacterial antigens, a cycle of chronic immune stimulation and inflammation is set up.

Enteric microflora
Resident gut microflora are likely to be a major environmental factor in the pathogenesis of IBD. Clinical and experimental evidence highlights the importance of the faecal stream in driving mucosal inflammation. Patients with active IBD show loss of immunologic tolerance to intestinal microflora. Diversion of the faecal stream by formation of an ileostomy can lead to attenuation of colonic and perianal inflammation in Crohn's disease, which often recurs when the faecal stream is recontinued by closing the ileostomy.

In addition, the presence of gut flora is required for the full expression of enterocolitis in genetic and induced animal models of IBD. Animals kept in a germ-free environment do not develop inflammation.

Work from several research groups has linked Crohn's disease with a virulent form of enteroadherent *E. coli*. Furthermore, there is intriguing evidence linking defective innate immunity with an altered microbiota (Sartor and Muehlbauer, 2007). Lastly, antibiotics, and possibly, probiotics have a therapeutic role in IBD.

Dysregulation of the mucosal immune system
Two principle subtypes of T-cell have been identified according to their primary role and profile of cytokine release. These are T-helper (Th1 and Th2) cells (Table 1.1). Th1 cells are important in cell-mediated immunity and release predominantly IL-2, interferon γ, TNFβ and IL-12. Th2 cells are important in the humoral immune response and secrete mainly IL-4, IL-5 and IL-10. The profile of Th cells present in the mucosa differs between Crohn's disease (mainly Th 1) and ulcerative colitis (mainly Th2). Ulcerative colitis has traditionally and simplistically been described as a non-TH1 pattern, whereas that of Crohn's disease has been considered to be a typical TH1 pattern.

This distinction has become the focus for developing treatments which target individual cytokines, and explains why such treatments may not be uniformly effective in Crohn's disease and ulcerative colitis (e.g. anti-TNF α antibody).

More recently, the TH17 effector cell and associated cytokine profile have been linked with several immune-mediated disorders, including Crohn's disease. This is a CD4+ T cell lineage which is generated in response to IL-23. They are counter-regulated in a complex manner by both the TH1 and TH2 pathways. The balance of effector cells in the mucosa is subject to several regulatory constraints which include regulatory T cells (Treg). In the presence of inflammatory cytokines such as IL-6, TGF-β induces the differentiation of TH17 cells which produce IL-17. In the absence of inflammatory signals, transforming growth factor (TGF)-β tends to promote the development of Tregs which suppress inflammatory responses. The IL-23–TH17 pathway is now under investigation as a therapeutic target in IBD.

Epithelial cells themselves are able to secrete pro-inflammatory cytokines and chemokines such as IL-8 in response to pathogenic micro-organisms (Mahida *et al.*, 1996; Sanfilippo *et al.*, 2000). It is likely that in health this helps initiate an appropriate acute inflammatory response to protect the host from pathogenic bacteria or their products. If there is failure of regulation of such a response then inflammation may intensify inappropriately and/or continue unchecked after the initiating pathogen has been cleared.

Deficiency in the innate immune response

When bacteria escape from the lumen of the bowel into the bowel wall, the mucosal immune system rapidly kills the bacteria. However, in Crohn's disease there is compelling evidence that this response may be ineffective allowing the bacteria to survive causing a prolonged inflammatory response. An increased bacterial load in the mucosa of patients with Crohn's disease has been well demonstrated. This may be secondary to defective processing of intracellular bacteria, related to variant genes such as NOD2 or autophagy genes (see above). Reduced production of defensins, a group of antimicrobial peptides secreted into the lumen by Paneth cells in the small bowel epithelium, has also been linked with Crohn's disease and may be a contributory factor. In addition, defective phagocyte function, unrelated to NOD2 function, has been described in patients with Crohn's disease (Wehkamp and Stange, 2006) lending further support for the concept of an immune deficiency state rather than an immunoregulatory disorder.

The appendix

Previous appendicectomy, particularly if done before the age of 20, seems to be protective against developing UC. It has been suggested that T cells in an inflamed appendix could trigger inflammation (ulcerative colitis) in the more distal large bowel in genetically predisposed individuals (Rutgeerts *et al.*, 1994).

Stress

Psychological stress has been suspected of inducing exacerbations of IBD, but, as in other contexts, the possible pathophysiological mechanisms are not yet clear. There has been a recent surge of interest in psychoneuroimmunology, that is, study of the ways by which behavioural factors and central nervous system (CNS) function can influence inflammation and immunity at both systemic and local tissue levels (Anton and Shanahan, 1998; Ader *et al.*, 1995; Reichlin, 1993). Both systemic and tissue neural-immune interactions occur via two pathways linking the brain and the immune system: the autonomic nervous system (ANS) and neuroendocrine outflow via the pituitary gland.

Nerve fibres of the ANS form close junctions with white blood cells in lymph glands, bone marrow, thymus, spleen and mucosa-associated lymphoid tissue. Neurotransmitters released at these sites include catecholamines, substance P, vasoactive intestinal polypeptide (VIP), angiotensin II and somatostatin. These can interact with lymphocytes, macrophages, neutrophils, mast cells and other inflammatory cells which all bear specific receptors for these neurotransmitters (Anton and Shanahan, 1998; Ader *et al.*, 1995).

Lymphocytes and other inflammatory cells also carry receptors for hormones and neuropeptides of the neuroendocrine system. These include growth hormone, prolactin, corticotrophin-releasing factor (CRF), ACTH, corticosteroids, catecholamines and endogenous opioids (endorphins, enkephalins); the release of each is influenced by stress (Ader *et al.*, 1995; Reichlin, 1993). Clearly, the existence of these neuro-immune and endocrine-immune pathways provides a mechanism by which psychological stress may alter inflammatory and immune responses at both systemic and tissue levels by the modulation of cytokine release by lymphocytes, macrophages, neutrophils, and other inflammatory cells.

Vascular factors

Histological changes in the microvasculature, with small vessel occlusion, were noted in ulcerative colitis as long ago as 1966 (Donnellan, 1966). More recently, Crohn's disease has been described as a mesenteric vasculitis, based on light and electron microscopic examination of intestinal resection specimens revealing focal vascular injury with necrosis and fibrosis (Wakefield *et al.*, 1989). In later studies, granulomata in the vascular endothelium were associated with thromboses even in normal tissue from patients with Crohn's disease (Wakefield *et al.*, 1991).

Vascular abnormalities may contribute to, and may be exacerbated by, the hypercoagulable state that exists in IBD. This involves all components of the clotting system with elevations of fibrinogen, factor V, and factor VIII, and reduction of antithrombin III. Abnormalities of platelets are also described in IBD; these include thrombocytosis and increased platelet activation and aggregation (Collins *et al.*, 1994).

Conclusion

Inflammatory bowel disease (IBD) comprises two idiopathic chronic relapsing and remitting inflammatory disorders of the gastrointestinal tract: ulcerative colitis and Crohn's disease. Ulcerative colitis affects only the colon and rectum, while Crohn's disease may involve any part of the digestive tract from mouth to anus.

The cause of IBD remains unknown, but increasing evidence suggests that in addition to genetic predisposition, various environmental and host factors play a major role. Like many other chronic inflammatory disorders, pathogenesis involves tissue damage due to aggressive cellular immune responses, in this case, to a subset of luminal bacteria. Commensal bacteria (or their products), rather than conventional pathogens, appear to act as drivers of dysregulated immunity in IBD. Susceptibility to disease is in part, thereby, determined by genes encoding immune responses which are triggered by variable environmental stimuli. Discovery of several susceptibility genes has shown the importance of epithelial barrier function, and innate and adaptive immunity in disease pathogenesis. A number of host and environmental factors are described, but whether they are primary or secondary phenomena remains unclear.

References

Ader. R., Cohen, N. and Felten, D. (1995) Psychoneuroimmunology: interactions between the nervous system and the immune system. *Lancet*, **345**(8942), 99–103.

Almer, S., Franzen, L., Olaison, G., Smedh, K. and Strom, M. (1993) Increased absorption of polyethylene glycol 600 deposited in the colon in active ulcerative colitis. *Gut*, **34**(4), 509–13.

Anton, P. A. and Shanahan, F. (1998) Neuroimmunomodulation in inflammatory bowel disease. How far from 'bench' to 'bedside'? *Ann. NY Acad. Sci.*, **840**, 723–34.

Bettelli, E., Oukka, M. and Kuchroo, V. K. (2007) T(H)-17 cells in the circle of immunity and autoimmunity. *Nat. Immunol.*, **8**(4), 345–50.

Calkins, B. M. (1989) A meta-analysis of the role of smoking in inflammatory bowel disease. *Dig. Dis. Sci.*, **34**(12), 1841–54.

Cavanaugh, J. (2001) Consortium IBDIG. International collaboration provides convincing linkage replication in complex disease through analysis of a large pooled data set: Crohn's disease and chromosome 16. *Am. J. Hum. Genet.*, **68**(5), 1165–71.

Chiba, M., Fukushima, T., Horie, Y., Iizuka, M. and Masamune, O. (1998) No *Mycobacterium paratuberculosis* detected in intestinal tissue, including Peyer's patches and lymph follicles, of Crohn's disease. *J. Gastroenterol.*, **33**(4), 482–7.

Clarkston, W. K., Presti, M. E., Petersen, P. F., Zachary, P. E. Jr, Fan, W. X., Leonardi, C. L. *et al.* (1998) Role of *Mycobacterium paratuberculosis* in Crohn's disease: a prospective, controlled study using polymerase chain reaction. *Dis. Colon Rectum.*, **41**(2), 195–9.

Collins, C. E., Cahill, M. R., Newland, A. C. and Rampton, D. S. (1994) Platelets circulate in an activated state in inflammatory bowel disease. *Gastroenterology*, **106**(4), 840–5.

Cornish, J. A., Tan, E., Simillis, C., Clark, S. K., Teare, J. and Tekkis, P. P. (2008) The risk of oral contraceptives in the etiology of inflammatory bowel disease: a meta-analysis. *Am. J. Gastroenterol.* **103**(9), 2394–400.

Consortium UIG, Barrett, J. C., Lee, J. C., Lees, C. W., Prescott, N. J., Anderson, C. A. *et al.* (2009) Genome-wide association study of ulcerative colitis identifies three new susceptibility loci, including the HNF4A region. *Nat. Genet.*, **41**(12), 1330–4.

Cosnes, J., Beaugerie, L., Carbonnel, F. and Gendre, J. P. (2001) Smoking cessation and the course of Crohn's disease: an intervention study. *Gastroenterology*, **120**(5), 1093–9.

D'Inca, R., Di Leo, V., Corrao, G., Martines, D., D'Odorico, A., Mestriner, C. *et al.* (1999) Intestinal permeability test as a predictor of clinical course in Crohn's disease. *Am. J. Gastroenterol.*, **94**(10), 2956–60.

Donnellan, W. L. (1966) Early histological changes in ulcerative colitis. A light and electron microscopic study. *Gastroenterology*, **50**(4), 519–40.

Dubinsky, M. C., Wang, D., Picornell, Y., Wrobel, I., Katzir, L., Quiros, A. *et al.* (2007) IL-23 receptor (IL-23R) gene protects against pediatric Crohn's disease. *Inflamm. Bowel Dis.* **13**(5), 511–15.

Duchmann, R., Kaiser, I., Hermann, E., Mayet, W., Ewe, K., Meyer zum Buschenfelde, K. H. (1995) Tolerance exists towards resident intestinal flora but is broken in active inflammatory bowel disease (IBD). *Clin. Exp. Immunol.*, **102**(3), 448–55.

Duffy, L. C., Zielezny, M. A., Marshall, J. R., Weiser, M. M., Byers, T. E., Phillips, J. F. *et al.* (1990) Cigarette smoking and risk of clinical relapse in patients with Crohn's disease. *Am. J. Prev. Med.*, **6**(3), 161–6.

Galvez, J., Rodriguez-Cabezas, M. E. and Zarzuelo, A. (2005) Effects of dietary fiber on inflammatory bowel disease. *Mol. Nutr. Food Res.*, **49**(6), 601–8.

Hampe, J., Franke, A., Rosenstiel, P., Till, A., Teuber, M., Huse, K. *et al.* (2007) A genome-wide association scan of nonsynonymous SNPs identifies a susceptibility variant for Crohn disease in ATG16L1. *Nat. Genet.*, **39**(2), 207–11.

Hilsden, R. J., Meddings, J. B. and Sutherland, L. R. (1996) Intestinal permeability changes in response to acetylsalicylic acid in relatives of patients with Crohn's disease. *Gastroenterology*, **110**(5), 1395–403.

Hunter, J. O. (1998) Nutritional factors in inflammatory bowel disease. *Eur. J. Gastroenterol. Hepatol.*, **10**(3), 235–7.

Kanazawa, K., Haga, Y., Funakoshi, O., Nakajima, H., Munakata, A. and Yoshida, Y. (1999) Absence of *Mycobacterium paratuberculosis* DNA in intestinal tissues from Crohn's disease by nested polymerase chain reaction. *J. Gastroenterol.*, **34**(2), 200–6.

Kefalakes, H., Stylianides, T. J., Amanakis, G. and Kolios, G. (2009) Exacerbation of inflammatory bowel diseases associated with the use of nonsteroidal anti-inflammatory drugs: myth or reality? *Eur. J. Clin. Pharmacol.*, **65**(10), 963–70.

Kolls, J. K. and Linden, A. (2004) Interleukin-17 family members and inflammation. *Immunity*, **21**(4), 467–76.

Mahida, Y. R., Makh, S., Hyde, S., Gray, T. and Borriello, S. P. (1996) Effect of *Clostridium difficile* toxin A on human intestinal epithelial cells: induction of interleukin 8 production and apoptosis after cell detachment. *Gut*, **38**(3), 337–47.

Massey, D. C. and Parkes, M. (2007) Genome-wide association scanning highlights two autophagy genes, ATG16L1 and IRGM, as being significantly associated with Crohn's disease. *Autophagy*, **3**(6), 649–51.

Mayberry, J. F., Rhodes, J., Allan, R., Newcombe, R. G., Regan, G. M., Chamberlain, L. M. *et al.* (1981) Diet in Crohn's disease two studies of current and previous habits in newly diagnosed patients. *Dig. Dis. Sci.*, **26**(5), 444–8.

MacLean, C. H., Mojica, W. A., Newberry, S. J., Pencharz, J., Garland, R. H., Tu, W. *et al.* (2005) Systematic review of the effects of n-3 fatty acids in inflammatory bowel disease. *Am. J. Clin. Nutr.*, **82**(3), 611–19.

McFadden, J. J., Butcher, P. D., Chiodini, R. J. and Hermon-Taylor, J. (1987) Determination of genome size and DNA homology between an unclassified *Mycobacterium* species isolated from patients with Crohn's disease and other mycobacteria. *J. Gen. Microbiol.*, **133**(1), 211–14.

Ogura, Y., Bonen, D. K., Inohara, N., Nicolae, D. L., Chen, F. F., Ramos, R. *et al.* (2001) A frameshift mutation in NOD2 associated with susceptibility to Crohn's disease. *Nature*, **411**(6837), 603–6.

Reichlin, S. (1993) Neuroendocrine-immune interactions. *N. Engl. J. Med.*, **329**(17), 1246–53.

Rhodes, J. M. (2007) The role of *Escherichia coli* in inflammatory bowel disease. *Gut*, **56**(5), 610–12.

Rutgeerts, P., D'Haens, G., Hiele, M., Geboes, K. and Vantrappen, G. (1994) Appendectomy protects against ulcerative colitis. *Gastroenterology*, **106**(5), 1251–3.

Selby, W., Pavli, P., Crotty, B., Florin, T., Radford-Smith, G., Gibson, P. *et al.* (2007) Two-year combination antibiotic therapy with clarithromycin, rifabutin, and clofazimine for Crohn's disease. *Gastroenterology*, **132**(7), 2313–19.

Sanderson, J. D., Moss, M. T., Tizard, M. L. and Hermon-Taylor, J. (1992) *Mycobacterium paratuberculosis* DNA in Crohn's disease tissue. *Gut*, **33**(7), 890–6.

Sanfilippo, L., Li, C. K., Seth, R., Balwin, T. J., Menozzi, M. G. and Mahida, Y. R. (2000) *Bacteroides fragilis* enterotoxin induces the expression of IL-8 and transforming growth factor-beta (TGF-beta) by human colonic epithelial cells. *Clin. Exp. Immunol.*, **119**(3), 456–63.

Sartor, R. B. and Muehlbauer, M. (2007) Microbial host interactions in IBD: implications for pathogenesis and therapy. *Curr. Gastroenterol. Rep.*, **9**(6), 497–507.

Soderholm, J. D., Olaison, G., Lindberg, E., Hannestad, U., Vindels, A., Tysk, C. *et al.* (1999) Different intestinal permeability patterns in relatives and spouses of patients with Crohn's disease: an inherited defect in mucosal defence? *Gut*, **44**(1), 96–100.

Sutherland, L. R., Ramcharan, S., Bryant, H. and Fick, G. (1990) Effect of cigarette smoking on recurrence of Crohn's disease. *Gastroenterology*, **98**(5 Pt 1), 1123–8.

Wakefield, A. J., Sankey, E. A., Dhillon, A. P., Sawyer, A. M., More, L., Sim, R. *et al.* (1991) Granulomatous vasculitis in Crohn's disease. *Gastroenterology*, **100**(5 Pt 1), 1279–87.

Wakefield, A. J., Sawyerr, A. M., Dhillon, A. P., Pittilo, R. M., Rowles, P. M., Lewis, A. A. *et al.* (1989) Pathogenesis of Crohn's disease: multifocal gastrointestinal infarction. *Lancet*, **2**(8671), 1057–62.

Wehkamp, J. and Stange, E. F. (2006) A new look at Crohn's disease: breakdown of the mucosal antibacterial defense. *Ann. NY Acad. Sci.*, **1072**, 321–31.

Wright, R. and Truelove, S. C. (1965) A controlled therapeutic trial of various diets in ulcerative colitis. *Br. Med. J.*, **2**(5454), 138–41.

CHAPTER 2

Epidemiology

Clive Onnie

Introduction

Studying the epidemiology of ulcerative colitis (UC) and Crohn's disease (CD) is challenging because of the nature of the diseases. The clinical presentation of IBD may be insidious, with (for example) the time between onset of symptoms in a patient with CD and a definitive diagnosis often spanning several years. In some patients with CD, extra-intestinal manifestations can precede the onset of intestinal disease by years. Some affected persons may be asymptomatic or have only mild symptoms, so that they may either not seek medical advice or escape detection, as seen in the Nottingham faecal occult blood trial, which detected 52 cases of previously undiagnosed UC (Howarth et al., 2002). In addition, comparative studies of the incidence of IBD between geographical centres have been hampered by the lack of universally adopted diagnostic criteria.

Geographical trends

The prevalence of IBD is high in North America and Northern and Western Europe; less so in South Africa, Australia, and South and Mid-Europe; and rare in Asia and Africa (Karlinger et al., 2000). The annual incidence of UC is considered to be around 7 per 100,000 in Europe and North America, although higher figures are seen in regions more distant from the Equator, the reasons for this being unclear; Moum et al. (1997) recorded an incidence of 12.8 per 100,000 in southern Norway and Bernstein et al. (1999) found 14.3 per 100,000 in Canada. The incidence of CD has generally been lower than that of UC, but has risen to approach it in those regions in which it has been studied over time (see below). Studies from Europe (Munkholm et al., 1992) and North America (Loftus et al., 1998) yield annual incidences for CD of below 4 per 100,000 until 1970, rising in the 1970s and 1980s to around 5 per 100,000. The incidence of IBD in the early 1990s in the

United Kingdom, as represented by the indigenous population of Leicester, was 9.2 per 100,000 for UC and 3.8 per 100,000 for CD (Shivananda *et al.*, 1996).

Evidence for a North–South gradient in the incidence of IBD has been demonstrated in several studies. For example, the incidence of UC over a similar time period in Copenhagen, Denmark (8.1 per 100,000; Binder *et al.*, 1982) was four times that in Bologna, Italy (1.9 per 100,000; Lanfranchi *et al.*, 1976). For CD, Binder *et al.* (1982) showed that the incidence in Copenhagen of 4.1 per 100,000 was five times that of Galicia in northwest Spain (Ruiz, 1989). The reasons for these observed differences are unclear. Although such differences could be due to different study designs, this pattern of a North–South difference was further examined in a prospective study by a European collaborative study using a standardised protocol for case ascertainment and data analysis (Shivananda *et al.*, 1996). They observed an excess incidence of both UC and CD in northern European centres compared to those in southern Europe that did not seem to be explained by differences in tobacco consumption or education.

Time trends

Ulcerative colitis
Within individual population groups in northern Europe and America the incidence of ulcerative colitis is generally regarded now as being relatively constant over time, having increased in the first half of the 20th century (Logan, 1998). The most detailed American study available, examining the incidence rates of UC over a 54 year period from 1940 in Rochester, Minnesota, identified an increase from under 4 per 100,000 between 1940 and 1953 to peak at 9.4 in the 1970s before slipping back slightly to 8.3 for the 1980s and early 1990s (Loftus *et al.*, 2000). This picture of the 1970s and 1980s is also seen in the European studies with the incidence of UC in Cardiff, Wales, remaining constant at 6.4 per 100,000 population in 1968–77 and 6.3 for the period 1978–87 (Srivastava *et al.*, 1992). Similar trends are seen in the Swedish study between 1965 and 1983, which reached a peak incidence of almost 13 per 100,000 in 1980 (Ekbom *et al.*, 1991). Interestingly almost all the increase in incidence observed by Ekbom *et al.* (1991) was due to an increase in ulcerative proctitis, although this was not seen in the Rochester study by Loftus *et al.* (2000).

Crohn's disease
It is clear that throughout the 1950s and 1960s there was a noticeable increase in the incidence of CD in Western Europe and North America. Although some

of this increase may be explained by better case ascertainment and perhaps a reclassification of some patient's colitic illness that was once thought to be UC, it is unlikely to account for all of the increase, especially since the incidence of UC has remained broadly constant over the last 30 years. As for UC, the Rochester, Minnesota, study of the incidence of CD between 1940 and 1993 showed an increase from 3 cases per 100,000 between 1954 and 1963 to a peak of 7.8 between 1964 and 1973 (Loftus *et al.*, 1998). A similar picture was seen in Cardiff over a 60 year period with a steep rise in incidence between 1955 and 1985 that has started to plateau (Yapp *et al.*, 2000). However, increases are still being reported in high incidence areas such as Denmark (Fonager *et al.*, 1997) and Northern Scotland (Armitage *et al.*, 2001) and in Northern France the incidence of CD increased by 23% between 1988 and 1999 (Molinie *et al.*, 2004).

In general, the overall pattern of IBD incidence supports a significant role for environmental factors playing a role in the aetiology of the disease, possibly related to economic development and industrialisation.

Age and sex trends

IBD has classically been thought to demonstrate a bimodal age distribution with two separate age cohorts demonstrating an increased incidence of developing disease. Most cohort studies show a peak in the incidence of UC and CD in persons between the ages of 15 and 30 (Loftus *et al.*, 1998; Lapidus *et al.*, 1997; Loftus *et al.*, 2000; Ekbom *et al.*, 1991). However, although a second smaller peak has been observed in persons between ages 60 and 80, a finding which seems to occur more consistently in CD than UC (Kyle *et al.*, 1992; Rose *et al.*, 1988; Ekbom *et al.*, 1991), this does not appear to be a uniform finding (Lapidus *et al.*, 1997; Loftus *et al.*, 2000). At present it remains unknown whether these differences in age distribution are a real phenomenon or instead represent differences in diagnostic criteria or classification.

There are small gender differences in IBD incidence, with most studies having a small excess of females with CD, although males with CD may predominate in lower incidence areas (Trallori *et al.*, 1991). Whether the excess of females in CD is due to hormonal factors playing a role in disease expression or to the general female predominance in auto-immune influenced conditions remains unclear. In contrast, in UC most studies reveal a male-to-female ratio that is close to 1 with, if anything, a slight excess in males which becomes more pronounced with increasing age (Shivananda *et al.*, 1996; Ekbom *et al.*, 1991; Loftus *et al.*, 1998, 2000).

Urban–rural differences

Several studies have found a trend towards increased incidence rates of IBD in urban compared to rural communities (Ekbom *et al.*, 1991; Karlinger *et al.*, 2000; Loftus *et al.*, 2000). Although such observed differences may be disputed on the basis of unequal access to care within urban and rural areas, Sonnenberg *et al.* (1991) confirmed the trend in a study of Medicare beneficiaries across the USA.

Socioeconomic class and occupation

IBD occurs more frequently in populations of higher socioeconomic class and white collar occupations than in those of lower socioeconomic class and blue collar occupations. The most detailed analysis of this was performed by Sonnenberg (1990) who identified 12,014 patients with IBD from German social security statistics over a six-year period in the 1980s who had been granted disability. A low incidence of IBD was observed amongst men who were bricklayers, unskilled workers or road-construction workers, as well as women who were employed in cleaning. In contrast, a higher rate of IBD was found in men who worked as electricians, bakers and technical assistants as well as women who were office workers, sales representatives or healthcare workers. From this, Sonnenberg (1990) suggested that work involving physical activity or outdoor exposure was protective, whereas jobs in an air-conditioned environment or with irregular and prolonged shift-work conferred an increased risk. This theory would be consistent with not only the observed North–South gradient in the geographical distribution of IBD but also urban–rural differences.

Environmental risk factors

Smoking

Cigarette smoking is the most extensively investigated environmental factor associated with IBD. The effects of smoking on CD and UC are strikingly different. The first report, a retrospective study from South Wales (Harries *et al.*, 1982) showed that smoking is less common in UC than in healthy controls, with the highest frequency of UC being found in ex-smokers (Lindberg *et al.*, 1988), a finding that was subsequently confirmed in a prospective study (Vessey *et al.*, 1986). Results from a meta-analysis suggest that the risk of developing UC amongst smokers is approximately 40% that of non-smokers (Calkins, 1989). Although not consistently reproducible, a dose–response relationship between the number of cigarettes smoked and the risk of developing UC has been described by Boyko *et al.* (1987), suggesting a cause-and-effect relationship. Smoking also has an effect on the course of UC. Boyko *et al.* (1988) reported a lower rate of hospitalisation for UC in smokers. A study of smokers with UC in France showed that patients who stopped smoking developed an increase in disease activity together with a greater need for corticosteroids and immunosuppressive therapy compared with those who continued to smoke (Beaugerie *et al.*, 2001). In patients undergoing colectomy and ileoanal pouch formation, smoking is also associated with a decreased rate of pouchitis. Interestingly, ex-smokers have an increased risk of developing UC relative to those who have never smoked, with a meta-analysis by Calkins (1989) suggesting that ex-smokers are 70% more likely than those who have never smoked to develop UC.

In contrast to UC, smoking is associated with a twofold increase in the risk of CD (Tobin *et al.*, 1987), with a meta-analysis of existing studies suggesting that smokers are more than twice as likely as non-smokers to develop disease (Calkins, 1989). Tobin *et al.* (1987) found that ex-smokers are also at risk, although the relative risk of CD decreases to 1.6 that of the non-smoking population, significantly less than that of their smoking counterparts. However, unlike UC, a dose–response relationship between the number of cigarettes smoked per day and the risk of CD has not been observed. Apart from being over-represented in CD, Sutherland *et al.* (1990) showed that smokers have a worse prognosis, being associated with more frequent relapses, especially in female smokers, in whom the risk of disease recurrence was four times greater than that of non-smokers. A French retrospective study by Cosnes *et al.* (1996) of more than 400 patients followed for a mean of over 8 years showed that sites of intestinal involvement were similar between smokers and non-smokers, as was the age at diagnosis. Although there was a higher but non-significant frequency of repeated surgery in smokers compared to non-smokers (20% vs. 11%), there was a statistically significant greater use of corticosteroids and immunosuppressants in the smokers, which again was more pronounced in females. Ex-smokers behaved like non-smokers, with fewer exacerbations and use of less immunosuppressant therapy to control disease compared to patients who continued to smoke. Although similar findings have been observed in other studies (Breuer-Katschinski *et al.*, 1996; Florent *et al.*, 1996), the association between smoking and CD may not apply to all ethnic groups and geographical regions as several Israeli studies and a smaller Spanish study failed to demonstrate that smoking was a risk factor (Reif *et al.*, 2000; Fich *et al.*, 1997; Fraga *et al.*, 1997).

The results of passive smoking in childhood and the risk of IBD are conflicting. Lashner *et al.* (1993) observed that in children of parents who smoked, the risks of developing CD and UC were increased five-fold and two-fold respectively over those of age-matched controls. However, a Swedish group found that childhood exposure to smoking increased the risk of developing CD but not UC (Lindberg *et al.*, 1992), whereas Sandler *et al.* (1992) observed that children exposed to passive smoking were half as likely compared to controls to develop UC in adulthood. A recent meta-analysis on this subject, however, did not identify a significant positive relationship between childhood passive smoke exposure and CD, or that it exerted a protective effect against developing UC (Jones *et al.*, 2008)

Appendicectomy

Appendicectomy appears to be protective for the development of UC. Gilat *et al.* (1987) were the first to show an inverse relationship between appendicectomy and risk of UC. In their case-control study of childhood risk factors and development of IBD, a prevalence of appendicectomy was found in 3% of UC patients compared with 10% of controls, a statistically significant finding. A more striking observation in a case-control study by Rutgeerts *et al.* (1994) found that only 0.6% of UC patients had undergone an appendicectomy compared with 25.4% of controls. This highly significant association suggested an almost 60-fold lower risk for UC for patients who had had a previous appendicectomy. Similar findings of such an inverse relationship have now been found in more than ten studies. A subsequent recent meta-analysis of 17 case-control studies comprising a total of 3594 cases and 4638 controls showed that appendicectomy was associated with a 69% reduction in the risk of developing UC (Koutroubakis *et al.*, 2002).

More recent analysis suggests that the protective effect from appendicectomy appears to be conferred on those patients who are actually found to have an inflamed appendix at the time of operation (Frisch *et al.*, 2009). In addition, studies from France and Australia suggest that patients with UC who had undergone appendicectomy prior to diagnosis were significantly less likely to undergo colectomy (Radford-Smith *et al.*, 2002; Cosnes *et al.*, 2002) and less likely to require immunosuppressive therapy to control disease (Radford-Smith *et al.*, 2002).

It remains unclear why appendicectomy appears to be protective against developing UC, although several hypotheses have been generated: firstly, patients who have an appendicectomy may differ from those who develop UC in terms of genetic or environmental risk factors, or alternatively, early appendicectomy may modify the intestinal immune response to protect against the development of UC (Radford-Smith *et al.*, 2002).

The effect of appendicectomy on the future risk of CD is less clear cut. Evidence for an association has been examined in at least 11 studies. Although eight of these showed a positive association of a previous appendicectomy on later development of CD, in only one study was this statistically significant. One study has suggested a small protective effect of appendicectomy on the development of CD (Radford-Smith *et al.*, 2002). A large Swedish cohort study observed an increased risk of developing CD following appendicectomy even after excluding a diagnosis within one year of the procedure (thus excluding the risk that appendicectomy was performed because of undiagnosed CD rather than appendicitis). However, children who underwent an appendicectomy before the age of 10 were less likely to develop CD (Andersson *et al.*, 2003).

Oral contraceptive
There have been several reports linking the use of oral contraceptives and the development of CD. In a case-control study, Lesko *et al.* (1985) compared a group of 57 women hospitalised for CD with 2,189 patients in hospital for other illnesses and found that the relative risk of CD for oral contraceptive users was 1.9 (with 95% confidence intervals 1.0 to 3.5) compared to women who had never been on these drugs. In addition, the magnitude of risk was proportional to the duration of use of the contraceptive pill. In a prospective study of 17,032 women from the Oxford Family Planning Association contraceptive study, Vessey *et al.* (1986) also documented an increased risk of CD in women using oral contraceptives, although the difference did not reach statistical significance. A 1995 meta-analysis by Godet *et al.* (1995) pooling the results of two cohort studies and seven case-control studies derived an odds ratio for CD among users of the oral contraceptive pill after adjusting for smoking of 1.4 (with 95% confidence intervals 1.1–1.9). A more recent meta-analysis by Cornish *et al.* (2008) analysed the results of studies which investigated the use of lower contraceptive pill oestrogen doses on the development of IBD. This also identified an increased risk for developing CD, which reversed after stopping use of the drug. It should be emphasized, however that the association between contraceptive pill use and IBD is only modest, and at present it is not advocated that female patients should stop using the contraceptive pill.

The data for UC are less clear. Although the meta-analysis by Godet *et al.* (1995) did not find evidence of a statistical association between women taking oral contraceptives and development of UC, the more recent analysis by Cornish *et al.* (2008) has suggested a link, although the risk is smaller than for CD.

Non-steroidal anti-inflammatory drugs (NSAIDs)
NSAIDs have been implicated in case reports in the aetiology of IBD (Gibson *et al.*, 1992; Gleeson *et al.*, 1994). A case-control study by Evans *et al.* (1997) examined

the case records of over 319,000 residents from Tayside, Scotland. They identified that patients taking NSAIDs at some point in the previous 6 months resulted in an increased risk of admission to hospital due to IBD. Although NSAIDs may have been used by patients to treat symptoms of an associated arthropathy before diagnosis, it is rare for patients to have arthritic symptoms before onset of intestinal symptoms (Evans *et al.*, 1997), therefore suggesting a possible causal link between NSAID use of development of IBD. A smaller but prospective study by Gleeson *et al.* (1996) suggested a much stronger association between NSAID use and the development of colitis, with an odds ratio of 33.1 (95% confidence intervals 17.31 to 63), although to date this has only been published in abstract form. Recent evidence suggests that the newer cyclooxygenase -2 (COX-2) inhibitors are also associated with a high incidence of exacerbation of IBD symptoms (Matuk *et al.*, 2004).

Diet

The response of patients with CD to treatment with exclusive liquid polymeric diets has led to speculation that interaction between certain dietary particles and the intestinal mucosa may be a contributing cause of IBD. Studies investigating associations between diet and disease are difficult to perform because of poor recall and the possibility that diet has been altered before diagnosis of IBD in response to gastrointestinal symptoms. The most consistent association has been the link between increased carbohydrate consumption, especially sucrose, and CD (Riordan *et al.*, 1998). A low fibre, refined food diet appears to be a risk factor for the development of IBD with a high fruit, fibre and vegetable diet being protective (Reif *et al.*, 1997). Similar findings of an association between high intake of mono- and polyunsaturated fat and the development of UC have been made (Geerling *et al.*, 2000).

There has been some interest in the role of dietary inert microparticles which occur naturally as soil particles but are also added to food. A low microparticle diet was shown in a pilot study to be effective in the treatment of Crohn's (Lomer *et al.*, 2001). However, results from a more recent randomised trial found no evidence that reducing microparticle intake aids remission in active CD (Lomer *et al.*, 2005). Data on the use of omega-3 fatty acids in IBD is also inconsistent with both protective and risk associations being proposed (Molodecky and Kaplan, 2010).

Infection

An infective aetiology has long been suggested as a cause for CD, with several organisms suggested as being pathogenic. A case-control study by Gent *et al.*

(1994) examined childhood socioeconomic circumstances of patients with IBD in comparison to age- and sex-matched controls. They found that access to hot running water and a separate bathroom in the first five years of life were associated with a greatly increased risk of CD but not UC. The authors hypothesised that better hygiene and access to household amenities limits the exposure of children to common environmental organisms in early childhood, rendering some individuals more susceptible to CD later on in life. In support of this hypothesis is the observation by Montgomery *et al.* (1997) that countries with a high mortality from childhood diarrhoeal illnesses consistently have a low incidence of IBD. More recently, helminth (a parasitic worm) infestation, which is rare in highly industrialised Western countries in contrast to less developed areas of the world, where most people carry worms, has been shown to reduce inflammation in experimental colitis, with clinical trials ongoing (Summers *et al.*, 2005).

On the other hand, Ekbom *et al.* (1990) identified from the medical records of IBD patients, compared to controls, that those patients with a recorded perinatal health event such as infection or serious illness had a four-fold increased risk for IBD. In addition, they showed that infants from families of low socioeconomic status were three times more likely to develop IBD in later life.

Mycobacteria

Mycobacterium paratuberculosis (MAP) has long been suspected of having a role in the aetiology of CD, because the appearances of CD closely resemble Johne's disease of cattle, a chronic wasting infective disease for which MAP is known to be the cause. MAP is present in cows' milk and may survive pasteurisation (Bull *et al.*, 2003). Initial studies of the prevalence of antibodies to MAP suggested higher rates in patients with CD, although subsequent studies have not replicated these findings (Sanderson, 1993; Van Kruiningen, 1999). Subsequent studies using polymerase chain reactions (PCR – a molecular biology technique to amplify the amount of DNA available to study) to recover MAP DNA from CD patients has shown considerable variation in the rate of detection amongst both CD cases and unaffected controls (Van Kruiningen, 1999). However, recently, Bull *et al.* (2003) identified MAP DNA from mucosal specimens of 92% of CD patients compared with 26% of controls ($p = 0.0002$). Although there is no evidence of MAP infection in cattle in Sweden, yet there is a high incidence of CD in that country, Pickup *et al.* (2005) demonstrated that MAP could be cultured from lake water and that the high incidence of CD in certain geographical areas of Cardiff may be due to wind carriage of aerosols containing MAP from the river (Hermon-Taylor, 1993). However, if MAP were a significant and active pathogen in CD, then antimycobacterial therapy should be of benefit. Although open-label studies have suggested a clinical improvement (Shafran *et al.*, 2002; Borody *et al.*, 2002), results from clinical trials have been disappointing (Balfour Sartor, 2005, Selby *et al.*, 2007).

Measles

Initial observations by Wakefield *et al.* (1993) suggested that measles virus is capable of causing persistent infection of the intestine, and that CD may be caused by a granulomatous vasculitis in response to this virus. However, other studies using both immunohistochemistry and PCR have not confirmed these findings (Iizuka *et al.*, 1995; Haga *et al.*, 1996; Chadwick *et al.*, 1998). More recently, Afzal *et al.* (2000), using full thickness intestinal specimens from CD cases, examined all samples with primers for the three different gene regions of the measles virus genome (N, H and M) to exclude the possibility that one part of the genome was less suitable for amplification than others. Again no evidence of measles-specific nucleic acid was found in any specimen.

Epidemiological evidence for a link between CD and measles came from a study by Ekbom *et al.* (1996), who investigated the absolute risk of developing Crohn's following *in utero* exposure of measles. Four such cases were found out of 25,000 deliveries over a 9 year period between 1940 and 1949. Three out of four of the children developed CD, leading the authors to suggest that exposure to measles virus *in utero* is a major risk factor for the development of Crohn's later in life. However, attempts to replicate the findings of Ekbom *et al.* (1996) in other European populations have failed to show any association (Nielsen *et al.*, 1998; Haslam *et al.*, 2000).

Thompson *et al.* (1995) also examined the prevalence of CD in a cohort of people who had originally received the live measles vaccine in 1964 as part of a vaccine trial, compared to a cohort of unvaccinated controls, and demonstrated a statistically significant threefold relative risk of developing CD compared to the control cohort. However, concerns have been raised about this study's methodology because the means by which IBD cases were identified in these two cohorts differed considerably. Interestingly, the difference in reported actual measles infection in the control versus the vaccination group was approximately 85% versus 0% (Farrington and Miller, 1995). The finding that infection with the wild-type virus was associated with a significantly lower risk of IBD is not consistent with the original hypothesis, especially in view of the study by Ekbom *et al.* (1996). Other case-control studies have not demonstrated any significant differences in vaccination rates among IBD cases and unaffected controls (Feeney *et al.*, 1997; Morris *et al.*, 2000). A recent Cochrane Database review found no evidence that the measles, mumps and rubella (MMR) vaccination increased the risk of developing IBD (Demicheli *et al.*, 2005).

Other micro-organisms

Others have suggested *Listeria* and *Yersinia* species being associated with CD. These bacteria have been suggested as part of the 'cold chain' hypothesis, whereby CD is a result of an excessive response to pathogenic psychotrophic bacteria which can exist and grow at temperatures between -1 °C and 10 °C (Hugot *et al.*, 2003). Using this hypothesis, Hugot *et al.* (2003) suggested that the advent of domestic refrigeration contributed to the outbreak of CD in the 20th century.

Conclusion

There are significant limitations and difficulties in the study of the epidemiology of IBD. There has been a worldwide increase in the incidence and prevalence of IBD throughout most of the last century, with a relative stabilisation of numbers over the last two decades. Several environmental risk factors have been identified, with the most consistent risk factor – smoking – having a paradoxical influence on CD and UC. However, even smoking only contributes partially to disease pathogenesis, and there is a need to further understand the environmental determinants of IBD and how they may interact with the genetic factors that have been identified over the past decade.

Patient translation summary

■ The number of new cases of both UC and CD has risen over the last half of the 20th century, with higher numbers observed in North European countries. The reasons for this are unclear.

■ There is a paradoxical effect from smoking: it appears protective against developing UC but increases the likelihood of developing CD, as well as the need for surgery and recurrent disease post-surgery.

■ Having an appendicectomy for appendicitis is protective against developing UC.

■ The combined oral contraceptive appears to increase the risk of developing IBD, although this is modest and patients at present are advised not to discontinue taking the pill. NSAIDs may be associated with a flare of IBD.

■ There has been much research into possible infections and other environmental factors that may trigger IBD, with results often being inconclusive.

References

Afzal, M. A., Armitage, E., Ghosh, S., Williams, L. C. and Minor, P. D. (200) Further evidence of the absence of measles virus genome sequence in full thickness intestinal specimens from patients with Crohn's disease. *J. Med. Virol.*, **62**(3), 377–82.

Andersson, R. E., Olaison. G., Tysk, C. and Ekbom, A. (2003) Appendectomy is followed by increased risk of Crohn's disease. *Gastroenterology*, **124**(1), 40–6.

Armitage, E., Drummond, H. E., Wilson, D. C. and Ghosh, S. (2001) Increasing incidence of both juvenile-onset Crohn's disease and ulcerative colitis in Scotland. *Eur. J. Gastroenterol. Hepatol.*, **13**(12), 1439–47.

Balfour Sartor, R. (2005) Does *Mycobacterium avium* subspecies *paratuberculosis* cause Crohn's disease? *Gut*, **54**, 896–8.

Beaugerie, L., Massot, N., Carbonnel, F., Cattan, S., Gendre, J. P. and Cosnes, J. (2001). Impact of cessation of smoking on the course of ulcerative colitis. *Am. J. Gastroenterol.*, **96**(7), 2113–16.

Bernstein, C. N., Blanchard, J. F., Rawsthorne, P. and Wajda, A. (1999). Epidemiology of Crohn's disease and ulcerative colitis in a central Canadian province: a population-based study. Am. J. Epidemiol., **149**(10), 916–24.

Binder, V., Both, H., Hansen, P. K., Hendriksen, C., Kreiner, S. and Torp-Pedersen, K. (1982) Incidence and prevalence of ulcerative colitis and Crohn's disease in the County of Copenhagen, 1962 to 1978. *Gastroenterology*, **83**(3), 563–8.

Borody, T. J., Leis, S., Warren, E. F. and Surace, R. (2002) Treatment of severe Crohn's disease using antimycobacterial triple therapy – approaching a cure? *Dig. Liver Dis.*, **34**(1), 29–38.

Boyko, E. J., Koepsell, T. D., Perera, D. R. and Inui, T. S. (1987) Risk of ulcerative colitis among former and current cigarette smokers. *N. Engl. J. Med.*, **316**(12), 707–10.

Boyko, E. J., Perera, D. R., Koepsell, T. D., Keane, E. M. and Inui, T. S. (1988) Effects of cigarette smoking on the clinical course of ulcerative colitis. *Scand. J. Gastroenterol.*, **23**(9), 1147–52.

Breuer-Katschinski, B. D., Hollander, N. and Goebell, H. (1996) Effect of cigarette smoking on the course of Crohn's disease. *Eur. J. Gastroenterol. Hepatol.*, **8**(3), 225–8.

Bull, T. J., McMinn, E. J., Sidi-Boumedine, K., Skull, A., Durkin, D., Neild, P., Rhodes, G., Pickup, R. and Hermon-Taylor. J. (2003) Detection and verification of *Mycobacterium avium* subsp. *paratuberculosis* in fresh ileocolonic mucosal biopsy specimens from individuals with and without Crohn's disease. *J. Clin. Microbiol.*, **41**(7), 2915–23.

Calkins, B. M. (1989) A meta-analysis of the role of smoking in inflammatory bowel disease. *Dig. Dis. Sci.*, **34**(12), 1841–54.

Chadwick, N., Bruce, I. J., Schepelmann, S., Pounder, R. E. and Wakefield, A. J. (1998) Measles virus RNA is not detected in inflammatory bowel disease using hybrid capture and reverse transcription followed by the polymerase chain reaction. *J. Med. Virol.*, **55**(4), 305–11.

Cornish, J. A., Tan, E., Simillis, C., Clark, S. K., Teare, J. and Tekkis, P. P. (2008) The risk of oral contraceptives in the etiology of inflammatory bowel disease: a meta-analysis. *Am. J. Gastroenterol.*, **103**(9), 2394–400.

Cosnes, J., Carbonnel, F., Beaugerie, L., Le Quintrec, Y. and Gendre, J. P. (1996) Effects of cigarette smoking on the long-term course of Crohn's disease. *Gastroenterology*, **110**(2), 424–31.

Cosnes, J., Carbonnel, F., Beaugerie, L., Blain, A., Reijasse, D. and Gendre, J. P. (2002) Effects of appendicectomy on the course of ulcerative colitis. *Gut*, **51**(6), 803–7.

Demicheli, V., Jefferson, T., Rivetti, A. and Price, D. (2005) Vaccines for measles, mumps and rubella in children. *Cochrane Database Syst. Rev.* 2005(4):CD004407.

Ekbom, A., Adami, H. O., Helmick, C. G., Jonzon, A. and Zack, M. M. (1990) Perinatal risk factors for inflammatory bowel disease: a case-control study. *Am. J. Epidemiol.*, **132**(6), 1111–19.

Ekbom, A., Helmick, C., Zack, M. and Adami, H.O. (1991) The epidemiology of inflammatory bowel disease: a large, population-based study in Sweden. *Gastroenterology*, **100**(2), 350–8.

Ekbom, A., Daszak, P., Kraaz, W. and Wakefield, A. J. (1996) Crohn's disease after *in utero* measles virus exposure. *Lancet*, **348**(9026), 515–17.

Evans, J. M., McMahon, A. D., Murray, F. E., McDevitt, D. G. and MacDonald, T. M. (1997) Non-steroidal anti-inflammatory drugs are associated with emergency admission to hospital for colitis due to inflammatory bowel disease. *Gut*, **40**(5), 619–22.

Farrington, P. and Miller, E. (1995) Measles vaccination as a risk factor for inflammatory bowel disease. *Lancet*, **345**(8961), 1362.

Feeney, M., Ciegg, A., Winwood, P. and Snook, J. (1997) A case-control study of measles vaccination and inflammatory bowel disease. The East Dorset Gastroenterology Group. *Lancet*, **350**(9080), 764–6.

Fich, A., Eliakim, R., Sperber, A. D., Carel, R. S. and Rachmilewitz, D. (1997) The association between smoking and inflammatory bowel disease among Israeli Jewish patients. *Inflamm. Bowel Dis.*, **3**, 6–9.

Fraga, X. F., Vergara, M., Medina, C., Casellas, F., Bermejo, B. and Malagelada, J. R. (1997) Effects of smoking on the presentation and clinical course of inflammatory bowel disease. *Eur. J. Gastroenterol. Hepatol.*, **9**(7), 683–7.

Florent, C., Cortot, A., Quandale, P., Sahmound, T., Modigliani, R., Sarfaty, E., Valleur, P., Dupas, J. L., Daurat, M., Faucheron, J. L., Lerebours, E., Michot, F., Belaiche, J., Jacquet, N., Soule, J. C., Rothman, N., Gendre, J. P. and Malafosse, M. (1996) Placebo-controlled clinical trial of mesalazine in the prevention of early endoscopic recurrences after resection for Crohn's disease. Groupe d'Etudes Therapeutiques des Affections Inflammatoires Digestives (GETAID). *Eur. J. Gastroenterol. Hepatol.*, **8**(3), 229–33.

Fonager, K., Sorensen, H. T. and Olsen, J. (1997) Change in incidence of Crohn's disease and ulcerative colitis in Denmark. A study based on the National Registry of Patients, 1981–1992. *Int. J. Epidemiol.*, **26**(5), 1003–8.

Frisch, M., Pederson, B. and Andersson, R. E. (2009) Appendicitis, mesenteric lymphadenitis, and subsequent risk of developing ulcerative colitis: cohort studies in Sweden and Denmark. *Br. Med. J.*, **338**, b716.

Geerling, B. J., Dagnelie, P. C., Badart-Smook, A., Russel, M. G., Stockbrugger, R. W. and Brummer, R. M. (2000) Diet as a risk factor for the development of ulcerative colitis. *Am. J. Gastroenterol.*, **95**(5), 1008–13.

Gent, A. E., Hellier, M. D., Grace, R. H., Swarbrick, E. T. and Coggon, D. Inflammatory bowel disease and domestic hygiene in infancy. *Lancet*, **343**(8900), 766–7.

Gibson, G. R., Whitacre, E. B. and Ricotti, C. A. (1992) Colitis induced by nonsteroidal anti-inflammatory drugs. Report of four cases and review of the literature. *Arch. Intern. Med.*, **152**(3), 625–32.

Gilat, T., Hacohen, D., Lilos, P. and Langman, M. J. (1987) Childhood factors in ulcerative colitis and Crohn's disease. An international cooperative study. *Scand. J. Gastroenterol.*, **22**(8), 1009–24.

Gleeson, M. H. and Warren, B. F. (1998) Emergency admission to hospital for colitis due to inflammatory bowel disease. *Gut*, **42**(1), 144.

Gleeson, M., Ramsay, D., Hutchinson, S., Spencer, D. and Monteith, G. (1994) Colitis associated with non-steroidal anti-inflammatory drugs. *Lancet*, **344**(8928), 1028.

Godet, P. G., May, G. R. and Sutherland, L. R. (1995) Meta-analysis of the role of oral contraceptive agents in inflammatory bowel disease. *Gut*, **37**(5), 668–73.

Haga, Y., Funakoshi, O., Kuroe, K., Kanazawa, K., Nakajima, H., Saito, H., Murata, Y., Munakata, A. and Yoshida, Y. (1996) Absence of measles viral genomic sequence in intestinal tissues from Crohn's disease by nested polymerase chain reaction. *Gut*, **38**(2), 211–15.

Harries, A. D., Jones, L., Heatley, R. V. and Rhodes, J. (1982) Smoking habits and inflammatory bowel disease: effect on nutrition. *Br. Med. J. (Clin. Res. Ed.)*, **284**(6323), 1161.

Haslam, N., Mayberry, J. F., Hawthorne, A. B., Newcombe, R. G., Holmes, G. K. and Probert, C. S. (2000) Measles, month of birth, and Crohn's disease. *Gut*, **47**(6), 801–3.

Hermon-Taylor, J. (1993) Causation of Crohn's disease: the impact of clusters. *Gastroenterology*, **104**(2), 643–6.

Howarth, G. F., Robinson, M. H., Jenkins, D., Hardcastle, J. D. and Logan, R. F. (2002) High prevalence of undetected ulcerative colitis: data from the Nottingham fecal occult blood screening trial. *Am. J. Gastroenterol.*, **97**(3), 690–4.

Hugot, J. P., Alberti, C., Berrebi, D., Bingen, E. and Cezard, J. P. (2003) Crohn's disease: the cold chain hypothesis. *Lancet*, **362**(9400), 2012–15.

Iizuka, M., Nakagomi, O., Chiba, M., Ueda, S, and Masamune, O. (1995) Absence of measles virus in Crohn's disease. *Lancet*, **345**(8943), 199.

Jones, B. T., Osterman, M. T., Bewtra, M. and Lewis, J. D. (2008) Passive smoking and inflammatory bowel disease: a meta-analysis. *Am. J. Gastroenterol.*, **103**(9), 2382–93.

Karlinger, K., Gyorke, T., Mako, E., Mester, A. and Tarjan, Z. (2000) The epidemiology and the pathogenesis of inflammatory bowel disease. *Eur. J. Radiol.*, **35**(3), 154–67.

Koutroubakis, I. E., Vlachonikolis, I. G. and Kouroumalis, E. A. (2000) Role of appendicitis and appendectomy in the pathogenesis of ulcerative colitis: a critical review. *Inflamm. Bowel. Dis.*, **8**(4), 277–86.

Kyle, J. (1992) Crohn's disease in the northeastern and northern Isles of Scotland: an epidemiological review. *Gastroenterology*, **103**(2)392–9.

Lapidus, A., Bernell, O., Hellers, G., Persson, P. G. and Lofberg, R. (1997) Incidence of Crohn's disease in Stockholm County 1955–1989. *Gut*, **41**(4), 480–6.

Lanfranchi, G., Paladini, I., Pallone, F., Ponti, V. *et al.* (1994) Oral mesalazine (5-aminosalicylic acid; Asacol) for the prevention of post-operative recurrence of Crohn's disease. Gruppo Italiano per lo Studio del Colon e del Retto (GISC). *Aliment. Pharmacol. Ther.*, **8**(1), 35–43.

Lashner, B. A., Shaheen. N. J., Hanauer, S. B. and Kirschner, B. S. (1993) Passive smoking is associated with an increased risk of developing inflammatory bowel disease in children. *Am. J. Gastroenterol.*, **88**(3), 356–9.

Lesko, S. M., Kaufman, D. W., Rosenberg, L., Helmrich, S. P., Miller, D. R., Stolley, P. D. and Shapiro, S. (1985) Evidence for an increased risk of Crohn's disease in oral contraceptive users. *Gastroenterology*, **89**(5), 1046–9.

Lindberg, E., Jarnerot, G. and Huitfeldt, B. (1992) Smoking in Crohn's disease: effect on localisation and clinical course. *Gut*, **33**(6), 779–82.

Lindberg, E., Tysk, C., Andersson, K. and Jarnerot, G. (1988) Smoking and inflammatory bowel disease. A case control study. *Gut*, **29**(3), 352–7.

Loftus, E. V., Jr, Silverstein, M. D., Sandborn, W. J., Tremaine, W. J., Harmsen, W. S. and Zinsmeister, A. R. (1998) Crohn's disease in Olmsted County, Minnesota, 1940–1993: incidence, prevalence, and survival. *Gastroenterology*, **114**(6), 1161–8.

Loftus, E. V., Jr, Silverstein, M. D., Sandborn, W. J., Tremaine, W. J., Harmsen, W. S., Zinsmeister, A. R. (2000) Ulcerative colitis in Olmsted County, Minnesota, 1940–1993: incidence, prevalence, and survival. *Gut*, **46**(3), 336–43.

Logan, R. F. (1998) Inflammatory bowel disease incidence: up, down or unchanged? *Gut*, **42**(3), 309–11.

Lomer, M. C., Harvey, R. S., Evans, S. M., Thompson, R. P. and Powell, J. J. (2001) Efficacy and tolerability of a low microparticle diet in a double blind, randomized, pilot study in Crohn's disease. *Eur. J. Gastroenterol. Hepatol.*, **13**(2), 101–6.

Lomer, M. C., Grainger, S. L., Ede, R., Catterall, A. P., Greenfield, S. M., Cowan, R. E., Vicary, F. R., Jenkins, A. P., Fidler, H., Harvey, R. S., Ellis, R., McNair, A., Ainley, C. C., Thompson, R. P. and Powell, J. J. (2005) Lack of efficacy of a reduced microparticle diet in a multi-centred trial of patients with active Crohn's disease. *Eur. J. Gastroenterol. Hepatol.*, **17**(3), 377–84.

Matuk, R., Crawford, J., Abreu, M. T., Targan, S. R., Vasiliauskas, E. A. and Papadakis, K. A. (2004) The spectrum of gastrointestinal toxicity and effect on disease activity of selective cyclooxygenase-2 inhibitors in patients with inflammatory bowel disease. *Inflamm. Bowel. Dis.*, **10**(4), 352–6.

Molinie, F., Gower-Rousseau, C., Yzet, T., Merle, V., Grandbastien, B., Marti, R., Lerebours, E., Dupas, J. L., Colombel, J. F., Salomez, J. L. and Cortot, A. (2004) Opposite evolution in incidence of Crohn's disease and ulcerative colitis in Northern France (1988–1999). *Gut*, **53**(6), 843–8.

Molodecky, N. A. and Kaplan, G. G. (2010) Environmental risk factors for inflammatory bowel disease. *Gastroenterol. and Hepatol.*, **6**(5), 339–46.

Montgomery, S. M., Pounder, R. E. and Wakefield, A. J. (1997) Infant mortality and the incidence of inflammatory bowel disease. *Lancet*, **349**(9050), 472–3.

Morris, D. L., Montgomery, S. M., Thompson, N. P., Ebrahim, S., Pounder, R. E. and Wakefield, A. J. (2000) Measles vaccination and inflammatory bowel disease: a national British cohort study. *Am. J. Gastroenterol.*, **95**(12), 3507–12.

Moum, B., Ekbom, A., Vatn, M. H., Aadland, E., Sauar, J., Lygren, I., Schulz, T., Stray, N. and Fausa, O. (1997) Inflammatory bowel disease: re-evaluation of the diagnosis in a prospective population based study in south eastern Norway. *Gut*, **40**(3), 328–32.

Munkholm, P., Langholz, E., Nielsen, O. H., Kreiner, S. and Binder, V. (1992) Incidence and prevalence of Crohn's disease in the county of Copenhagen, 1962–87: a sixfold increase in incidence. *Scand. J. Gastroenterol.*, **27**(7), 609–14.

Nielsen, L., Nielsen, N., Melbye, M., Sodermann, M., Jacobsen, M. and Aaby, P. (1998) Exposure to measles *in utero* and Crohn's disease: Danish register study. *Br. Med. J.*, **316**, 196–7.

Pickup, R. and Hermon-Taylor, J. (2003) Detection and verification of *Mycobacterium avium* subsp. *paratuberculosis* in fresh ileocolonic mucosal biopsy specimens from individuals with and without Crohn's disease. *J. Clin. Microbiol.*, **41**(7), 2915–23.

Radford-Smith, G. L., Edwards, J. E., Purdie, D. M., Pandeya, N., Watson, M., Martin, N. G., Green, A., Newman, B., Florin, T. H. (2002) Protective role of appendicectomy on onset and severity of ulcerative colitis and Crohn's disease. *Gut*, **51**(6), 808–13.

Reif, S., Klein, I., Lubin, F., Farbstein, M., Hallak, A. and Gilat, T. (1997) Pre-illness dietary factors in inflammatory bowel disease. *Gut*, **40**(6), 754–60.

Riordan, A. M., Ruxton, C. H. and Hunter, J. O. (1998) A review of associations between Crohn's disease and consumption of sugars. *Eur. J. Clin. Nutr.*, **52**(4), 229–38.

Rose, J. D., Roberts, G. M., Williams, G., Mayberry, J. F. and Rhodes, J. (1988) Cardiff Crohn's disease jubilee: the incidence over 50 years. *Gut*, **29**(3), 346–51.

Ruiz, V. (1989) Crohn's disease in Galicia, Spain. *Scand. J. Gastroenterol.*, **24**(s170), 29–31.

Rutgeerts, P., D'Haens, G., Hiele, M., Geboes, K. and Vantrappen, G. (1994) Appendectomy protects against ulcerative colitis. *Gastroenterology*, **106**(5), 1251–3.

Sanderson, J. D. (1993) Mycobacteria in Crohn's disease. *Br. Med. J.*, **306**(6885), 1131.

Sandler, R. S., Sandler, D. P., McDonnell, C. W. and Wurzelmann, J. I. (1992) Childhood exposure to environmental tobacco smoke and the risk of ulcerative colitis. *Am. J. Epidemiol.*, **135**(6), 603–8.

Selby, W., Pavli, P., Crotty, B., Florin, T., Radford-Smith, G., Gibson, P., Mitchell, B., Connell, W., Read, R., Merrett, M., Ee, H. and Hetzel, D. (2007) Antibiotics in Crohn's Disease Study Group. Two-year combination antibiotic therapy with clarithromycin, rifabutin, and clofazimine for Crohn's disease. *Gastroenterology*, **132**(7), 2313–19.

Shafran, I., Kugler, L., El-Zaatari, F. A., Naser, S. A. and Sandoval, J. (2002) Open clinical trial of rifabutin and clarithromycin therapy in Crohn's disease. *Dig. Liver. Dis.*, **34**(1), 22–8.

Shivananda, S., Lennard-Jones, J., Logan, R., Fear, N., Price, A., Carpenter, L. and van Blankenstein, M. (1996) Incidence of inflammatory bowel disease across Europe: is there a difference between north and south? Results of the European Collaborative Study on Inflammatory Bowel Disease (EC-IBD). *Gut*, **39**(5), 690–7.

Sonnenberg, A., McCarty, D. J. and Jacobsen, S. J. (1991) Geographic variation of inflammatory bowel disease within the United States. *Gastroenterology*, **100**(1), 143–9.

Sonnenberg, A. (1990) Occupational distribution of inflammatory bowel disease among German employees. *Gut*, **31**(9), 1037–40.

Srivastava, E. D., Mayberry, J. F., Morris, T. J., Smith, P. M., Williams, G. T., Roberts, G. M., Newcombe, R. G. and Rhodes, J. (1992) Incidence of ulcerative colitis in Cardiff over 20 years: 1968–87. *Gut*, **33**(2), 256–8.

Summers, R. W., Elliott, D. E., Urban, J. F., Jr, Thompson, R. and Weinstock, J. V. (2005) Trichuris suis therapy in Crohn's disease. *Gut*, **54**(1), 87–90.

Sutherland, L. R., Ramcharan, S., Bryant, H. and Fick, G. (1990) Effect of cigarette smoking on recurrence of Crohn's disease. *Gastroenterology*, **98**(5 Pt 1), 1123–8.

Thompson, N. P., Montgomery, S. M., Pounder, R. E., Wakefield, A. J. (1995) Is measles vaccination a risk factor for inflammatory bowel disease? *Lancet*, **345**(8957), 1071–4.

Tobin, M. V., Logan, R. F., Langman, M. J., McConnell, R. B. and Gilmore, I. T. (1987)

Cigarette smoking and inflammatory bowel disease. *Gastroenterology*, **93**(2), 316–21.

Trallori, G., d'Albasio, G., Palli, D., Bardazzi, G., Cipriani, F., Frittelli, G., Russo, A., Vannozzi, G. and Morettini, A. (1991) Epidemiology of inflammatory bowel disease over a 10-year period in Florence (1978–87). *Ital. J. Gastroenterol.*, **23**(9), 559–63.

Van Kruiningen, H. J. (1999) Lack of support for a common etiology in Johne's disease of animals and Crohn's disease in humans. *Inflamm. Bowel. Dis.*, **5**(3), 183–91.

Vessey, M., Jewell, D., Smith, A., Yeates, D. and McPherson, K. (1986) Chronic inflammatory bowel disease, cigarette smoking, and use of oral contraceptives: findings in a large cohort study of women of childbearing age. *Br. Med. J. (Clin. Res. Ed.)*, **292**(6528), 1101–3.

Wakefield, A. J., Pittilo, R. M., Sim, R., Cosby, S. L., Stephenson, J. R., Dhillon, A. P. and Pounder, R. E. (1993) Evidence of persistent measles virus infection in Crohn's disease. *J. Med. Virol.*, **39**(4), 345–53.

Yapp, T. R., Stenson, R., Thomas, G. A., Lawrie, B. W., Williams, G. T., and Hawthorne, A. B. (2000) Crohn's disease incidence in Cardiff from 1930: an update for 1991–1995. *Eur. J. Gastroenterol. Hepatol.*, **12**(8), 907–11.

CHAPTER 3

Clinical features

Ailsa L. Hart

Introduction

Crohn's disease and ulcerative colitis are inflammatory bowel diseases of unknown cause (idiopathic) that affect about 1 person in every 250 in the UK. Ulcerative colitis affects up to 120,000 people in the UK with between 6,000 and 12,000 new cases being diagnosed each year. Crohn's disease affects about 60,000 people in the UK with up to 6,000 new cases diagnosed each year. The number of people with Crohn's disease has been steadily increasing, particularly amongst young people. Both diseases can be diagnosed at any age but IBD is most commonly diagnosed between 10 and 40 years of age (Stowe *et al.*, 1990).

Case study 1
A 20-year-old man had an eight week history of bloody diarrhoea, opening his bowels up to five times a day, with faecal urgency and abdominal cramps. He also had noticed joint pains particularly in his ankles and wrists. He was otherwise well, took no regular medications, was a non-smoker and there was no family history of intestinal disease. On examination, there was tenderness in the left side of the abdomen. Blood tests showed raised inflammatory markers and platelets. Stool testing for infection was negative. Colonoscopy showed marked erythema and friability up to the sigmoid colon. Biopsies showed diffuse crypt architectural distortion and diffuse acute and chronic inflammation. The diagnosis was left-sided ulcerative colitis.

Clinical presentation of ulcerative colitis
The principal symptoms of ulcerative colitis include diarrhoea with rectal bleeding, abdominal pain and cramps, usually relieved by defecation. Symptoms

are dependent on the extent and severity of disease. Patients with disease limited to the rectum (proctitis) tend to present with rectal bleeding and mucus discharge. Diarrhoea is not always a feature of ulcerative colitis, in particular when the disease is limited to the rectum, and a proportion of these patients complain of constipation and passage of hard stools. When disease extends beyond the rectum and involves a much greater extent of the colon a greater proportion of patients complain of diarrhoea (often with blood and mucus), faecal urgency and faecal incontinence. Patients with a more severe colitis have associated systemic symptoms of fever, vomiting and anorexia. One way of classifying ulcerative colitis is using the Montreal classification (Table 3.1) which takes into account the part of the colon affected (Silverberg *et al.*, 2005).

Table 3.1 Montreal classification of ulcerative colitis (Silverberg *et al.*, 2005).

E1	Limited to rectum
E2	Colorectum distal to splenic flexure
E3	Involvement extends proximal to splenic flexure

The severity of disease can be assessed on the basis of symptoms, clinical observations and laboratory tests. The Truelove and Witts criteria (Truelove and Witts, 1954) provide a practical guide to the clinical assessment of severity (see Table 3.2).

Table 3.2 Truelove and Witt's criteria (Truelove and Witts, 1954) – severity of ulcerative colitis.

	Mild	Moderate	Severe
Number of bloody stools per day	< 4	4–6	> 6
Temperature (°C)	afebrile	intermediate	> 37.8
Heart rate (bpm)	normal	intermediate	> 90
Haemoglobin (g/dl)	> 11	10.5–11	< 10.5
ESR (mm/h)	< 20	20–30	> 30

At presentation a majority of patients have clinically mild to moderate disease. Severe or fulminant colitis is seen in approximately 10–20% at presentation (Edwards and Truelove, 1963).

Clinical course of ulcerative colitis

Ulcerative colitis tends to begin in the rectum and extends proximally affecting the bowel in a continuous fashion. Approximately one third of patients have disease confined to the rectum (proctitis) or the rectum and sigmoid (proctosigmoiditis) at the time of diagnosis. Approximately one third of patients will have a pancolitis at diagnosis. Disease can progress and extend, so that patients who have rectal or rectosigmoid involvement at presentation can progress to have disease affecting the proximal colon in 10–30% of patients at ten years follow-up and in up to 50% at 25 years follow-up (Ayres *et al.*, 1996; Langholz *et al.*, 1994).

The pattern of disease can follow a number of different courses. The majority of patients have a chronic intermittent course with remissions and relapses (Langholz *et al.*, 1994); a cumulative relapse rate in the first year after diagnosis is about 50% irrespective of disease extent. Other patients can have chronic continuous symptoms. Some patients have a single attack and subsequent remission. Some patients have a fulminant course leading to colectomy within the first disease episode. About 10% of patients have long-term remission after the initial disease episode. The extent of disease at diagnosis does not seem to affect the subsequent disease activity. When patients are followed up long-term, disease activity in the previous year appears to be a good indicator of the subsequent course of disease 1994). For example a full year in remission is prognostically favourable and predicts an 80% probability of staying in remission for another year. The more years in remission, the higher the probability of experiencing yet

Case study 2

A 36-year-old woman had a 10 week history of abdominal pain, weight loss and non-bloody diarrhoea, opening her bowels 3–4 times a day. She had also noticed some soreness around the perianal area. She was otherwise well, took no regular medications and in her family history a paternal aunt had Crohn's disease. She was a smoker. On examination, there was tenderness on the right side of the abdomen and a perianal abscess. Blood tests showed a low haemoglobin, increased platelet count, decreased albumin and raised inflammatory markers. Colonoscopy showed ileocaecal inflammation and proctitis. Biopsies showed granulomatous patchy inflammation. Small bowel imaging revealed 30 cm of terminal ileal disease. MRI of the perianal area showed a perianal abscess and a fistula tract. The diagnosis was ileocolonic and perianal Crohn's disease.

another year in remission. On the other hand, relapse in the previous year predicts a 70% probability of relapse in the subsequent year.

Clinical presentation of Crohn's disease

Crohn's disease can affect any part of the gastrointestinal tract, from the mouth to the anus, in contrast with UC which affects the colon alone (occasionally with backwash ileitis, which is when there is some inflammation at the end of the ileum in UC patients). Most CD patients will have ileocaecal disease or involvement of the colon only. Crohn's disease has been classified using the Montreal classification (Table 3.3) which takes into account the location of disease, in addition to the behaviour of the disease (inflammatory; structuring or penetrating) and the age at diagnosis (Silverberg *et al.*, 2005).

The clinical features depend on the location on the disease in the gastrointestinal tract. The symptoms may present insidiously or acutely. The majority of patients have diarrhoea (70–90%); abdominal pain (45–66%); weight loss (65–70%). Rectal bleeding is more common in patients with rectal involvement. Obstructive symptoms of nausea/vomiting and abdominal pain/fullness are more common in patients with ileal disease, when stricturing occurs. The mouth can be affected by Crohn's disease and a distinction needs to be made between true oral Crohn's disease and oral manifestations of Crohn's disease. True oral Crohn's disease is rare (about 1%) and tends to affect children and young adults. It presents with lip swelling and fissures, gingivitis, buccal cobblestoning and nodularity. Oral manifestations of Crohn's disease include aphthous ulcers, glossitis and angular cheilitis and are more common, occurring in about 20% of patients with Crohn's disease (Basu and Asquith, 1980). Perianal fistulae are a common complication of Crohn's disease occurring in around a third of patients with Crohn's disease (Tozer *et al.*, 2009). In a recent community-based study there was a cumulative risk of developing a perianal fistula in 26% at 20 years. Some patients are diagnosed with perianal fistulae before or at the time of diagnosis of Crohn's disease.

Table 3.3 Montreal classification of Crohn's disease (Silverberg *et al.*, 2005).

Age at diagnosis	Location	Behaviour
A1 < 16 years	L1 ileal	B1 inflammatory
A2 17–40 years	L2 colonic	B2 stricturing
A3 > 40 years	L3 ileocolonic	B3 penetrating
	*L4 isolated upper GI disease	†p perianal disease

*L4 is a modifier that can be added to L1–L3
†p is a modifier that can be added to B1–B3

Perianal disease generally denotes a more aggressive Crohn's disease phenotype (Beaugerie *et al.*, 2006). If perianal disease is present at initial diagnosis, the disease is more likely to require several medical therapies and surgical interventions. Colonic disease is associated with perianal disease in up to a third of patients. The types of perianal lesions in patients with Crohn's disease include skin tags, fissures, anal ulcers, fistulae (including recto-vaginal fistulae), perianal abscesses, anorectal strictures and cancer.

The age at diagnosis influences disease location with jejuno-ileal disease being more common in children and adolescents compared with adults in whom colonic disease is more common (Harper *et al.*, 1986; Polito *et al.*, 1996).

Clinical course of Crohn's disease

There can be a significant change in disease behaviour over time, whereas disease location remains relatively stable. Behaviour of disease progresses from inflammatory disease to structuring disease to penetrating disease (Cosnes *et al.*, 2002). This means that with time, complications such as strictures, perforations, abscesses and fistulae (entero-enteric, entero-cutaneous, entero-vesical) become more common.

In the first year after diagnosis, 50% of all Crohn's patients will experience a flare of disease, irrespective of the site of disease (Moum *et al.*, 1997). Of these about one third will have a single flare and two thirds will have at least two relapses. Overall, over 80% of Crohn's patients will need surgery at some time.

Smoking adversely influences the course of disease in Crohn's disease patients. Patients who smoke have an increased risk of developing severe disease needing immunomodulating drugs. Women who smoke are particularly at risk (Cosnes *et al.*, 1996; Cosnes *et al.*, 1999; Cosnes *et al.*, 2001).

IBD (unclassified)

In about 10–15% of cases of IBD, a diagnosis of UC or Crohn's disease cannot be established and the term IBD (unclassified) (IBD-U) is used. With time, over 50% will be reclassified as UC or Crohn's disease. The term Indeterminate Colitis (IC) is sometimes used interchangeably with IBD-U. The term IC was first used by Price at St Mark's Hospital when colectomy specimens were examined and difficulties in diagnosing UC or Crohn's disease were noted (Price, 1978). The term IC should now be restricted to Price's original intentions, to classify colonic resections (Martland and Shepherd, 2007). However, IBD-U now refers to a diagnosis based on a composite of clinical, endoscopic, radiologic and histologic parameters and probably represents part of the spectrum of IBD.

Extra-intestinal manifestations of IBD

Extra-intestinal manifestations (EIM) affect organs outside the gut; joints (peripheral arthritis, ankylosing spondylitis, sacroiliitis), skin (pyoderma gangrenosum, erythema nodosum), eyes (uveitis, episcleritis), hepatobiliary system (primary sclerosing cholangitis (PSC). The overall incidence of such manifestations is about 25–30% with joints being most commonly involved, followed by skin, eye and hepatobiliary involvement (Bouhnik *et al.*, 1993; Monsen *et al.*, 1990). EIM are most common when the colon is inflamed (as opposed to the small bowel). Some of the EIM appear directly related to the activity of the bowel disease, e.g. erythema nodosum. Other EIM appear to follow a distinct course, e.g. PSC and ankylosing spondylitis/sacroiliitis.

Joints

Arthritis is the most common extra-intestinal manifestation of inflammatory bowel disease occurring in 10–20% of patients with IBD (Gravallese and Kantrowitz, 1988). There are two clinical patterns of joint disease in IBD: axial disease and peripheral arthritis. Peripheral arthritis is divided into types 1 and 2 (Table 3.4) (Orchard *et al.*, 1998). Axial disease includes ankylosing spondylitis, which occurs in 3–6% of patients with IBD. Large joint arthritis tends to respond to treatment of the underlying inflammatory bowel disease; however, small joint polyarthritis tends to be more difficult to treat and may require longer-term treatment with immunomodulators.

Table 3.4 Types of peripheral arthritis.

Type 1	Less than 5 joints affected; parallels activity of bowel disease; attacks last less than ten weeks
Type 2	Greater than 5 joints affected; independent of bowel disease; tends to last months to year

Skin

The most common skin conditions related to IBD are pyoderma gangrenosum and erythema nodosum (Tavarela, 2004). Pyoderma gangrenosum occurs in 1–2% of patients with inflammatory bowel disease. Pyoderma gangrenosum may first appear as a blister, red lump or pustule, and eventually forms an ulcer with purplish-coloured, indistinct edges (Figure 3.1). The ulcers may appear alone or in a group, and are commonly found on the extremities. The lesions tend to be painful as well as slow to heal. At times, the occurrence of these ulcers corresponds to an active

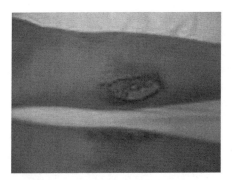

Figure 3.1 Pyoderma gangrenosum.

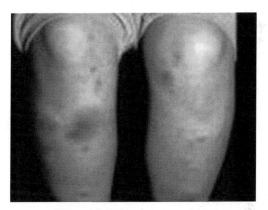

Figure 3.2 Erythema nodosum.

flare-up of IBD, and may respond when the underlying IBD is treated. Other cases, however, do not appear to be directly related to disease activity, and pyoderma gangrenosum may begin or even worsen when the IBD is quiescent.

Erythema nodosum (Figure 3.2) is a skin condition that most often affects people with Crohn's disease, but can also develop in those who have ulcerative colitis. It can occur in 10–15% of people with IBD. The lesions present as painful red nodules that most often develop on the arms or lower legs, but may also appear in other places on the body. This condition is more prevalent in adults than children and women than men. The lesions first appear as tender, red nodules, becoming hard and painful in the first week. The lesions themselves each last for about two weeks, but may be replaced by new lesions when they resolve. In IBD, erythema nodosum may appear during a flare-up and follow the course of IBD, and improve when the flare-up is better controlled.

Eyes

Ocular manifestations occur in about 5% of patients with IBD (Soukiasian *et al.*, 1994). Anterior uveitis is a serious eye complication with an incidence of up to 3% in patients with ulcerative colitis, needing ophthalmic expertise and prompt treatment. The milder eye conditions, scleritis and episcleritis, which involve inflammation of the sclera, occur more frequently in Crohn's disease.

Liver

Primary sclerosing cholangitis complicates approximately 2–5% of cases of ulcerative colitis. It is less commonly associated with Crohn's disease. Although it may be asymptomatic for years, it is a progressive cholestatic liver disease, which is characterised by obliterative fibrosis and biliary strictures and can eventually result in cirrhosis and cholangiocarcinoma. Medium survival from diagnosis to death or liver transplantation is around eighteen years. Imaging with MRCP is usually sufficient to diagnose primary sclerosing cholangitis (Vitellas *et al.*, 2002), sometimes making liver biopsy unnecessary. Patients with PSC and IBD have a higher risk of colorectal cancer and should be offered colonoscopic surveillance.

Colorectal cancer

Patients with longstanding ulcerative colitis and Crohn's colitis have an increased risk of colorectal cancer (Bernstein *et al.*, 2001; Eaden *et al.*, 2001). Factors associated with this increased risk include disease duration, disease extent, the presence of PSC, a family history of colorectal cancer and the presence of ongoing inflammation in the colon (at a microscopic level) (Rutter *et al.*, 2004). Patients with risk factors for developing colitis-associated colorectal cancers are advised to have regular surveillance colonoscopies.

Other extra-intestinal complications of IBD

Patients with IBD have an increased risk of developing renal calculi (particularly urate stones in patients with ileostomy and proctocolectomy and oxalate stones in patients with ileocaecal resections). Additionally IBD patients have an increased risk of gallstones. In particular patients with extensive ileal Crohn's disease or extensive small bowel resections have an increased incidence of gallstones.

The risk of thrombo-embolism is increased in patients with IBD particularly during active disease and compounded by dehydration, immobilisation and sepsis. In-patients with IBD need to be given prophylactic low molecular weight heparin.

Due to multiple factors including underlying disease activity, therapy with corticosteroids, poor nutritional intake and/or absorption of vitamin D and calcium, low body mass index, low physical activity, IBD patients are at increased risk of developing osteoporosis. All of these factors need to be taken into account when managing osteoporosis/osteopaenia in IBD patients.

Conclusion

Crohn's disease and ulcerative colitis are chronic inflammatory bowel diseases of unknown cause that affect about 1 in 250 people in the UK. Whereas Crohn's disease can affect any part of the gastrointestinal tract from the mouth to the anus and the full thickness of the bowel wall, ulcerative colitis predominantly affects the colon and the more superficial layers of the bowel wall. Both are associated with extraintestinal manifestations that can affect the skin, joints, eyes and liver. There is also an increased risk of osteoporosis in IBD, particularly in active disease and where corticosteroids have been used; and an increased risk of colorectal cancer in long-standing extensive UC and Crohn's. IBD-U accounts for approximately 10% of IBD and is a clinical, endoscopic, radiologic and histologic diagnosis which may evolve to become UC or Crohn's disease. The clinical symptoms that the patient reports determines the investigations planned for the patient.

Patient translation summary

Crohn's disease and ulcerative colitis are diseases characterised by inflammation in the gut. Crohn's disease affects any part of the gut from the mouth to the anus, whereas ulcerative colitis affects the colon or large bowel. The inflammation in Crohn's disease goes all the way through the bowel wall and this can lead to complications such as fistulae (communications), perforations and abscesses. In contrast, the inflammation in ulcerative colitis affects the more superficial parts of the bowel wall and does not tend to cause such complications. Crohn's disease tends to present with symptoms of abdominal pain, diarrhoea and weight loss, but the symptoms depend on which part of the gut is affected; ulcerative colitis tends to present with bloody diarrhoea and faecal urgency. Other parts of the body can also be affected, for example skin, joints, eye or liver. There is an increased risk of bowel cancer in patients with inflammatory bowel disease, in particular in patients with longstanding ulcerative colitis that has involved the whole colon for a long duration.

References

Ayres, R. C., Gillen, C. D., Walmsley, R. S. and Allan, R. N. (1996) Progression of ulcerative proctosigmoiditis: incidence and factors influencing progression. *Eur. J. Gastroenterol. Hepatol.*, **8**, 555–8.

Basu, M. K. and Asquith, P. (1980) Oral manifestations of inflammatory bowel disease. *Clin. Gastroenterol.*, **9**, 307–21.

Beaugerie, L., Seksik, P., Nion-Larmurier, I., Gendre, J. P. and Cosnes, J. (2006) Predictors of Crohn's disease. *Gastroenterology*, **130**, 650–6.

Bernstein, C. N., Blanchard, J. F., Kliewer, E. and Wajda, A. (2001) Cancer risk in patients with inflammatory bowel disease: a population-based study. *Cancer*, **91**, 854–62.

Bouhnik, Y., Benamouzig, R., Rybojad, M., Matuchansky, C. and Rambaud, J. C. (1993) [Systemic manifestations associated with chronic inflammatory bowel diseases]. *Gastroenterol. Clin. Biol.*, **17**, 121–9.

Cosnes, J., Carbonnel, F., Beaugerie, L., Le, Q. Y. and Gendre, J. P. (1996) Effects of cigarette smoking on the long-term course of Crohn's disease. *Gastroenterology*, **110**, 424–31.

Cosnes, J., Carbonnel, F., Carrat, F., Beaugerie, L., Cattan, S. and Gendre, J. (1999) Effects of current and former cigarette smoking on the clinical course of Crohn's disease. *Aliment. Pharmacol. Ther.*, **13**, 1403–11.

Cosnes, J., Beaugerie, L., Carbonnel, F. and Gendre, J. P. (2001) Smoking cessation and the course of Crohn's disease: an intervention study. *Gastroenterology*, **120**, 1093–9.

Cosnes, J., Cattan, S., Blain, A. *et al.* (2002) Long-term evolution of disease behavior of Crohn's disease. *Inflamm. Bowel Dis.*, **8**, 244–50.

Eaden, J. A., Abrams, K. R. and Mayberry, J. F. (2001) The risk of colorectal cancer in ulcerative colitis: a meta-analysis. *Gut*, **48**, 526–35.

Edwards, F. C. and Truelove, S. C. (1963) The course and prognosis of ulcerative colitis. *Gut*, **4**, 299–315.

Gravallese, E. M. and Kantrowitz, F. G. (1988) Arthritic manifestations of inflammatory bowel disease. *Am. J. Gastroenterol.*, **83**, 703–9.

Harper, P. C., McAuliffe, T. L. and Beeken, W. L. (1986) Crohn's disease in the elderly. A statistical comparison with younger patients matched for sex and duration of disease. *Arch. Intern. Med.*, **146**, 753–5.

Langholz, E., Munkholm, P., Davidsen, M. and Binder, V. (1994) Course of ulcerative colitis: analysis of changes in disease activity over years. *Gastroenterology*, **107**, 3–11.

Martland, G. T. and Shepherd, N. A. (2007) Indeterminate colitis: definition, diagnosis, implications and a plea for nosological sanity. *Histopathology*, **50**, 83–96.

Monsen, U., Sorstad, J., Hellers, G. and Johansson, C. (1990) Extracolonic diagnoses in ulcerative colitis: an epidemiological study. *Am. J. Gastroenterol.*, **85**, 711–16.

Moum, B., Ekbom, A., Vatn, M. H. *et al.* (1997) Clinical course during the 1st year after diagnosis in ulcerative colitis and Crohn's disease. Results of a large, prospective population-based study in southeastern Norway, 1990–93. *Scand. J. Gastroenterol.*, **32**, 1005–12.

Orchard, T. R., Wordsworth, B. P. and Jewell, D. P. (1998) Peripheral arthropathies in inflammatory bowel disease: their articular distribution and natural history. *Gut*, **42**, 387–91.

Polito, J. M., Childs, B., Mellits, E. D., Tokayer, A. Z., Harris, M. L. and Bayless, T. M. (1996) Crohn's disease: influence of age at diagnosis on site and clinical type of disease. *Gastroenterology*, **111**, 580–6.

Price, A. B. (1978) Overlap in the spectrum of non-specific inflammatory bowel disease: colitis indeterminate. *J. Clin. Pathology*, **31**, 567–77.

Rutter, M., Saunders, B., Wilkinson, K. *et al.* (2004) Severity of inflammation is a risk factor for colorectal neoplasia in ulcerative colitis. *Gastroenterology*, **126**, 451–9.

Silverberg, M. S., Satsangi, J., Ahmad, T. *et al.* (2005) Toward an integrated clinical, molecular and serological classification of inflammatory bowel disease: report of a Working Party of the 2005 Montreal World Congress of Gastroenterology. *Can. J. Gastroenterol.*, **19**(suppl. A), 5–36.

Soukiasian, S. H., Foster, C. S. and Raizman, M. B. (1994) Treatment strategies for scleritis and uveitis associated with inflammatory bowel disease. *Am. J. Ophthalmol.*, **118**, 601–11.

Stowe, S. P., Redmond, S. R., Stormont, J. M. *et al.* (1990) An epidemiologic study of inflammatory bowel disease in Rochester, New York. Hospital incidence. *Gastroenterology*, **98**, 104–10.

Tavarela, V. F. (2004) Review article: skin complications associated with inflammatory bowel disease. *Aliment. Pharmacol. Ther.*, **20**(suppl. 4), 50–3.

Tozer, P. J., Whelan, K., Phillips, R. K. and Hart, A. L. (2009) Etiology of perianal Crohn's disease: role of genetic, microbiological, and immunological factors. *Inflamm. Bowel Dis.*, **15**, 1591–8.

Truelove, S. C. and Witts, L. J. (1954) Cortisone in ulcerative colitis; preliminary report on a therapeutic trial. *Br. Med. J.*, **2**(4884), 375–8.

Vitellas, K. M., Enns, R. A., Keogan, M. T. *et al.* (2002) Comparison of MR cholangiopancreatographic techniques with contrast-enhanced cholangiography in the evaluation of sclerosing cholangitis. *Am. J. Roentgenol.*, **178**, 327–34.

PART 2

Clinical management

CHAPTER 4

Investigating inflammatory bowel disease

Siew C. Ng and Nisha Patel

Case study

A 26-year-old woman presented to Accident and Emergency with a three-day history of bloody diarrhoea. Her bowels were opening at least 12 times a day with blood each time and she felt faint and hot. She suffered from nocturnal symptoms and had a one-week history of anorexia and weight loss. She had a similar episode three years ago after returning from a trip to India and was diagnosed with infective colitis. Treatment with metronidazole and ciprofloxacin settled her symptoms immediately. Since then she has experienced soft stool with normal bowel frequency once every month. She did not have any eye, skin or joint complaints and had no relevant past medical history, social or drug history. She was a non-smoker with no family history of inflammatory bowel disease (IBD) or colorectal carcinoma. On examination she was haemodynamically stable, afebrile and had a soft abdomen with some minimal left iliac fossa tenderness but no rebound tenderness or guarding. Bowel sounds were present. Laboratory investigations revealed the following values; haemoglobin 11.1 (normal range, 11.5–15.5 g/dL), white cell count 13.1 ($4-10 \times 10^9$ cells/litre units), albumin 25 (36–52 g/L), CRP 102 (< 5 mg/L), ESR 72 (0–10 mm/hr), with normal renal and liver function tests. A plain abdominal radiograph showed bowel wall thickening but no evidence of colon dilatation. Four stool samples for microscopy, culture and clostridium difficile toxin were negative. A flexible sigmoidoscopy showed active confluent erythematous ulceration to the sigmoid colon. Biopsies confirmed active ulcerative colitis. The patient was commenced on intravenous steroids, oral and rectal 5-aminosalicylic acid preparations, and her symptoms resolved within three days.

Introduction

Inflammatory bowel disease (IBD) comprises two main subtypes: ulcerative colitis (UC) and Crohn's disease (CD). The incidence is increasing and approximately 240,000 people in the UK have IBD. Men and women are equally affected. It is a lifelong chronic relapsing and remitting disorder that primarily affects the young. Patients with IBD will benefit from a multidisciplinary approach in investigating and managing their disease, which involves gastroenterologists, radiologists, histopathologists, IBD nurse specialists, dietitians, psychologists and in some cases surgeons. The diagnosis can be made from history, examination, laboratory tests, stool tests, radiological, endoscopic and histological examinations.

Differential diagnosis

There are a number of differential diagnoses that should be considered when investigating bloody diarrhoea (Table 4.1). Infectious and malignant causes should always be included in the differentials. The main differential diagnoses have been described below and these are primarily dependent on the history, examination and blood tests.

Endoscopy

Ileocolonoscopy

In patients with suspected ulcerative colitis (UC), a flexible sigmoidoscopy with biopsies can be performed initially to establish the diagnosis, followed by a subsequent colonoscopy to assess the disease extent. In patients with suspected Crohn's disease (CD), the first line investigation is colonoscopy with visualisation of the terminal ileum. Typical endoscopic features of UC are continuous, confluent and concentric colonic inflammation from the rectum with proximal extension whereas the most useful endoscopic features of CD include patchy involvement, cobblestoning, anal lesions, and ileal inflammation or ulceration. Multiple biopsies with a minimum of two samples from each colonic segment should be obtained (Bentley *et al.*, 2002; Pera *et al.*, 1987). In patients in whom there is severe active colonic disease, an initial flexible sigmoidoscopy is recommended instead of a full colonoscopy to limit the risk of bowel perforation (Carter *et al.*, 2004). Gastroduodenoscopy is only recommended in patients with CD who have upper gastrointestinal symptoms (Travis *et al.*, 2006). Figure 4.1 shows endoscopic features suggestive of CD and UC.

Once CD is assessed on ileocolonoscopy and confirmed on histology, further investigations are recommended to assess the extent, severity and the site of

Table 4.1 Differential diagnosis of bloody diarrhoea.

Inflammatory bowel disease	Crohn's disease
	Ulcerative colitis
Infectious colitis	*Shigella*
	Campylobacter jejuni
	Escherichia coli
	Salmonella
	Yersinia enterocolitica
	Mycobacteria tuberculosis
	Protoza and worms: *Entamoeba histolytica, Giardia lamblia, Strongyloides stercoralis, Isoporidia belli, Cryptosporidia*
	Amoebae
	Cytomegalovirus
	Human immunodeficiency virus
	Rotavirus
	Herpes viruses
	Actinomycosis
	Neisseria gonorrhoeae – mainly proctitis
	Chlamydia trachomatis – mainly proctitis
	Treponema pallidum – mainly proctitis
	Clostridium difficile
	Henoch–Schoenlein disease
Antibiotics	
Vasculitis	
Neutropenic colitis	
Radiation-induced bowel injury	
Coeliac sprue	
Sarcoidosis	
Ischaemic colitis	
Amyloidosis	
Carcinoma	Primary colorectal carcinoma
	Lymphomas
	Metastatic carcinoma
	Carcinoid

small bowel disease. Several modalities, including small bowel follow through, transabdominal ultrasound (USS), computed tomography (CT) enterography/enteroclysis and magnetic resonant (MR) enterography/enteroclysis may have a

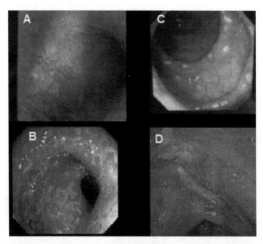

Figure 4.1 Endoscopic diagnosis of IBD. A: mild UC: Loss of vascular pattern and erythema; B: moderate/severe UC – mucosa friability with severe inflammation and ulceration; C: colonic CD – patchy aphthous ulcers; D: severe ileal CD – deep ulceration and cobblestoning.

role. The benefits and limitations of these modalities are discussed in the next section. The decision on the types of investigations will depend on the patient history, local radiological availability and expertise.

In patients with UC and CD, colonoscopy is recommended to monitor disease activity, mucosal healing and response to therapy following an initial diagnosis.

Wireless capsule endoscopy (WCE) and small bowel enteroscopy

WCE is a novel minimally invasive modality that allows complete visualisation of the small intestinal mucosa (Iddan *et al.*, 2000). It is useful in symptomatic patients with suspected CD of the small intestine where initial evaluation with traditional radiographic and endoscopic studies has failed to establish the diagnosis and in whom stricture or stenosis has been excluded (Papadakis *et al.*, 2005).The diagnostic yield of WCE in suspected CD patients varies from 43% to 71%, and WCE appears to be superior to small bowel follow through, CT enterography (Fireman *et al.*, 2003), and MR enteroclysis (Albert *et al.*, 2005) in the diagnosis of small bowel CD. However CD-associated lesions seen on WCE need to be better characterised and larger prospective studies are necessary to determine the precise role of WCE on the diagnostic algorithm of CD. Contraindications for

WCE include intestinal obstruction, stenosis/strictures, swallowing disorders and pacemakers/implanted electromedical devices.

In selected patients with suspected CD in whom conventional radiology and endoscopy fail to provide a diagnosis, enteroscopy (single or double balloon) with a push endoscope is a safe and useful procedure to obtain biopsies in order to confirm the diagnosis (Bourreille *et al.*, 2009; Pasha and Leighton, 2009).

Radiology

Radiographic imaging has an important role in the workup of patients with suspected IBD and in the differentiation of UC and CD. These tests are performed in conjunction with the history, examination and laboratory tests to reach a diagnosis. Methods of minimising radiation exposure should be considered in the predominantly younger population group in whom given the chronicity of IBD may be exposed to recurrent radiation-associated investigations.

Plain radiograph

Plain abdominal X-rays are quick, effective and an inexpensive way of investigating IBD. They are not diagnostic tests for IBD but may show small or large bowel inflammation, dilatation or obstruction. In patients with UC, toxic megacolon, which is easily diagnosed on a plain abdominal radiograph, should be excluded. These can be used along with an erect chest radiograph to look for free air suggestive of a perforation. In patients with suspected severe CD, there may be evidence of small bowel dilatation on plain abdominal radiograph. Complications of IBD such as osteopenia, renal stones (calcium oxalate stones in CD) or sacroilitis may also be detected. Figure 4.2 demonstrates an abdominal radiograph suggestive of left-sided UC.

Ultrasound

Increasingly ultrasound is becoming an indispensable tool with significant improvements in resolution, playing a role in the monitoring of disease activity and with the added benefit of no ionizing radiation. When performed by specialists, sonographic changes consistent with IBD can be found in up to 90% of patients with CD (Sheridan *et al.*, 1993; Tarjan *et al.*, 2000).

Sonographic findings suggestive of IBD such as bowel wall thickening should prompt endoscopy and a histological diagnosis. In CD, characteristically long segments of bowel are affected involving the terminal ileum and caecum and there may be narrowing of the lumen and stenosis. Complications of IBD such as toxic megacolon, perforation, abscesses, fistulae and ileus may be detected.

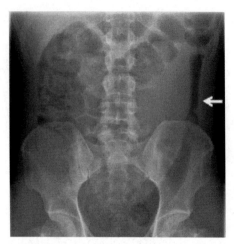

Figure 4.2 Abdominal radiograph showing featureless left colon and lead piping (arrow) with faecal residue in the transverse colon and right colon, suggestive of left-sided ulcerative colitis.

Limitations of ultrasound include the need for an experienced operator; body habitus and overlying bowel or air can lead to poor images of the underlying organs. There is no continuous visualisation of the GI tract and these changes are non-specific.

Contrast studies

Investigation of the small bowel using contrast can be performed by two methods: barium follow-through or enteroclysis. Double-contrast (barium and air) barium enema is a valuable tool in differentiating between UC and CD. Early inflammatory changes may be suggested by fine granular mucosa which becomes coarsely granular when ulcers become established and granulation tissue develops. The whole colon may be affected or changes may be segmental (usually in the left colon) with rarely rectal sparing. Benign strictures predominantly in the left colon occur in up to 11% of patients with chronic UC but malignant lesions must be excluded. However, contrast studies can be time-consuming, require large amounts of bowel cleansing to ensure adequate visualisation of the mucosa, and may precipitate toxic megacolon. Findings on contrast studies suggestive of IBD have been described in Table 4.2.

Table 4.2 Findings on barium follow-though, CT and MRI scans suggestive of IBD.

Imaging modality	Ulcerative colitis	Crohn's disease
Barium follow-through	■ Pseudopolyposis (appear as filling defects) ■ Backwater ileitis ■ Mucosal bridges ■ Narrow colon associated with incomplete filling	■ Skip lesions ■ Cobblestoning ■ Loss of colonic haustra ■ Patulous ileocaecal valve ■ Collar-button ulcers and double-tracking ulcers ■ Thumbprinting
CT scan	■ Bowel wall thickening ■ Colonic dilatation ■ Toxic megacolon ■ Rectal and presacral space narrowing ■ Mucosal bridges ■ Intra-abdominal abscesses ■ No faecal residue in inflamed bowel ■ Submucosal fat deposition ■ Narrow colon	■ Bowel wall thickening – eccentric and segmental ■ Fistulae ■ Strictures ■ Sinus tracks – extraluminal air bubbles most commonly associated with sinus track formation (entero-cutaneously or entero-sinus track) ■ Perforation and pneumoperitoneum ■ Shortened colon ■ Loss of colonic haustra ■ Intra-abdominal abscesses ■ No faecal residue in inflamed bowel ■ Submucosal fat deposition
MRI	■ Diffuse bowel wall thickening ■ Colonic dilatation ■ Rectal and presacral space narrowing ■ No faecal residue in inflamed bowel ■ Submucosal fat deposition ■ Halo sign ■ Target sign – peri-rectal fat proliferation ■ Narrow colon	■ Bowel wall thickening – eccentric and segmental ■ Fistulae ■ Strictures ■ Sinus tracks – extraluminal air bubbles Most commonly associated with sinus track formation (entero-cutaneously or entero-sinus track) and may also be formed by gas forming bacteria ■ 'Vascular jejunisation' – hypervascularity of mesentery and ileum or 'comb sign'

Imaging modality	Ulcerative colitis	Crohn's disease
MRI (*continued*)		■ Loss of colonic haustra ■ Patulous ileocaecal valve ■ No faecal residue in inflamed bowel ■ Submucosal fat deposition ■ Halo sign ■ Target sign – peri-rectal fat proliferation

Computed tomography (CT) scans

Cross-sectional imaging in the form of CT scans (CT enterography or enteroclysis) is used primarily to evaluate the complications of IBD included in Table 4.2. It also provides extra information on bowel wall thickening and changes in vascularity, but early disease may be missed on a CT scan and mucosal and transmural thickening is a non-specific finding. Nonetheless, CT scans are useful in the differential diagnosis of IBD, the acute abdomen and mesenteric abnormalities. CT scan can be used to percutaneously drain abscesses or fluid collections, thereby avoiding the need for surgery. CT scans are fast and inexpensive methods of detecting small or large bowel inflammation (although this is non-specific), but can also be useful to eliminate other differential diagnoses such as appendicitis, abscesses and renal stones. However, its radiation burden should be taken into account in young patients. CT enteroclysis involves the placement of a nasojejunal tube to ensure adequate distension of the small bowel for accurate assessment of strictures. Figures 4.3–4.5 show examples of complications of CD on CT imaging.

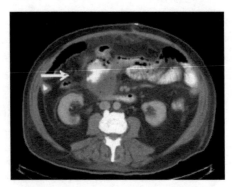

Figure 4.3 CT scan: focal inflammatory collection suggestive of abscess formation (arrow) in a patient with background Crohn's disease.

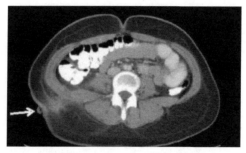

Figure 4.4 Enterocutaneous fistula (arrow) in a patient with complex CD on a CT scan.

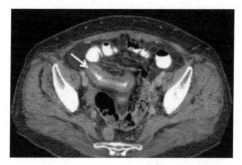

Figure 4.5 Ileal thickening (arrow) in CD on a CT scan.

Magnetic resonance imaging (MRI)

Magnetic resonance imaging (MRI) plays an increasing role in the investigation of both luminal and perianal CD (Rimola *et al.*, 2008, 2009; Schwartz *et al.*, 2001). Technical developments have now allowed for higher quality images of the abdomen with improved transmural assessments. MR enterography is complementary to ileocolonoscopy for assessing the site, extent and disease activity of CD (Maccioni *et al.*, 2000). It is also useful to identify extramural complications, such as internal fistula, abscess, gallstones, renal calculi and sacroiliitis. MRI enteroclysis produces clear images enabling radiologists to detect both transmural and extramural disease, but this technique involves intravenous, oral and rectal contrast as well as intravenous anti-peristaltic agents. Contrast is instilled via a nasogastric tube directly onto small bowel mucosa leading to distension and accurate visualisation of complications including stenoses. The

69

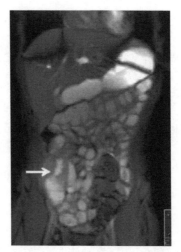

Figure 4.6 Coronal MRI: terminal ileal stricture (arrow) in CD.

lack of ionising radiation makes it a desirable test in young patients. Findings on cross-sectional imaging suggestive of IBD have been described in Table 4.2. Figure 4.6 shows an ileal stricture in a patient with CD seen on MRI scan.

Nuclear medicine

Leukocyte scintigraphy or 'tagged white blood cell (WBC) scan' detects white blood cell accumulation in inflamed tissue. The indium-111 (^{111}In) WBC study can be used to detect the location and extent of bowel inflammation and to evaluate treatment response. Labelled white blood cells travel through the bloodstream and migrate into inflamed tissue including diverticulitis, abscesses and ischaemic bowel where they accumulate and become visible on the scan. Altogether leukocyte scintigraphy is a relatively safe test which entails less radiation exposure than contrast barium X-ray or CT scans and does not involve any preparation, however it lacks specificity (Giaffer *et al.*, 1996). It is also not useful in defining anatomy or in assessing rectal inflammation.

A variety of techniques are available for imaging the small bowel. No single procedure can be recommended and the decision of the investigations should be a decision made in the context of the clinical history, patient age and local radiological expertise and resource (Carter *et al.*, 2004).

Pathology

Blood tests

Laboratory tests are integral in the investigation of IBD. They provide complementary information to radiological and endoscopic studies such as an objective measure of disease activity and severity. Serial laboratory patterns can be useful to predict an imminent flare despite the absence of clinical symptoms. Patients with weight loss, malabsorption and fatigue indicating severe IBD will generally show a wide derangement of laboratory tests. Many of the serum laboratory values are, however, non-specific and do not differentiate between CD and UC. Table 4.3 outlines some of the more useful laboratory tests and trends expected in IBD.

Acute phase proteins are produced primarily by the liver and are released during infection, tissue destruction, tumour growth and immunological diseases. Their production leads to a cascade of events resulting in a systemic and local response including platelet aggregation and increased capillary permeability. A number of acute phase proteins can be quantitatively measured as serum proteins using immunological techniques and a current disruption of homeostasis such as bowel inflammation can be reflected in their concentrations. Their serum values hence provide valuable information on the current state of inflammatory process. However, their response to inflammation is non-specific. Raised serum values may also be seen in other inflammatory processes such as bacterial infections,

Table 4.3 Useful laboratory tests and trends associated with IBD.

Serum sample	Trend in IBD
Haemoglobin	Decreased – often anaemic in chronic disease
Platelets	Increased – in chronic disease
White cells	Increased – if active inflammation or infection
Albumin	Decreased – reflecting poor nutritional state, malabsorption, acute infection or inflammation
CRP	Increased
ESR	Increased
Iron studies	Decreased – may reflect malnutrition or chronic inflammation
Folate	Decreased – may reflect malnutrition
Vitamin B$_{12}$	Decreased – may reflect malnutrition

diverticulitis, vasculitis and pancreatitis. Their role is most useful in quantifying the acute inflammatory condition once the diagnosis has been established.

The most widely used parameter of inflammation is C-reactive protein (CRP). CRP increases and decreases at times of acute inflammation and resolution, respectively, because of its short half-life of 19 hours (Nielsen *et al.*, 2000; Vermeire *et al.*, 2004). CD is associated with higher CRP levels than UC (Shine *et al.*, 1985). Asymptomatic patients with raised serum CRP levels have a higher rate of relapse (Boirivant *et al.*, 1988). There is a relatively good correlation between the levels of acute phase proteins and clinical findings in patients with CD (Meryn *et al.*, 1985). CRP is also useful in guiding therapy and follow-up.

Erythrocyte sedimentation rate (ESR) is a non-specific marker of inflammation. It increases with age and is higher in females. It should be used in conjunction with other laboratory values, as normal values may not necessary indicate remission. Occult bleeding in chronic inflammation, acute bleeding and poor oral intake may lead to iron deficiency anaemia. Extensive small bowel CD or short bowel syndrome post extensive small bowel resection may lead to iron deficiency anaemia. Vitamin B_{12} deficiency may be due to terminal ileal resection, ileal inflammation or malabsorption. Anaemia may also be caused by bone marrow suppression secondary to inflammation or immunosuppressive medication. In an acute disease flare, serum haemoglobin may decrease in conjunction with deranged CRP, ESR and albumin indicating an acute inflammatory process. Haematocrit is the only laboratory value that is included in the Crohn's disease activity index (CDAI), a scoring system generally used in clinical trials of CD (Best *et al.*, 1976). Acute flare of disease may also be accompanied by raised platelet count, often with values $> 600,000/mm^3$.

White cell and neutrophil counts can be elevated in the presence of inflammation. Liver function tests should be performed to assess for primary sclerosing cholangitis (PSC) particularly in patients with UC. Renal function should be monitored for interstitial nephritis associated with CD, or as an adverse effect of medication such as mesalazine. Albumin produced in the liver has a half-life of 19 days and patterns of changes in its levels are important prognostic markers. Albumin levels also drop due to the catabolic state associated with inflammation.

Stool tests

Stool samples should be sent for culture, microscopy and sensitivities, and *Clostridium difficile* toxin to exclude an infectious cause. If there is a history of foreign travel, samples should be sent for ova, cysts and parasites. Faecal calprotectin (a neutrophilic calcium-binding protein) or lacteferrin is elevated in intestinal mucosa inflammation and their values are related to the extent of ulcerated intestinal mucosa. These stool markers may be useful in the initial diagnosis or in predicting disease flares in specialised centres. Protein levels > 50 mg/l are considered abnormal with a 90% sensitivity and an 83% specificity in predicting disease recurrence (Tibble *et al.*, 2000a,b). However, there is currently no evidence-based recommendation to implement the routine use of these stool markers in the diagnosis of IBD, and adequately powered studies are required to confirm their role in clinical practice.

Histology

Histological examination is routinely used to establish the diagnosis of CD and UC. Histological features used to diagnose colonic CD include focal or patchy chronic inflammation with increased plasma cells and lymphocytes, focal crypt irregularity and the presence of granulomas in the lamina propria not associated with crypt injury. The presence of the above features together with irregular villous architecture is diagnostic of ileal CD. Typical pathologic findings for UC include widespread crypt architectural distortion (crypt atrophy, cryptitis and crypt abscess) and diffuse lamina propria cell neutrophilic or lymphocytic infiltration, and basal plasmacytosis.

Genetic and serological tests

There is currently no evidence to recommend the use of genetic testing, such as nucleotide-binding oligomerisation domain (NOD) 2/CARD 15, organic cation transporter (OCTN) 1 and 2 or DLG5, in routine clinical practice because individual predictive value remains low, and if genetic tests are positive, no therapeutic strategies exist to prevent disease (Stange *et al.*, 2006). Serology tests including anti-*Saccharomyces cerevisiae* antibody (ASCA) or anti-neutrophilic cytoplasmic antibody (ANCA) have shown a high sensitivity for the diagnosis of CD but carry a low predictive value and they are therefore not helpful for routine use (Peeters *et al.*, 2001). Perinuclear (p)-ANCA is present in most patients with UC or colonic CD and coexisting primary sclerosing cholangitis (Saxon *et al.*, 1990).

Special considerations

Perianal fistulising Crohn's disease

In patients with perianal fistulising CD, initial assessment should include (1) sigmoidoscopy or colonoscopy, to assess proximal disease and specifically assess for the presence and extent of rectal disease, (2) pelvic floor imaging with MRI pelvis or anal endosonography (AES) to delineate fistula anatomy, extent and relationship of the tracks to the sphincter muscles, and identify complicating factors such as an abscess; and (3) examination under anaesthetic (EUA), to include surgical drainage, and/or seton placement if necessary (Kamm and Ng, 2008; Ng *et al.*, 2009).

Pregnant women
Investigation of IBD in pregnancy should include history, examination, laboratory tests and limited radiology. Active disease in the mother will have an adverse effect on the foetus and hence investigation cannot be delayed. Given the risk of ionising radiation to the foetus, safer forms of radiology such as USS or MRI could be used to evaluate bowel wall thickness, disease extent, severity and complications. In severe cases, or in emergencies such as perforation, toxic megacolon or obstruction, such contrast studies may not be avoided. In these cases, plain abdominal films with lower radiation are preferable to CT scans or barium studies.

Children
Initial investigations of a child suspected of UC or CD should include a colonoscopy with terminal ileal intubation multiple biopsies; this is best carried out under general anaesthesia. In addition, upper gastrointestinal endoscopy and small bowel radiology should be preformed. Studies have shown that histology from upper GI endoscopy can confirm the diagnosis of CD that might have been missed in up to one third of cases, whereas small bowel radiology may demonstrate abnormal small bowel even though terminal ileum is normal, and exclude complications such as internal fistula and strictures. Complete examination at diagnosis in children is necessary to establish the type of disease, severity, location and extent of disease before treatment is commenced (Caprilli *et al.*, 2006). In children with suspected IBD, a CRP of more than 10 times the normal value will suggest a bacterial super infection with abscess formation or fistulae.

Elderly patients
The elderly may not be able to tolerate endoscopic procedures to diagnose or assess their disease. Cross-sectional imaging and contrast studies should be used to examine the bowel lumen instead. Their performance status should be assessed whilst they are an in-patient or in out-patient visits and documented to ensure they do not undergo invasive, lengthy, time-consuming investigations.

Conclusion

Figure 4.7 illustrates a proposed diagnostic algorithm for patients with suspected IBD.

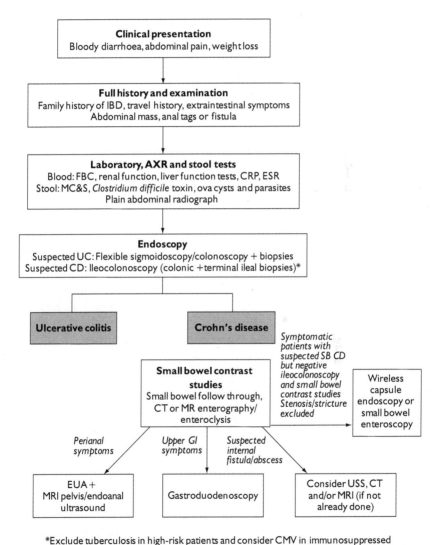

Figure 4.7 Proposed diagnostic algorithm for patients with suspected IBD.

Prior to a diagnosis of IBD, a number of differentials need to be excluded: namely infective and malignant causes of intestinal inflammation. A diagnosis of IBD is based on a combination of clinical assessment, laboratory, endoscopic, histological and radiological investigations. Ileocolonoscopy with biopsies is the first line investigation to establish the diagnosis of UC and CD (with the exception of isolated proximal small bowel CD). Small bowel capsule endoscopy (SBCE) is reserved for patients in whom the clinical suspicion for CD remains high despite negative ileocolonoscopy and radiological imaging. Double balloon enteroscopy (DBE) can be used to obtain biopsies from involved areas of small bowel for the diagnosis of CD, or for the dilatation of small bowel strictures. In CD, further investigations, including small bowel follow-through, US, CT, or MR enterography or enteroclysis are recommended to assess the extent and involved site of small bowel disease. The choice of examination is dependent on local expertise and availability.

Key points

- Initial laboratory investigations should include FBC, renal function, liver function, CRP and/or ESR.
- Stool tests should be sent for bacteria pathogens, *Clostridium difficile* toxin, and ova, cysts and parasites.
- First line investigations include flexible sigmoidoscopy/colonoscopy for suspected ulcerative colitis and ileocolonoscopy with biopsies for suspected Crohn's disease.
- In Crohn's disease, further investigations (small bowel follow-through, USS, CT or MRI) are recommended to examine the extent and location of small bowel disease.
- Suspected perianal Crohn's disease should be investigated with examination under anaesthesia and MRI pelvis or endoanal ultrasound.
- Once diagnosis of IBD has been confirmed, disease activity and extent can be monitored with colonoscopy.

Patient translation summary
The diagnosis and activity of UC and CD is confirmed by clinical evaluation (patient history and physical examination) and a combination of laboratory tests, endoscopic, histological and radiological investigations, incorporating a discussion between patient, physician, histopathologist and radiologist.

References

Albert, J. G., Martiny, F., Krummenerl, A., Stock, K., Lesske, J., Gobel, C. M., Lotterer, E., Nietsch, H. H., Behrmann, C. and Fleig, W. E. (2005) Diagnosis of small bowel Crohn's disease: a prospective comparison of capsule endoscopy with magnetic resonance imaging and fluoroscopic enteroclysis. *Gut*, **54**, 1721–7.

Bentley, E., Jenkins, D., Campbell, F. and Warren, B. (2002) How could pathologists improve the initial diagnosis of colitis? Evidence from an international workshop. *J. Clin. Pathol.*, **55**, 955–60.

Best, W. R., Becktel, J. M., Singleton, J. W. and Kern, F., Jr (1976) Development of a Crohn's disease activity index. National Cooperative Crohn's Disease Study. *Gastroenterology*, **70**, 439–44.

Boirivant, M., Leoni, M., Tariciotti, D., Fais, S., Squarcia, O. and Pallone, F. (1988) The clinical significance of serum C reactive protein levels in Crohn's disease. Results of a prospective longitudinal study *J. Clin. Gastroenterol.*, **10**, 401–5.

Bourreille, A., Ignjatovic, A., Aabakken, L., Loftus, E. V., Jr, Eliakim, R., Pennazio, M., Bouhnik, Y., Seidman, E., Keuchel, M., Albert, J. G., Ardizzone, S., Bar-Meir, S., Bisschops, R., Despott, E. J., Fortun, P. F., Heuschkel, R., Kammermeier, J., Leighton, J. A., Mantzaris, G. J., Moussata, D., Lo, S., Paulsen, V., Panes, J., Radford-Smith, G., Reinisch, W., Rondonotti, E., Sanders, D. S., Swoger, J. M., Yamamoto, H., Travis, S., Colombel, J. F. and Van, G. A. (2009) Role of small-bowel endoscopy in the management of patients with inflammatory bowel disease: an international OMED-ECCO consensus. *Endoscopy*, **41**, 618–37.

Caprilli, R., Gassull, M. A., Escher, J. C., Moser, G., Munkholm, P., Forbes, A., Hommes, D. W., Lochs, H., Angelucci, E., Cocco, A., Vucelic, B., Hildebrand, H., Kolacek, S., Riis, L., Lukas, M. de F. R., Hamilton, M., Jantschek, G., Michetti, P., O'Morain, C., Anwar, M. M., Freitas, J. L., Mouzas, I. A., Baert, F., Mitchell, R. and Hawkey, C. J. (2006) European evidence based consensus on the diagnosis and management of Crohn's disease: special situations. *Gut*, **55**(suppl. 1), i36–i58.

Carter, M. J., Lobo, A. J. and Travis, S. P. (2004) Guidelines for the management of inflammatory bowel disease in adults. *Gut*, **53**(suppl. 5), V1–16.

Fireman, Z., Mahajna, E., Broide, E., Shapiro, M., Fich, L., Sternberg, A., Kopelman, Y. and Scapa, E. (2003) Diagnosing small bowel Crohn's disease with wireless capsule endoscopy. *Gut*, **52**, 390–2.

Giaffer, M. H., Tindale, W. B. and Holdsworth, D. (1996) Value of technetium-99m HM-PAO-labelled leucocyte scintigraphy as an initial screening test in patients suspected of having inflammatory bowel disease. *Eur. J. Gastroenterol. Hepatol.*, **8**, 1195–200.

Iddan, G., Meron, G., Glukhovsky, A. and Swain, P. (2000) Wireless capsule endoscopy. *Nature*, **405**, 417.

Kamm, M. A. and Ng, S. C. (2008) Perianal fistulizing Crohn's disease: a call to action. *Clin. Gastroenterol. Hepatol.*, **6**, 7–10.

Maccioni, F., Viscido, A., Broglia, L., Marrollo, M., Masciangelo, R., Caprilli, R. and Rossi, P. (2000) Evaluation of Crohn's disease activity with magnetic resonance imaging. *Abdom. Imaging*, **25**, 219–28.

Meryn, S., Lochs, H., Bettelheim, P., Sertl, K. and Mulak, K. (1985) [Blood protein concentrations – are they parameters of disease activity in Crohn's disease?] *Leber Magen Darm*, **15**, 160–4.

Ng, S. C., Plamondon, S., Gupta, A., Burling, D., Swatton, A., Vaizey, C. J. and Kamm, M. A. (2009) Prospective evaluation of anti-tumor necrosis factor therapy guided by magnetic resonance imaging for Crohn's perineal fistulas. *Am. J. Gastroenterol.*, **104**, 2973–86.

Nielsen, O. H., Vainer, B., Madsen, S. M., Seidelin, J. B. and Heegaard, N. H. (2000) Established and emerging biological activity markers of inflammatory bowel disease. *Am. J. Gastroenterol.*, **95**, 359–67.

Papadakis, K. A., Lo, S. K., Fireman, Z. and Hollerbach, S. (2005) Wireless capsule endoscopy in the evaluation of patients with suspected or known Crohn's disease. *Endoscopy*, **37**, 1018–22.

Pasha, S. F. and Leighton, J. A. (2009) Enteroscopy in the diagnosis and management of Crohn's disease. *Gastrointest. Endosc. Clin. N. Am.*, **19**, 427–44.

Peeters, M., Joossens, S., Vermeire, S., Vlietinck, R., Bossuyt, X. and Rutgeerts, P. (2001) Diagnostic value of anti-*Saccharomyces cerevisiae* and antineutrophil cytoplasmic autoantibodies in inflammatory bowel disease. *Am. J. Gastroenterol.*, **96**, 730–4.

Pera, A., Bellando, P., Caldera, D., Ponti, V., Astegiano, M., Barletti, C., David, E., Arrigoni, A., Rocca, G. and Verme, G. (1987) Colonoscopy in inflammatory bowel disease. Diagnostic accuracy and proposal of an endoscopic score. *Gastroenterology*, **92**, 181–5.

Rimola, J., Rodriguez, S. and Ayuso, C. (2008) [Magnetic resonance enterography in Crohn's disease: a new diagnostic tool?] *Med. Clin. (Barc.)*, **130**, 580–4.

Rimola, J., Rodriguez, S., Garcia-Bosch, O., Ordas, I., Ayala, E., Aceituno, M., Pellise, M., Ayuso, C., Ricart, E., Donoso, L. and Panes, J. (2009) Magnetic resonance for assessment of disease activity and severity in ileocolonic Crohn's disease. *Gut*, **58**, 1113–20.

Saxon, A., Shanahan, F., Landers, C., Ganz, T. and Targan, S. (1990) A distinct subset of antineutrophil cytoplasmic antibodies is associated with inflammatory bowel disease. *J. Allergy Clin. Immunol.*, **86**, 202–10.

Schwartz, D. A., Pemberton, J. H. and Sandborn, W. J. (2001) Diagnosis and treatment of per anal fistulas in Cohn's disease. *Ann. Intern. Med.*, **135**, 906–18.

Sheridan, M. B., Nicholson, D. A. and Martin, D. F. (1993) Trans-abdominal ultrasonography as the primary investigation in patients with suspected Crohn's disease or recurrence: a prospective study. *Clin. Radiol.*, **48**, 402–4.

Shine, B., Berghouse, L., Jones, J. E. and Landon, J. (1985) C-reactive protein as an aid in the differentiation of functional and inflammatory bowel disorders. *Clin. Chim. Acta*, **148**, 105–9.

Stange, E. F., Travis, S. P., Vermeire, S., Beglinger, C., Kupcinkas, L., Geboes, K., Barakauskiene, A., Villanacci, V., Von, H. A., Warren, B. F., Gasche, C., Tilg, H., Schreiber, S. W., Scholmerich, J. and Reinisch, W. (2006) European evidence based consensus on the diagnosis and management of Crohn's disease: definitions and diagnosis. *Gut*, **55**(suppl. 1), i1–i15.

Tarjan, Z., Toth, G., Gyorke, T., Mester, A., Karlinger, K. and Mako, E. K. (2000) Ultrasound in Crohn's disease of the small bowel. *Eur. J. Radiol.*, **35**, 176–82.

Tibble, J. A., Sigthorsson, G., Bridger, S., Fagerhol, M. K. and Bjarnason, I. (2000a) Surrogate markers of intestinal inflammation are predictive of relapse in patients with inflammatory bowel disease. *Gastroenterology*, **119**, 15–22.

Tibble, J., Teahon, K., Thjodleifsson, B., Roseth, A., Sigthorsson, G., Bridger, S., Foster, R., Sherwood, R., Fagerhol, M. and Bjarnason, I. (2000b) A simple method for assessing intestinal inflammation in Crohn's disease. *Gut*, **47**, 506–13.

Travis, S. P., Stange, E. F., Lemann, M., Oresland, T., Chowers, Y., Forbes, A., D'Haens, G., Kitis, G., Cortot, A., Prantera, C., Marteau, P., Colombel, J. F., Gionchetti, P., Bouhnik, Y., Tiret, E., Kroesen, J., Starlinger, M. and Mortensen, N. J. (2006) European evidence based consensus on the diagnosis and management of Crohn's disease: current management. *Gut*, **55**(suppl. 1), i16–i35.

Vermeire, S., Van, A. G. and Rutgeerts, P. (2004) C-reactive protein as a marker for inflammatory bowel disease. *Inflamm. Bowel. Dis.*, **10**, 661–5.

CHAPTER 5

Nursing assessment

Julie Duncan

Introduction

Nursing assessment is a constant process. It occurs, often unconsciously, in a variety of settings: in the outpatient clinic, over the telephone, by the bedside, even when you meet a patient in the corridor! Depending on the setting in which the assessment takes place, and the role of the nurse making the assessment, the purpose will be different and this will influence what, and why, you assess. This chapter will focus on the assessment process for the IBD Clinical Nurse Specialist (CNS) in the outpatient setting and aims to discuss the issues for consideration whilst faced with a patient with IBD rather than act as a comprehensive, didactic assessment tool. However, it should be said that the principles of good assessment are the same no matter what the clinical context.

What is assessment?

Essentially, assessment is information gathering. In the context of a health assessment it would involve gathering information about a patient's physical, psychological and social state, as well as significant lifestyle and environmental factors which may affect health (Walsh, 2000). It can be formal, in the context of a planned outpatient visit (e.g. assessing response to a new treatment) or completing a checklist prior to a procedure such as endoscopy; or informal, as in the example of meeting a patient in the corridor. In that instance the nurse makes observations and listens to the patient which results in making a clinical judgement. Depending on the role and experience of the nurse the purpose of the assessment may be to review progress in the immediate post-operative period by making clinical observations, including vital signs and verbal and non-verbal cues, or, in the instance of the advanced nurse practitioner (see Chapter 21), using advanced assessment skills to diagnose and treat conditions. Overall, the function of assessment in the context of IBD management is to:

- Ascertain actual *and* potential needs (physical, psychosocial or educational)
- Obtain information on which to plan interventions or treatments
- Provide a recorded baseline for later reassessment
- Evaluate response to treatments
- Evaluate effect of disease and treatments on quality of life

Case study 1

Matt, a 22-year-old man with longstanding ileocolonic and perianal Crohn's disease refractory to current immunomodulation, is considered appropriate for treatment with infliximab in combination with surgical drainage of his perianal fistula. Although initially keen on treatment he failed to attend appointments for pre-screening investigations. At first he was evasive about why he did not come for screening, despite clearly saying he was keen to start the medication. The IBD nurse picked up from non-verbal cues that he may have an unexpressed concern about the treatment and asked him very directly with closed questions about this. He asked how adrenaline would be administered should he have an anaphylactic reaction to infliximab. The CNS explained that, should this be necessary, it would be administered via a peripheral cannula. With palpable relief Matt described his fear that, having previously watched the film *Pulp Fiction*, adrenaline may have been administered through his breast bone directly into his heart.

Case study 2

Jasmine is a 19-year-old woman diagnosed with stricturing ileal and perianal Crohn's disease aged 12. She has had a complex course of disease with two previous ileal resections and several surgeries for her perianal disease. Over the years she has been prescribed most available immunomodulators and lost response to infliximab. She had an initial response to adalimumab 40 mg fortnightly, but this needed to be increased to weekly treatments a few months previously. Her disease course has been complicated by adherence and lifestyle issues, including an unwillingness to take responsibility for her disease management for prolonged periods. She lives a significant distance from her IBD team's location and often does not attend clinic appointments, although the same pattern was apparent to a previous local treatment team.

She failed to attend an appointment with her consultant gastroenterologist, but a week later contacted his secretary to request a telephone consultation. She was offered an appointment in the IBD nurse-led telephone clinic the following week. During that telephone consultation she stated her main problem was side-effects to adalimumab. She felt it was causing abdominal pain, especially after food, with nausea and vomiting. She had decided to stop the medication three weeks previously, but was not completely sure if there was a resolution to her symptoms. She was on no medication for her Crohn's disease other than occasional codeine phosphate for pain. Through advanced communication skills, knowledge of disease process and IBD treatments, along with Jasmine's past medical history of stricturing disease, the IBD CNS was able to hypothesise that the symptoms Jasmine was experiencing were most likely due to new ileal stricture(s), possibly requiring surgical resection, rather than to side-effects of adalimumab. Accordingly, and within local guidelines, she arranged a small bowel MRI scan and referral to an IBD surgeon. However, the CNS was aware that Jasmine had in the past refused referral to surgeons and explored the reasons for this. It became apparent that the main issue was a fear of stoma formation. She expressed that she would not attend a surgical appointment, or consent to surgery should the need arise, unless there were guarantees she could avoid a stoma. Clearly the CNS could not afford that guarantee but they discussed at length (the CNS using her knowledge of IBD, surgical management and anatomy and physiology) that if stoma formation was necessary then it would be temporary. Following this discussion Jasmine agreed to a surgical referral.

Both of these cases demonstrate the importance of communication, both verbal and non-verbal, including listening, demonstrating empathy and observation, and of having a therapeutic relationship with your patient which enables open and frank discussions. Therapeutic relationships are discussed in more detail in Chapter 16. By possessing these communication skills the CNS was able to assess that there were underlying problems which were barriers to Matt and Jasmine receiving appropriate treatment and change a situation which could have led to deterioration of their health status.

The Nursing Process

There are many models of nursing used in the assessment and planning of patient care. Possibly the most simple and commonly used is the Nursing Process (Rogers, 1989). This has five stages:

1. Assessment
2. Problem identification (diagnosing)
3. Planning (goal setting)
4. Implementation
5. Evaluation

Assessment is first and fundamental to the whole process, and, arguably, a good assessment is the most important aspect of health provision.

Assessment of the IBD patient

Assessment starts when you first meet your patient for a consultation. When you call their name in the waiting area you begin a process of assessment. You observe their posture whilst sitting in the waiting area, their gait when they walk towards the clinic room and even their face and mannerisms provide clues to their physical and psychological state. When introducing yourself and shaking hands you can obtain clues about a patient's strength and even their temperature (for example: do their hands feel cold or clammy?). In that brief encounter you can often assess that a patient is, for example, in pain, anxious or worried. Some of the techniques used in assessment are interview, direct observation and measurement.

The health history or health interview

Taking a holistic health history is essentially conducting an interview to elicit detailed and accurate information. It is a skilled task and not merely a matter of recording patient's responses to questions. Table 5.1 is an example of a system of gathering information (Ford *et al.*, 2005).

Table 5.1 The history taking process: system for gathering information (Ford *et al.*, 2005).

Listen	■ To patients' story in their own words ■ Encourage flow with verbal and non-verbal cues ■ Don't interrupt
Clarify	■ Any terms not understood or vague ■ Timing of events ■ Any inconsistencies or gaps in story
Question	■ Specific areas of relevance ■ Use open questions initially ■ Closed questions to understand specifics ■ Avoid leading questions
Summarise	■ Outline story as you understand it ■ Invite patient to correct inaccuracies

Firstly the nurse should establish the patients' *subjective* perceptions about health concerns and/or their feelings. For example ask 'What is the main problem?' or 'How do you feel?'. Information about established IBD diagnosis (and date of diagnosis) can be obtained from the patient, and medical notes, about previous treatments, allergies, surgeries, medications, along with relevant past medical history and family history (such as a family history of colorectal cancer). An assessment of current symptoms pertinent to IBD can follow. Figure 5.1 (overleaf) provides an example of an assessment proforma which can aid the nurse in clinic, although it should be pointed out that proforma are not comprehensive and do not replace clinical judgement or reasoning, but merely form a baseline in which to assess, and help maintain consistency. They can also aid a logical process in which to take a history. Table 5.2 takes the reader through the importance of the health questions outlined in Figure 5.1.

There should be a clear aim of the purpose of assessment and the patient should be made aware of this, for example: 'The purpose of this appointment is to assess your progress with Azathioprine'. If both nurse and patient are fully cognisant of the aim of the consultation it will make the assessment more efficient and effective (Baid, 2006). If a patient is unable to fully take part in a health history then other sources such as medical notes or accompanying family members can be used.

Also worth remembering is that many patients are expert in their disease and have a greater understanding of the significance of their individual symptoms than many healthcare professionals. Therefore it is useful to ask patients if they have experienced these symptoms in the same context before and what was the outcome, as this may enhance your assessment and clinical decision-making.

An important part of the history taking process should be to establish not just what medications the patient is on, but their actual adherence to this. Again, building a rapport and a trusting nurse–patient relationship is important to this. Adherence to medications is a significant facet of IBD care. It is known that adherence to treatment regimens is associated with improved health outcomes (Jackson *et al.*, 2010) and, non-adherence to 5-ASAs significantly increase the risk of relapse in patients with ulcerative colitis (Higgins *et al.*, 2009). If reasons for non-adherence, and other barriers to treatment, are identified then a solution can normally be found, as in the case of Matt and Jasmine.

Communication skills

Enhanced communication skills are arguably the greatest tool to obtaining a thorough and efficient assessment. It has been shown that clinicians who use effective communication skills identify their patients' actual problems more

IBD NURSING REVIEW		
Date: **Time:** **Reason for visit:** ☐ Clinical ☐ Education ☐ OPC ☐ Phone clinic	**Patient details**: (addressograph label) Hospital No: Name: DOB:	**Consultant:** ☐ Dr Smith ☐ Dr Brown ☐ Dr Jones ☐ Other: _____

Diagnosis and relevant history:	
☐ CD ☐ UC ☐ IBD-U ☐ OFG ☐ Other____ Disease location: Date of diagnosis: Smoker: **Yes / No** If yes, no. cigarettes: Alcohol (units):	Past medical, surgical & psychosocial history: Dietary history:

Current medications:

Presenting problem or concern:

Symptom profile:	

Frequency (24 hr):
 Consistency:
 Blood:
 Mucus:
 Pain: **Yes /No**
     ■ Location
     ■ Frequency
     ■ Duration
     ■ Severity
     ■ Precipitating factors
 	
 Nausea/Vomiting:
	Appetite:
	 Weight loss: **Yes / No** If yes: amount:
	 Fatigue:
	 Urgency:
	 Faecal incontinence: **Yes / No**
	     ■ UI
	     ■ Passive
	     ■ Flatus
	     ■ Frequency
	     ■ Pads
	
	 Evacuation difficulties: **Yes / No**

Most recent investigations:

Figure 5.1 An assessment proforma.

Disease activity score:	
Harvey Bradshaw Index (recorded over last 24 hrs)	**Simple Clinical Colitis Activity Index** (recorded over last 24 hrs)

Harvey Bradshaw Index		Simple Clinical Colitis Activity Index	
No. of **liquid** stools in last 24 hrs:		Bowel frequency: (daytime)	0 = 1–3× 1 = 4–6× 2 = 7–9× 3 = >9×
Abdominal pain:	0 = none 1 = mild 2 = moderate 3 = severe	Nocturnal frequency:	1 = 1–3× 2 = 4–6×
General well being:	0 = very well 1 = slightly below par 2 = poor 3 = very poor 4 = terrible	Urgency	1 = hurry 2 = immediate 3 = incontinence
		Blood in stool:	1 = trace 2 = occasionally frank 3 = usually frank
Abdominal mass:	0 = no mass 1 = dubious 2 = definite 3 = definite + tender	General well being:	0 = very well 1 = slightly below par 2 = poor 3 = very poor 4 = terrible
Extracolonic features: (1 each)	Arthralgia Pyoderma Erythema nodosum Aphthous ulcers Fissure New fistula Abscess	Extracolonic features: (1 each)	Arthralgia Pyoderma Erythema Nodosum Aphthous ulcers Fissure New fistula Abscess
Total:		**Total:**	

Summary of discussion and advice

Discussed with:	Action taken:
☐ Dr Brown ☐ Not discussed ☐ Dr Jones ☐ Dr Smith ☐ Registrar: _____ ☐ Other : _____	☐ Discussion and advice ☐ Referral ☐ Investigations arranged ☐ Secretarial action ☐ Medication initiated ☐ VBIC discussion ☐ Medication changed ☐ MDM discussion ☐ NACC new pt pack ☐ NACC info ☐ IBD advice service info ☐ Other _____
Practitioner: (sign and print)	**Date and time of completion:**

Figure 5.1 (*continued*)

Table 5.2 Nursing considerations whilst assessing the patient with IBD.

Assessment point	Nursing considerations
Diagnosis and relevant history	■ Differentiate whether the patient has CD, UC or IBD-unclassified. This is important in determining the current clinical condition, but also to identify treatment options and patient education needs.
Disease location	■ This is important for the reasons above, providing further clues for clinical decision making. Using disease classification tools such as the Montreal classification of IBD (see Chapter 3) can be useful (Satsangi et al., 2006).
Date of diagnosis	■ How long since diagnosis is important to determine the course of disease (e.g. how aggressive) and to trigger considerations such as timing and frequency of cancer surveillance in patients with UC or colonic CD.
Past medical and surgical history	■ Previous and current relevant medical and surgical events including dates. Timings of surgery can be particularly pertinent in the assessment of post-operative recurrence in CD as this may drive the level of intervention (for example, may be an indication to escalate medical therapy to biological drugs if seen to have earlier than expected recurrence).
Psychosocial and family history	■ Relevant psychological or psychiatric history ■ Health-related quality of life ■ Social circumstances relevant to ability to manage IBD or barriers to treatments (e.g. work, family, dependents) ■ Lifestyle issues such as stress or smoking ■ Relevant family history (e.g. first line relatives with colorectal cancer)
Dietary history	■ Current dietary intake and any restrictions (either as a result of IBD or reasons independent of this) ■ Use of dietary supplementation including vitamins or high-calorie drinks ■ Any current or previous dietary interventions (see Chapter 8)
Current medications	■ Include all prescribed, herbal and over the counter medications, including dosage and frequency of use. ■ Record any known drug allergies
Presenting problem	■ This is the patient's subjective perceptions about health concerns.

Table 5.2 (*continued*)

Assessment point	Nursing considerations
Symptom profile	
Bowel frequency	■ Frequency of bowel actions per 24 hour period ■ What is normal frequency for the individual patient? ■ This helps to assess current disease activity
Stool consistency	■ Often helpful to use Bristol stool form chart (Lewis and Heaton, 1997) to aid patient's interpretation of this.
Blood	■ If passes blood per rectum, how frequently and type (e.g. bright, dark, clots, on wiping, in toilet pan etc.), with stool or on its own.
Mucus	■ With stool, blood or on its own, frequency.
Pain	■ Location: abdominal (specific or general)/rectal/both ■ Frequency: how often does the pain occur ■ Duration: how long does the episode of pain last ■ Severity: mild, moderate or severe. Often useful to use a rating scale (e.g. 0 = no pain, 10 = worst imaginable) ■ Precipitating factors: is the pain associated with any particular activity such as defecation or eating ■ Resolution: does anything in particular resolve the pain (e.g. medication, defecation, hot water bottle)
Appetite and weight loss	■ Has appetite changed? ■ Has there been a change in weight? ■ If there is weight loss establish how much over what period of time. It's helpful if patients are weighed each time they attend clinic in order to look back and monitor this. ■ Some medications may alter weight and appetite (e.g. corticosteroids)
Urgency	■ Do you need to rush to the toilet? ■ How long can you wait?
Faecal incontinence	■ Does this relate to urgency (urge incontinence) ■ Does it just leak with no warning (passive incontinence) ■ Flatus incontinence ■ Need to wear pads or use other continence products ■ Any difficulties evacuating bowels such as straining or feeling of incomplete evacuation
Nausea or vomiting	■ Frequency, what triggers onset ■ What, if anything resolves it

Table 5.2 (*continued*)

Assessment point	Nursing considerations
Recent investigations	■ Date and results of last relevant investigations, e.g. colonoscopy, small bowel imaging, bone scan, blood testing. Along with providing the nurse information to build a clinical picture, knowing both the date of procedure and the ability to interpret results will, along with the current clinical story, aid decisions about timing any necessary reinvestigation or the need to conduct other investigations.

accurately (Maguire *et al.*, 1986). According to Maguire and Pitceathly (2002), key aspects of effective communication with patients include:

■ Identifying the patient's main problem(s) (including subjective perception and impact socially and on quality of life)
■ Tailoring information to personal needs (checking understanding)
■ Identifying how much the patient can, or wants to, participate in decision-making
■ Discussing treatment options in a way the patient understands the implications (e.g. risk/benefits)
■ Engaging the patient in decisions such that it can maximise adherence to treatments

Effective communication not only saves time due to its efficiency, it has been shown to increase patient satisfaction with their care and improve adherence to prescribed treatments and agreed lifestyle changes (e.g. smoking cessation) (Silverman *et al.*, 1998). An appropriate clinical area which affords privacy, comfort and dignity to the patient, free of interruption should be standard. Introducing one-self and establishing eye contact at the beginning of the health interview helps to establish a rapport, and re-establishing eye contact at regular intervals during the consultation show the clinician is interested (Maguire and Pitceathly, 2002). It can be useful to encourage the patient to be focused on the question at hand, gently bringing them back to the question asked in order that the clinician obtains the information needed. However, it is important not to interrupt before patients have completed important statements (Beckman and Frankel, 1984). Active listening clarifies and explores patients' concerns (Goldberg *et al.*, 1993). Briefly summarising the key points of the interview is useful to the clinician to clarify accurate identification of the issues, but also reinforce to the patient they

---

Box 5.1 Key skills for effective communication
- Provision of private, comfortable environment
- Establishing and maintaining eye contact
- Building rapport with patient
- Identify clear purpose for the health interview
- Identify patients subjective perceptions and beliefs
- Focused, relevant questioning
- Utilise closed and open questions
- Use active listening techniques
- Demonstrate empathy
- Use language your patient understands
- Summarise information to allow for clarification
- Engage patient in decision-making process

---

have been listened to and afford an opportunity to correct any misunderstandings. Some key skills required for effective communication are shown in Box 5.1.

Identifying patient understanding and what information they actually want helps individualise information-giving to their needs. Involving patients in decision making is more likely to result in adherence (Silverman *et al.*, 1998) and building a therapeutic relationship (see Chapter 16) with the patient facilitates that negotiation (Cutcliffe and McKenna, 2005).

Objective measurements

The next logical process in the assessment of the IBD patient is to identify objective clues to their health status. These would include most recent investigations, such as endoscopic procedures, blood tests and radiological examinations. The information gained from these investigations and the health history will direct the extent and nature of any physical examination undertaken with appropriate consent (Baid, 2006). Depending on the training and skill set of the CNS this will be carried out by her or by a medical colleague.

Scoring systems

Simple disease activity indices such as Simple Clinical Colitis Activity Index (SSCAI), (Walmsley *et al.*, 1998) and Harvey–Bradshaw Index (HBI), (Harvey and Bradshaw, 1980) are also useful assessment tools. These are 4–5 point indices which measure symptoms of disease activity over the previous 24 hours and thus give a snapshot of disease activity. Additionally the use of scoring systems in clinical practice is a useful baseline in the reassessment of disease, and assessment of response to treatment. They are often used, along with other subjective and objective measures, to justify the use of treatments (for example having an HBI greater than 8 is *one* justification for starting a biological in the author's hospital). The SSCAI and HBI are simple, quick tools and are included in the example assessment proforma in Figure 5.1. The Perianal Crohn's Disease Activity Index (PCDAI) is a useful tool in the assessment of perianal disease (Pikarsky *et al.*, 2002) and aims to assist in standardising assessment of perianal CD allowing more accurate use of surgery.

Physical assessment
The skill of clinical examination is one that is learned both academically and practically over a prolonged period, normally under medical and academic supervision. It is not the purpose of this chapter to explore this area of assessment in depth, but in IBD there are some general principles to consider. Table 5.3 lists potential systemic features of IBD which may be found during clinical examination. These systemic features are further explored in Chapter 3.

Following appropriate consent (Department of Health, 2009) and a general physical examination (Douglas *et al.*, 2005; Baid, 2006) the abdomen may be examined by inspection, palpation, percussion and auscultation, all of which are well described elsewhere (Douglas *et al.*, 2005; Ford *et al.*, 2005).

The knowledge gained from the health history and these objective measurements will allow the CNS to use his or her clinical reasoning to influence a diagnosis or clinical decision. This in turn allows an advanced nursing care plan to be developed. For example, it will allow consideration of the need for alteration of medication regimens, to request further investigation to assess disease activity or response to treatments, but also for the need to assess for potential complications of disease and its treatment, such as bone scanning in the patient exposed to steroids, or surveillance colonoscopy in the patient with UC 10 years

Table 5.3 Systemic features of IBD (Ford et al., 2005).

System	Clinical feature
General	Fever, malaise, weight loss
Eyes	Inflammation: conjunctivitis, iritis, episcleritis
Joints	Arthralgia of large joints, sacroileitis, ankylosing spondylitis
Skin	Mouth ulcers, pyoderma gangrenosum, erythema nodosum
Liver	Fatty liver, gallstones, sclerosing cholangitis

post diagnosis. It should be acknowledged that advanced interventions such as physical examination, non-medical prescribing or ordering investigations should only be undertaken following appropriate training and within local and national guidelines.

Chapters 4, 6, 7 and 8 fully explore investigating and medical management of IBD, and Chapter 21 further elucidates the role of advanced practice.

Conclusion

A good assessment is the cornerstone of any clinical intervention. It is important to remember the basics such as affording privacy, comfort and dignity, along with the more advanced aspects of history taking, expert communication and assessment of objective measures. To effectively assess and optimise the IBD patients clinical management, the IBD CNS needs to develop and utilise a combination of observational skills, effective communication, a good relationship with his or her patient and MDT along with sound knowledge of anatomy and physiology, IBD disease process and clinical management.

References

Baid, H. (2006) The process of conducting a physical assessment: a nursing perspective. *Br. J. Nursing,* 5(13), 710–14.

Beckman, A. B. and Frankel, R. M. (1984) The effect of physician behaviour on the collection of data. *Ann. Intern. Med.,* **101**, 692–6.

Cutcliffe, J. R. and McKenna, H. P. (2005) *The Essential Concepts of Nursing.* London: Elsevier.

Douglas, G., Nicol, F. and Robertson, C. (2005) *MacLeod's Clinical Examination,* 11th edn. Edinburgh: Elsevier Churchill Livingstone.

Department of Health (2009) *Reference Guide for Consent for Examination or Treatment,* 2nd edn. London: Department of Health.

Ford, M. J., Hennessey, I. and Japp, A. (2005) *Introduction to Clinical Examination,* 8th edn. Edinburgh: Elsevier Churchill Livingstone.

Goldberg, D. P., Jenkins, I., Miller, T. and Farrier, E. B. (1993) The ability of trainee general practitioners to identify psychological distress among their patients. *Psychological Medicine,* **23**, 185–93.

Harvey, R. F. and Bradshaw, J. M. (1980) A simple index of Crohn's disease activity. *Lancet,* **1**, 514.

Higgins, P. D. R., Rubin, D. T., Kaulback, K. *et al.* (2009) Systematic review: impact of non-adherence to 5-aminosalicylic acid products on the frequency and cost of ulcerative colitis flares. *Alimentary Pharmaceuticals and Therapeutics,* **29**, 247–57.

Jackson, C. A., Clatworthy, J., Robinson, A. and Horne, R. (2010) Factors associated with non-adherence to oral medication for inflammatory bowel disease: a systematic review. *American Journal of Gastroenterology*, **105**, 525–39.

Lewis, S. J. and Heaton, K. W. (1997) Stool form scale as a useful guide to intestinal transit time. *Scand. J. Gastroenterol.*, **32**, 920–4.

Maguire, P., Fairbairn, S. and Fletcher, C. (1986) Consultation skills of young doctors: benefits of feedback training in interviewing as students persist. *Br. Med. J.*, **292**, 1573–8.

Maguire, P. and Pitceathly, C. (2002) Key communication skills and how to acquire them. *Br. J. Med.*, **325**, 697–700.

Pikarsky, A. J., Gervaz, P. and Wexner, S. D. (2002) Perianal Crohn's disease. A new scoring system to evaluate and predict outcome of surgical intervention. *Archives of Surgery*, **137**, 774–8.

Rogers, M. E. (1989) Creating a climate for the implementation of a nursing conceptual framework. *J. Cont. Ed. Nursing*, **20**, 112–16.

Satsangi, J., Silverberg, M. S., Vermeire, S. *et al.* (2006) The Montreal classification of inflammatory bowel disease: controversies, consensus and implications. *Gut*, **55**, 749–53.

Silverman, J., Kurtz, S. and Draper, J. (1998) *Skills for Communicating with Patients*. Oxford: Radcliffe Medical Press.

Walmsley, R. S., Ayres, R. C. S., Punder, R. E. and Allan, R. N. (1998) A simple clinical colitis activity index. *Gut*, **43**, 29–32.

Walsh, M. (2000) *Watson's Clinical Nursing and Related Science*. London: Baillière Tindall.

CHAPTER 6

Medical management of inflammatory bowel disease in the adult general setting

Kirstin M. Taylor and Peter M. Irving

Introduction

The first step in managing patients with Crohn's disease and ulcerative colitis is a thorough assessment of the patient. This requires that a full history is taken from the patient, covering not only the history of their disease and its current state, but also any coexisting medical conditions and past medical problems. A full drug history must be taken which should include use of over the counter and complementary medicines as well as a list of allergies. Finally, the patient's social and family history should be recorded. This must be complemented by a thorough examination and appropriate investigations. Simple tests may include blood tests and stool cultures, the results of which will normally be available quickly, but imaging investigations and endoscopic examinations are more likely to be carried out at a separate visit (see Chapter 4).

Modern management of IBD uses a patient-focused approach, with the patient being at the centre of a multidisciplinary team (MDT). This team is likely to vary between institutions and will partly depend on local availability and skill mix. However, in addition to gastroenterologists and surgeons with a special interest in IBD, other key members of the team include dietitians, radiologists, histopathologists, pharmacists, primary care physicians and, of course, IBD nurses. At times it may also be appropriate to include other professionals, such as counsellors, psychologists, social workers and physiotherapists. Because the management of IBD is often complex, and can involve input from many members of the team, it is important to keep everyone updated; this is often a role that is fulfilled by IBD nurses who may be best placed to coordinate various aspects of the patient's care.

With regard to medical therapy, decisions about which drugs to use and when will often be based on information gained from a number of members of the MDT. Most importantly, however, these decisions must also be taken in conjunction with the central member of the team, namely the patient. Without their involvement, adherence to treatment, a well-recognised problem in IBD, is likely to be poor.

In this chapter we discuss the standard treatments used in the medical management of IBD, along with some of the newer and more unusual treatments that are available.

Factors influencing choice of treatments

Choice of medical therapy is based on a number of factors:

- patient-related
  - co-morbidities
  - tolerance
  - drug interactions
  - family planning
  - side-effects
  - patient preference
- disease-related
  - site of disease
  - severity of disease
  - complications
  - extra-intestinal manifestations
- local expertise
- funding issues

Most treatment is initiated in the outpatient setting, and many clinics are now nurse-led. An increasing number of nurses prescribe medication, although the majority of prescriptions are still written by doctors. However, IBD nurse specialists, whether able to prescribe or not, are often involved in educating patients in a number of areas related to prescribed medications. These include potential side-effects and how to deal with them, how to take medication, how to optimise adherence and, of increasing importance, how to choose between drugs when a choice is available. The role of monitoring for side-effects may also fall within the remit of the IBD nurse specialist.

Treatment aim

The aim of medical treatment is to achieve and maintain corticosteroid-free remission using a drug (or combination of drugs) with an acceptable safety and side-effect profile. Maintenance of remission is important to enable the patient to achieve as good a quality of life as possible, and, where appropriate, avoid surgery and its associated complications. The long-term use of corticosteroids is to be avoided due to the poor side-effect profile (as detailed later in this chapter).

The use of complementary and alternative medicine (CAM) is becoming widespread, although evidence for its use is limited, high quality trials being few in number. While some patients' symptoms may improve when using CAM, consideration must be given to the nature of IBD, which is relapsing and remitting (in other words the disease may have got better by itself), and the placebo effect. It goes without saying that the same consideration must also be given to all treatment, be it conventional or complementary.

There is an increased awareness of the effects of immunomodulatory therapy for IBD on the risk of developing opportunistic infections (e.g. hepatitis B, tuberculosis, chicken pox). There is a move towards screening for and vaccinating patients against such infections early in their diagnosis, before such medication is commenced. This is covered in more detail in Chapter 7.

Ulcerative colitis

5-aminosalicylates (5-ASAs)

5-ASAs are available in a number of different preparations. They can be taken orally as capsules, tablets or granules, or can be applied topically as suppositories, or enemas.

Case study

A 34-year-old man with pan-ulcerative colitis diagnosed five years ago had been maintained in remission with Asacol 1.2 g twice a day until six months ago when he had a flare of his disease. This initially responded to a course of oral steroids, but within a few months he was once again opening his bowels five times a day, passing loose bloody stool. Stool cultures were negative. Despite increasing his Asacol to 2.4 g twice a day, he required a further course of oral corticosteroids. After discussion in clinic, measurement of his thiopurine methyltransferase and screening for infection, he was commenced on azathioprine 2 mg/kg once a day in an attempt to maintain his steroid-induced remission.

Suppositories are first-line treatment for mild to moderate proctitis and are generally better tolerated than foam enemas, which treat the sigmoid and, in the case of liquid enemas, the descending colon. Combined topical and oral treatment is often more effective than either preparation alone (Marteau *et al.*, 2005), although patients with active disease sometimes have difficulty retaining topical preparations. They are normally easier to retain if used at night.

Oral preparations have various delivery systems that affect the location at which the active drug is released. This may, therefore, influence response depending on disease location: azo-bonded compounds (sulfasalazine, balsalazide) are released when they encounter bacteria in the colon, while controlled release preparations (Pentasa) are released throughout the bowel. The use of a pH-dependent coating (Asacol, Salofalk, Mezavant XL) targets release of the drug in the distal small bowel or the colon. High doses of 5-ASA (> 4 g/day) have been shown to be safe and effective in achieving and maintaining remission in mild to moderate UC (Sutherland *et al.*, 2000).

5-ASAs have a good safety profile. Diarrhoea, headache, nausea and abdominal pain are the most frequently reported side-effects and are generally dose-dependent. More serious complications, such as Stevens–Johnson syndrome (a systemic illness with fever, joint pains and blistering rash), hepatitis, pancreatitis, alveolitis, agranulocytosis, interstitial nephritis and nephrotic syndrome, are rare.

- *Dosage*: depends on formulation used. Oral preparations are unlikely to be effective at < 1 g a day. Higher doses (> 4 g a day) are used to achieve remission, while the dose is often reduced to maintain remission.
- *Monitoring*: yearly renal function and dipstick of urine (to detect proteinuria/ albuminuria indicative of renal disease).

Corticosteroids

Topical, oral and intravenous (iv) preparations are available. Topical corticosteroid treatment (suppositories and enemas) is less effective than topical 5-ASA (Marshall and Irvine, 1997) but can be used in combination with 5-ASA if the latter is unable to control disease. Oral corticosteroids are used when symptoms of active colitis do not respond quickly to 5-ASAs, when a patient has a flare whilst on treatment with higher doses of 5-ASAs or an immunomodulator, or when rapid symptom relief is needed. Oral prednisolone (for example, starting at 40 mg a day) is effective in inducing remission. Higher doses are associated with increased side-effects without additional clinical benefit, and doses of 15 mg a day or less are ineffective in active disease.

For severe disease of any extent, patients should be admitted to hospital for iv corticosteroids. This is covered later in the chapter.

The biggest problem with steroids relates to their side-effect profile. Steroid-induced side-effects include, acutely: sleep and mood disturbance, glucose intolerance, dyspepsia, and cosmetic effects (acne, moon face, fluid retention). In the longer-term, metabolic bone disease (osteoporosis, osteopenia, osteonecrosis), myopathy, cataracts, accelerated atherogenesis, impaired wound healing and increased risk of infection may occur. Sudden withdrawal may cause acute adrenal insufficiency. Accordingly, it is usual to decrease the dose gradually over a number of weeks. (Usually a course of prednisolone is tapered over at least 8 weeks; however, some patients may require a more protracted reduction.)

- *Dosage*: acute severe UC: hydrocortisone 100 mg every 6 hours iv or methylprednisolone 60 mg/day iv
  Oral dosing: prednisolone 40 mg once a day with tapering, commonly by 5 mg a week
  Remember concurrent calcium and vitamin D for bone protection
- *Monitoring*: if there is a history of prolonged or repeated exposure to corticosteroids, consider DEXA bone scan to look for osteopenia or osteoporosis

Thiopurines

Azathioprine (AZA) and 6-mercaptopurine (6MP) (both unlicensed for the treatment of IBD) act as steroid-sparing agents and should be considered in those who:

- have two or more courses of steroid within a year
- relapse when prednisolone is reduced below 15 mg
- relapse within three months of steroid cessation

Their onset of action, however, is slow, taking three to six months for full effect. No direct comparison between the two drugs has been made in UC, but approximately 60% of patients intolerant of AZA are able to tolerate 6MP (Lees *et al.*, 2008).

AZA is metabolised to 6MP and subsequently to 6-thioguanine nucleotides (6-TGN). Thiopurine methyltransferase (TPMT) is an enzyme that metabolizes thiopurines, and the activity of this enzyme or its genotype are usually measured prior to treatment. TPMT activity can be absent, low, high and very high. Genotype can be deficient (associated with absent TPMT activity), heterozygote (low TPMT activity) or homozygous wildtype (high and very high activity). The initial maintenance dose of AZA is 2–2.5 mg/kg/day and of 6MP, 1-1.5 mg/kg/day for patients with 'normal' to high levels of TPMT or a wildtype genotype. For those with low activity (or heterozygotes) a 50% dose reduction is recommended. With absent TPMT activity (deficient), thiopurines are generally avoided. If available, 6-TGN levels can be measured to assess therapeutic targets and compliance, and allow tailored treatment. Further discussion about optimising thiopurine treatment can be found in Chapter 7.

Significant leukopenia can develop at any time (whatever the TPMT genotype or activity) and it is important that patients are advised to seek medical help should a sore throat or other sign of infection occur. The most frequently reported side-effects are nausea and flu-like symptoms that occur early in the course of treatment. Hepatotoxicity and pancreatitis are uncommon (< 5%) (Fraser *et al.*, 1989; Present *et al.*, 1989). There is a 3–4-fold increased risk of lymphoma associated with the use of thiopurines and an increase in the risk of developing non-melanoma skin cancers. It is important to put these risks in context by expressing the absolute rather than the relative risk of developing these conditions. For example, the absolute risk of developing lymphoma for a person in their 20s is about 1:10,000/ year. Increasing this risk by a factor of 4 by taking thiopurines means that the absolute risk is still very small at 4:10,000/year. In comparison, expressing the relative risk of using thiopurines, namely that they are associated with a 4-fold increase in risk of developing lymphoma, may be interpreted very differently by patients.) The risk of taking thiopurines must also be compared with the risks of not using them (such as uncontrolled disease activity which is a risk factor for developing colorectal cancer.)

- *Dosage*: Azathioprine 2–2.5 mg/kg a day (50% reduction if low TPMT)
  6-mercaptopurine 1–1.5 mg/kg a day (50% reduction if low TPMT)
- *Monitoring*: The manufacturers recommend weekly full blood counts (FBCs) for the first eight weeks of treatment followed by blood tests at least every three months. Liver function should be measured at the same time. Individual hospital protocols may differ.

Methotrexate

Studies of methotrexate (MTX) for UC are small and inconsistent with variable outcomes. The only randomised controlled trial (RCT) for MTX in UC showed no benefit, although the dose was much lower than that found to be effective in Crohn's disease (Oren *et al.*, 1996). There are ongoing trials that should provide a better guide to the efficacy of MTX in UC; however, retrospective data suggest that approximately 50% of people who failed to respond to, or are intolerant of, thiopurines will respond to MTX. MTX for UC is unlicensed.

MTX is used for the same indications as thiopurines. The usual dosage is 25 mg once a week for 16 weeks to achieve remission, followed by 15 mg a week for those who respond. It can be given orally or by subcutaneous (SC) (unlicensed for any condition) or intramuscular (IM) injection.

Full blood counts should be measured every two weeks for the first two months, and thereafter 2–3 monthly. There are concerns regarding the risk of hepatitis following long-term treatment and if the serum aspartate amino transferase (AST) rises to twice the upper limit of normal, MTX should be withheld until it normalises, before re-challenging. Side-effects are predominantly gastrointestinal (nausea, vomiting, diarrhoea and stomatitis) and usually respond to folic acid. This should be prescribed to all people taking MTX. There is little evidence to guide dosing of folic acid; however, it should not be taken on the day of MTX. A minimum of 5 mg/week should be given. Lung fibrosis, a side-effect seen in people with rheumatoid arthritis taking methotrexate, is extremely rare in people with IBD. However, should a patient taking MTX develop respiratory symptoms, they should be investigated quickly, and may require temporary or permanent interruption of treatment.

MTX is contraindicated during conception and pregnancy due to its teratogenic effects or in women of childbearing age unless robust methods of contraception are in place and they are fully aware of these risks. Breast-feeding should also be avoided. It is advised that men whose partners are trying to conceive should not use methotrexate although there is little evidence to support this.

- *Dosage*: 25 mg once a week, IM/SC/oral, for 16 weeks and if remission, continue treatment at 15 mg a week. Co-prescribe folic acid.
- *Monitoring*: FBC every two weeks for first two months, then 2–3 monthly LFTs 2–3 monthly.

Patients and their healthcare providers should record results in a National Patient Safety Agency (NPSA) MTX monitoring booklet

Ciclosporin

Ciclosporin (CsA) can be considered as rescue therapy to avoid or delay colectomy in patients with severe UC who have not responded to intravenous steroids. They should be counselled about the risks and benefits of this treatment as well as the alternatives – colectomy or infliximab. In some countries the use of infliximab may be restricted in this setting. It is given intravenously at 2–4 mg/kg/day, aiming for serum trough levels of 200–300 ng/mL (Van Assche *et al.*, 2003). Ciclosporin should be stopped if there is no response after 5–7 days or if there is clinical deterioration. In those who respond, treatment is changed to the oral route started at 5 mg/kg/day in two divided doses, aiming for a serum trough concentration of 100–200 ng/mL. CsA has a high long-term failure rate and its main role is as a bridge to maintenance with thiopurines. Corticosteroids should be tapered following response.

CsA has a number of associated side-effects. The main concerns are renal dysfunction, opportunistic infection and seizures (especially in those with hypomagnesaemia and hypocholesterolaemia, measurement of which is mandatory before treatment is commenced). Other side-effects include gingival hyperplasia, hypertension, tremor, hirsutism, hyperkalaemia, headache and abnormal liver function tests. When used with concomitant immunomodulators, consideration should be given to prophylaxis against *Pneumocystis jirovecii* with co-trimoxazole.

- *Dosage*: intravenously at 2–4 mg/kg/day
  Orally at 5 mg/kg/day in two divided doses
- *Monitoring*: avoid if cholesterol < 3 mmol/L, magnesium < 0.7 mg/dL or renal impairment
  Ciclosporin trough levels (200–300 ng/mL for iv ideally measured daily, 100–200 ng/mL for oral ideally measured weekly until stable)
  Renal function
- Blood pressure (monitored several times a day whilst on iv therapy, and weekly while on oral therapy until stable – local protocols may vary)

Infliximab
Infliximab (IFX, Remicade) is a chimeric anti-tumour necrosis factor (TNF) monoclonal antibody. Administered initially at 5 mg/kg iv at 0, 2 and 6 weeks, it is effective at inducing remission in moderate to severe UC. Maintenance is with further infusions every 8 weeks.

It can be used in the acute setting, as rescue therapy in patients who have not responded to intravenous hydrocortisone as an alternative to ciclosporin. It should not, however, be used in people who have failed to respond to CsA, as this combination is associated with a high risk of septic complications (Maser *et al.*, 2008).

It may also be used in patients who have chronic active disease despite an immunomodulator. However, recently in the UK the National Institute for Health and Clinical Excellence (NICE) has advocated the use of IFX as a rescue therapy (NICE guidance TA163, 2008) but not for chronic active UC (NICE guidance

TA140, 2008). This may lead to difficulties in obtaining funding for treatment with IFX in UC.

There is a risk of serious infection and demyelinating disease with anti-TNF therapy (around 3.5%). Infusion reactions are not uncommon and usually respond to slowing down the rate of the infusion and treatment with antihistamines and/ or corticosteroids. However, there is also a risk of anaphylaxis that is highest in patients who have had a long delay between infusions, probably related to the development of antibodies to IFX. Hepatosplenic T-cell lymphoma (HSTCL) has been reported in a small number of predominantly young, male, patients treated with IFX and concomitant immunosuppression. Although this condition is almost universally fatal, it is extremely rare (15 cases reported in IBD patients treated with IFX up to September 2008 (Mackey *et al.*, 2009)) and it is not clear how important anti-TNF treatment is in its causation. It is likely that infliximab also slightly increases the risk of other forms of non-Hodgkin's lymphoma. While it is difficult exactly to quantify this, it is likely that anti-TNF therapy has a similar effect on lymphoma risk as thiopurines.

Treatment with IFX may reactivate latent tuberculosis (TB) and, therefore, prior to treatment it is important to assess the risk of TB by taking an accurate history of possible exposure and by screening as per local guidelines. Treatment of latent TB should be started before treatment. Active TB is a contraindication to treatment with IFX. Prophylactic treatment for high-risk groups may also be indicated (see ECCO guidelines on opportunistic infection – referenced in the further reading list at the end of this chapter).

- *Dosage*: 5 mg/kg intravenously at 0, 2 and 6 weeks for induction, then. Usually every 8 weeks for maintenance

  If loss of response, consider increasing to 10 mg/kg, or reducing the interval between infusions
- *Monitoring*: There is no recommended monitoring regimen. However, FBC, LFTs, renal function and C-reactive protein measured at the time of each infusion are reasonable.

Other treatments

Fish oil (omega-3 fatty acids)

Omega-3 fatty acids are thought to have anti-inflammatory properties through reduction of leucotriene. RCTs of patients with UC in remission showed a similar relapse rate in those treated with fish oil versus those treated with placebo. There do not appear to be any safety concerns (Turner *et al.*, 2007).

Trichuris suis ova

Trichuris suis (pig whipworm) transiently colonises the gut and is non-pathogenic in man. Treatment was developed following the observation that UC is uncommon where helminth infection is prevalent. A randomised trial of patients with mild–moderate UC showed no significant difference in remission but an improved response in those treated with *T. suis* versus those given placebo (Summers *et al.*, 2005a).

Probiotics

Probiotics are defined as 'live micro-organisms which when administered in adequate amounts confer a health benefit on the host'. The *Escherichia coli* strain Nissle 1917 has been compared to mesalazine for maintenance of remission in UC in 3 RCTs and was found to be an effective alternative to mesalazine. Other strains including a combination of *Bifidobacterium bifidum* Y/T 4007, *B. breve* Y/T 4065 and *L. acidophilus* Y/T 0168, and *Lactobacillus* GG may also be effective, but have not been subject to properly powered RCTs (Hedin *et al.*, 2007).

Prebiotics

Prebiotics are nondigestible dietary oligosaccharides (e.g. inulin and oligofructose) that affect the host by selectively stimulating growth, activity, or both of probiotic bacteria. Their benefit (if any) in UC is unclear; trials are small in number and sample size, and use a combination of pre- and probiotics (synbiotics) (Hedin *et al.*, 2007).

Aloe vera gel

A RCT showed aloe vera gel (100 ml, twice a day, for four weeks) given to patients with moderate UC produced a clinical response in significantly more patients compared to those treated with placebo (Langmead *et al.*, 2004).

Curcumin

Curcumin is the yellow pigment of turmeric (*curcuma longa*). A RCT compared curcumin (1 g, twice a day) and 5-ASA with placebo and 5-ASA in quiescent UC. The addition of curcumin seemed to reduce relapse rates, improve clinical activity index and improve endoscopic index (Hanai *et al.*, 2006). Further studies are required.

Nicotine

Transdermal nicotine is superior for induction of remission in UC compared with placebo, and has been subject to a Cochrane review. However, there are a significant number of adverse events reported with this treatment that may limit its use. There does not appear to be any benefit of transdermal nicotine over standard medical therapy (McGrath *et al.*, 2004).

Dietary therapies will be explored in Chapter 8.

Acute severe ulcerative colitis

Severe UC should be managed in the inpatient setting. Initial assessment includes history, examination and observations (blood pressure, pulse, oxygen saturations, respiratory rate and temperature). Stool should be sent for culture and *Clostridium difficile* toxin to exclude infection and an abdominal X-ray should be performed to look for evidence of toxic megacolon. A CT scan of the abdomen should be considered if there is a concern of bowel perforation. Intravenous hydrocortisone is given at 100 mg, four times a day. Treatment should not be delayed pending results of stool cultures, although if there is a high index of suspicion, antibiotics may also be prescribed. This is particularly important if there is a history of travel to an area where amoebic dysentery is endemic. All patients should be prescribed low molecular weight heparin prophylaxis against venous thromboembolism unless there is a catastrophic haemorrhage. Stool charts must be maintained in order to assess response.

Treatment response (bowel frequency, clinical observations, C-reactive protein) should be assessed at day 3 to decide whether rescue therapy with, for example, ciclosporin or infliximab is warranted. Extended therapy with iv hydrocortisone without response is potentially dangerous. Surgical options must also be considered and discussed with the patient. Early review by a colorectal surgeon and stoma nurse is important so that the patient has time ask questions about surgery. Indications for colectomy in the acute setting include failure to respond to medical therapy, toxic megacolon, bowel perforation and major colonic haemorrhage. This is covered in more detail in Chapter 9.

Crohn's disease

Many of the medications used for UC are also used in Crohn's disease (CD); however, there are some important differences and these are mentioned below.

5-aminosalicylates (5-ASAs)

Oral aminosalicylates were initially reported to be effective for induction and maintenance of remission for both ileal and colonic CD. However, over recent years, their value as a treatment for Crohn's disease has become less clear. For example, a meta-analysis of Pentasa 4 g daily for active CD showed a reduction in

> ## Case study
>
> A 45-year-old woman with Crohn's colitis had been well controlled on azathioprine for many years. Over the last year, she had a recurrence of her previous symptoms of bloody diarrhoea and had started passing faeculent matter per vaginam. A colonoscopy confirmed active patchy left-sided colitis and an MRI scan of her pelvis showed a recto-vaginal fistula with no evidence of pelvic collections or abscesses. After discussion in clinic and screening for infection, she was commenced on infliximab induction at 5 mg/kg at 0, 2 and 6 weeks. Her symptoms improved and MRI following induction showed improvement in the fistula. Infliximab was continued every eight weeks, and the azathioprine was continued as concomitant immunosuppression.

the Crohn's disease activity index (CDAI) compared with placebo (Hanauer *et al.*, 2004a). However, the clinical significance of this is unclear and there has been a move away from using 5-ASAs recently. Similarly, 5-ASAs have not been found to be effective for maintenance of medically induced remission in CD (Akobeng *et al.*, 2005). Asacol is the only 5-ASA licensed for CD in the UK.

There have been no RCTs of topical 5-ASA in distal colonic CD.

Corticosteroids

Budesonide 9 mg a day orally is more effective than placebo and high dose 5-ASA for induction of remission in mild to moderate active ileocaecal CD, but is less effective in patients with more extensive colitis. It has fewer side-effects than prednisolone but is less effective, particularly in people with extensive colonic disease (in whom prednisolone may be more appropriate). Severe disease should initially be treated with intravenous corticosteroids.

- *Dosage*: Budesonide 9 mg controlled release, once a day, with tapering after response.

  Prednisolone 40 mg once a day with tapering, commonly by 5 mg a week.

  Remember concurrent calcium and vitamin D for bone protection.
- *Monitoring*: If there is a history of prolonged or repeated exposure to corticosteroids, consider DEXA bone scan to look for osteopenia or osteoporosis. (Prolonged and recurrent courses of budesonide can result in systemic side-effects.)

Antibiotics

Metronidazole and ciprofloxacin have been shown to be modestly effective in mildly active ileocaecal CD in small trials and case series. They are most useful for active perianal disease and if there is colonic involvement. Treatment needs to be long-term to achieve a response, but side-effects and complications often limit their use. For example, metronidazole often causes nausea and should not be taken in conjunction with alcohol. Long-term use of metronidazole can result in a peripheral neuropathy. Use of ciprofloxacin is associated with the development of *Clostridium difficile* colitis and, in the long-term, spontaneous rupture of the Achilles tendon (albeit rarely).

- *Dosage*: metronidazole 10–20 mg/kg a day, orally for up to 6 months. Ciprofloxacin 500 mg–1 g a day, orally for up to 6 months.
- *Monitoring*: stool cultures if concern of *Clostridium difficile* colitis.

Enteral nutrition

Elemental diets (based on amino acids, peptides and glucose) and more palatable polymeric diets (containing whole proteins, e.g. Modulen, Nestle) are predominantly used in children to induce remission in CD. Despite its limitations, nutritional therapy is normally used in preference to steroids in children because of the former's association with improved growth. A Cochrane review of nutritional therapy versus prednisolone showed corticosteroids to be slightly more effective for induction of remission. While controlled trials are few in adults, there is plenty of experience to suggest that enteral nutrition is also effective in older age groups.

Enteral nutrition (EN) is usually taken as sole nutrition for several weeks, followed by a gradual reintroduction of other food. The patient needs to be highly motivated, as many people find that the supplements are not very palatable, and complete abstinence from the usual diet can be very challenging. A dedicated dietitian is essential for initial nutritional assessment, follow-up and encouragement throughout the treatment course. IBD nurse specialists can support this role. EN is useful for induction of remission in patients who wish to avoid corticosteroids, but, as with steroids, is associated with a high risk of relapse on withdrawal of therapy (Akobeng *et al.*, 2007).

Nutritional therapies will be further explored in Chapter 8.

Thiopurines

Thiopurines are used as steroid-sparing agents to maintain remission of luminal Crohn's disease, as for UC (see UC section). They are also used in people with fistulising disease (Pearson *et al.*, 1995) and as post-operative prophylaxis of CD (Hanauer *et al.*, 2004b).

Methotrexate

RCTs have shown methotrexate (MTX) to be more effective than placebo at inducing and maintaining remission in CD. The starting dose is 25 mg a week (orally, SC or IM) for 16 weeks, continued at 15 mg a week for those who enter remission. MTX is used in a similar fashion to thiopurines: as a steroid-sparing agent (Patel *et al.*, 2009). It is generally used for those who are refractory or intolerant to AZA or 6MP (see UC section).

Biological therapy

In the UK, there are two biological drugs licensed for use in Crohn's disease: infliximab and adalimumab.

Infliximab (IFX; Remicade) is given as an intravenous infusion at a dose of 5 mg/kg iv at 0, 2 and 6 weeks to induce remission in active luminal Crohn's disease. It is also effective as a treatment for fistulising Crohn's disease; however, before using it in perianal disease, it is important to ensure no abscesses are present – by MRI, endoscopic ultrasound or examination under anaesthetic. For both indications maintenance of remission involves 8-weekly infusions. If response is lost, the dose of IFX can be increased to 10 mg/kg (sometimes temporarily), or the time between infusions decreased.

Adalimumab (Humira) is a fully human anti-TNF monoclonal antibody, administered by subcutaneous injection. This has the benefit that the patient does not need to attend hospital for treatment. It is given at an initial induction dose of 160 mg, followed by 80 mg at 2 weeks, or 80 mg followed by 40 mg at 2 weeks, to achieve remission, and continued at 40 mg a fortnight.

Although other biological drugs exist, currently adalimumab and infliximab are the only two available in the UK.

Certolizumab Pegol (Cimzia) is pegylated Fab fragment that binds TNF. It is also given subcutaneously. At a dose of 400 mg given at week 0, 2 and 6, and thereafter 4-weekly in moderate to severe CD, it was associated with an improvement in response rates at 26 weeks when compared with placebo, but not remission rates. However, of those who responded to induction therapy (week 6), maintained response and remission were more likely at week 26 with certolizumab pegol than those switched to placebo.

Natalizumab (Tysabri) is a monoclonal antibody against alpha 4 integrin and inhibits adhesion and migration of leucocytes to inflamed tissue within the gut.

A Cochrane review of natalizumab (300 mg or 3–4 mg/kg) versus placebo for moderate–severe CD showed it was effective for induction of clinical response and remission. Three patients treated with natalizumab (two with multiple sclerosis, also treated with interferon beta-1a, one with CD, also treated with AZA) developed progressive multifocal leukoencephalopathy (PML) resulting in two deaths. It may be possible to identify patients at risk for PML by testing blood for the JC virus (named after the initials of the first patient in whom it was described).

IBD nurse specialists are often involved in running or maintaining biological infusion services. For patients receiving infliximab, this all but guarantees 8-weekly assessment by a member of the team as well as confirming adherence with medication. This must be balanced with the convenience that self-administration at home allows with use of adalimumab. Until recently, there has been little in the way of patient choice between these two drugs, with the majority of patients receiving adalimumab being those who have lost response to or become intolerant of infliximab. However, the recently updated NICE guidance TA187 (National Institute of Clinical Excellence, 2010) has recommended that either adalimumab or IFX can be used as first line biological therapy, and this therefore opens up a choice for clinicians and patients. It is likely that IBD nurses will play a substantial role in educating patients about the benefits and disadvantages of each of these drugs. It is probably fair to say that their efficacy is broadly similar although there are no head-to-head trials to date.

Other treatments

Fish oil
A Cochrane review has shown that, as with UC, omega-3 fatty acids are safe but probably ineffective in maintaining remission in CD (Turner *et al.*, 2009).

Trichuris suis ova (see 'Other treatments' in UC section)
Ingestion of *T. suis* ova may lead to a response in CD, supported by an open label trial. However, there are no RCTs supporting this (Summers *et al.*, 2005b).

Probiotics
Saccharomyces boulardii in combination with 5-ASA, compared with 5-ASA alone, was more effective at maintaining remission in a small clinical trial. Work is ongoing into the gut microbiota in relation to both CD and UC. Of particular interest are the bacteria of the Firmicutes, especially *Faecalibacterium prausnitzii*, whose numbers are low in active IBD, and leads to reduction in inflammation in experimental colitis (Hedin *et al.*, 2007).

Prebiotics

A small open-label trial of 10 patients with active ileocolonic CD, who were treated with fructo-oligosaccharides for three weeks, showed a significant clinical response as measured by the Harvey–Bradshaw index, and a significant increase in faecal bifidobacteria. However, a subsequent randomised controlled trial failed to show benefit of this treatment (Hedin *et al.*, 2007).

Naltrexone

Naltrexone is an opioid antagonist and plays a role in the healing and repair of tissues. An open label trial showed remission rates of 67% in patients with Crohn's disease treated with oral low dose naltrexone (4.5 mg per day) with no adverse events. Sleep disturbance was the most common side-effect. A randomised controlled trial is awaited (Smith *et al.*, 2007).

Smoking cessation

Smoking significantly worsens the prognosis of CD. All patients should therefore be advised and encouraged to stop smoking, with support such as smoking cessation clinics and nicotine replacement therapy.

Extraintestinal manifestations

Extraintestinal manifestations (EIMs) are commonly encountered in IBD. They are particularly associated with extensive colonic disease. Clinical features of EIMs are discussed in Chapter 3.

Disorders that parallel disease activity

These include pyoderma gangrenosum, erythema nodosum, peripheral arthritis, aphthous stomatitis and episcleritis. Treatment of the underlying CD or UC often leads to an improvement in these EIMs. Arthritis tends to involve the large joints, and is usually acute and self-limiting. Pyoderma gangrenosum may respond to corticosteroids. In refractory cases infliximab has been shown to be effective in an RCT. Ciclosporin, tacrolimus and mycophenolate mofetil are also sometimes used to treat this condition.

Disorders associated with IBD but not related to disease activity

These include primary sclerosing cholangitis (PSC), ankylosing spondylitis, sacroiliitis and uveitis.

Ankylosing spondylitis and sacroiliitis should be treated with physiotherapy with or without disease-modifying drugs such as sulphasalazine and methotrexate.

Non-steroidal anti-inflammatory drugs can be effective, but may exacerbate the underlying IBD. Biological therapy with IFX, adalimumab and etanercept (another anti-TNF agent, used in rheumatological disease) is effective and recommended for treatment of severe active disease. However, etanercept, despite acting on TNF, is not an effective treatment for Crohn's disease.

PSC is a risk factor for cholangiocarcinoma and colon cancer (necessitating more frequent surveillance). It should be managed in conjunction with a hepatologist. The use of ursodeoxycholic acid in people with PSC has recently been questioned based on the results of a trial showing adverse outcomes associated with its use.

Patients with suspected uveitis should be referred urgently to an ophthalmologist and are treated with topical corticosteroids, sometimes requiring systemic corticosteroids. Resistant cases may need immunomodulation with AZA, MTX or even IFX.

Disorders resulting from the consequences of small bowel disease or active inflammation

Malabsorption due to active disease or ileal resection may produce deficiencies of fat-soluble vitamins, vitamin B_{12} or minerals, and can lead to anaemia, neurological disorders, clotting disorders and bone demineralisation amongst others. Active inflammation may lead to growth failure in children, and bone resorption, leading to osteoporosis. Renal stones can be a consequence of increased oxalate absorption, and gallstones can develop from impaired ileal resorption of bile salts.

Treatment of these conditions usually involves induction and maintenance of remission of the CD or UC, enteral or parenteral vitamin and mineral supplementation, and, for osteoporosis, calcium and vitamin D with or without a bisphosphonate.

Conclusion

A patient-centred approach to the management of IBD is essential. Good adherence to treatment is more likely if patients are engaged in decisions regarding their care. It is important to have outlined the potential side-effects and risks involved with treatment, as well as the benefits and alternative strategies. In particular, patients must be made aware of monitoring requirements and what action they should take if they experience side-effects.

In complex cases, discussion at a multidisciplinary meeting is often useful. When a patient is apparently not responding, or losing response, to a therapy it is important to address adherence issues. At this point, the disease may need to be reassessed either endoscopically, radiologically or by examination under anaesthetic. Alternative treatment, including surgery, should be considered, discussed and initiated without undue delay.

Patient translation summary

■ Ensure the patient has understood all the available treatment options – encourage them to ask questions if unsure.

■ Crohn's and Colitis UK (http://www.crohnsandcolitis.org.uk/) provides helpful advice on its website and is an important source of support for patients and their relatives. The organisation also funds research, but relies on subscriptions and donations to survive.

■ Inform patients that they must report a sore throat or other symptoms of infection while on an immunomodulator

■ Advise patients to plan ahead with prescriptions so doses are not missed, and that they understand the monitoring requirements of their medication.

■ Ask about plans for pregnancy so that medication issues can be addressed in good time.

References

Akobeng, A. K. and Gardener, E. (2005) Oral 5-aminosalicylate acid for maintenance of medically-induced remission in Crohn's disease. *Cochrane Database Syst. Rev.*, **(1)**:CD003715.

Akobeng, A. K. and Thomas, A. G. (2007) Enteral nutrition for maintenance of remission in Crohn's disease. *Cochrane Database Syst. Rev.*, **(3)**:CD005984.

Fraser, A. G., Orchard, T. R. and Jewell, D. P. (2002) The efficacy of azathioprine for the treatment of inflammatory bowel disease: a 30 year review. *Gut*, **50**, 485–9.

Hanai, H., Iida, T., Takeuchi, F. *et al.* (2006) Curcumin maintenance therapy for ulcerative colitis: randomised, multicenter, double-blind, placebo-controlled trial. *Clin. Gastro. Hepatol.*, **4**, 1502–6.

Hanauer, S. B. and Stromberg, U. (2004a) Oral Pentasa in the treatment of active Crohn's disease: a meta-analysis of double-blind; placebo-controlled trials. *Clin. Gastroenterol. Hepatol.*, **2**, 379–88.

Hanauer, S. B., Korelitz, B. I., Rutgeerts, P. *et al.* (2004b) Post-operative maintenance of Crohn's disease remission with 6-mercaptopurine, mesalamine or placebo: a 2 year trial. *Gastroenterology*, **127**, 723–9.

Hedin, C., Whelan, K. and Linday, J. O. (2007) Evidence for the use of probiotics and prebiotics in inflammatory bowel disease: a review of clinical trials. *Proc. Nutr. Soc.*, **66**, 307–15.

Langmead, L., Feakins, R. M., Goldthorpe, S. *et al.* (2004) Randomized, double-blind, placebo-controlled trial of oral aloe vera gel for active ulcerative colitis. *Aliment Pharmacol. Ther.*, **19**, 739–47.

Lees, C. W., Maan, A. K., Hansoti, B. *et al.* (2008) Tolerability and safety of mercaptopurine in azathioprine-intolerant patients with inflammatory bowel disease. *Aliment Pharmacol. Ther.*, **27**, 220–7.

Mackey, A. C., Green, L., Leptak, C. *et al.* (2009) Hepatosplenic T cell lymphoma associated with infliximab use in young patients treated for inflammatory bowel disease: update. *J. Pediatr. Gastroenterol. Nutr.*, **48**, 386–8.

Marshall, J. K. and Irvine, E. J. (1997) Rectal aminosalicylate therapy for distal ulcerative colitis: a meta-analysis. *Gut*, **40**, 775–81.

Marteau, P., Probert, C. S., Lindgren, S. *et al.* (2005) Combined oral and enema treatment with Pentasa (mesalazine) is superior to oral therapy alone in patients with extensive mild/moderate active ulcerative colitis: a randomised, double blind, placebo controlled study. *Gut*, **54**, 960–5.

Maser, E. A., Deconda, D., Lichtiger, S. *et al.* (2008) Cyclosporine and infliximab as rescue therapy for each other in patients with steroid-refractory ulcerative colitis. *Clin. Gastroenterol. Hepatol.*, **6**, 1112–16.

McGrath, J., McDonald, J. W. D. and Macdonald, J. K. (2004) Transdermal nicotine for induction of remission in ulcerative colitis. *Cochrane Database Syst. Rev.* **(4)**:CD004722.

National Institute for Health and Clinical Excellence (2008) *Infliximab for the Treatment of Subacute Manifestations of Ulcerative Colitis.* http://www.guidance.nice.org.uk/TA140 (accessed May 2010).

National Institute for Health and Clinical Excellence (2008) *Infliximab for the Treatment of Acute Exacerbations of Ulcerative Colitis.* http://www.guidance.nice.org.uk/TA163 (accessed May 2010).

National Institute of Clinical Excellence (2010) TA187 *Crohn's Disease – Infliximab (Review) and Adalimumab (Review of TA40): Guidance.* http://guidance.nice.org.uk/TA187/Guidance/pdf/English (accessed 30/11/10).

Oren, R., Arber, N., Odes, S. *et al.* (1996) Methotrexate in chronic active ulcerative colitis: a double-blind randomised, Israeli multicenter trial. *Gastroenterology*, **110**, 1416–21.

Patel, V., Macdonald, J. K., McDonald, J. W. and Chande, N. (2009) Methotrexate for maintenance of remission in Crohn's disease. *Cochrane Database Syst. Rev.*, **(4)**:CD006884.

Pearson, D. C., May, G. R., Fick, G. H. *et al.* (1995) Azathioprine and 6-mercaptopurine in Crohn's disease. A meta-analysis. *Ann. Intern. Med.*, **122**, 132–42.

113

Present, D. H., Meltzer, S. J., Krumholz, M. P. *et al.* (1989) 6-mercaptopurine in the management of inflammatory bowel disease: short- and long-term toxicity. *Ann. Intern. Med.*, **111**, 641–9.

Smith, A. P., Stock, H., Bingaman, S. *et al.* (2007) Low-dose naltrexone therapy improves active Crohn's disease. *Am. J. Gastroenterol.*, **102**, 820–8.

Summers, R. W., Elliott, D. E., Urban, J. F., Jr *et al.* (2005a) *Trichuris suis* therapy for active ulcerative colitis: a randomized controlled trial. *Gastroenterology*, **128**, 825–32.

Summers, R. W., Elliott, D. E., Urban, J. F., Jr *et al.* (2005b) *Trichuris suis* therapy in Crohn's disease. *Gut*, **54**, 87–90.

Sutherland, L., Roth, D., Beck, P. *et al.* (2000) Oral 5-aminosalicylic acid for inducing remission in ulcerative colitis. *Cochrane Database Syst. Rev.* (**2**):CD000543.

Turner, D., Steinhart, A. and Griffiths, A. (2007) Omega 3 fatty acids (fish oil) for maintenance of remission in ulcerative colitis. *Cochrane Database Syst. Rev.*, (**3**): CD006443.

Turner, D., Zlotkin, S. H., Shah, P. S., Griffiths, A. M. (2009) Omega 3 fatty acids (fish oil) for maintenance of remission in Crohn's disease. *Cochrane Database Syst. Rev.* (**1**):CD006320.

Van Assche, G., D'Haens, G., Noman, M. *et al.* (2003) Intravenous cyclosporine vs intravenous corticosteroids as single therapy for severe attacks of ulcerative colitis. *Gastroenterology*, **125**, 1025–31.

Further reading

The **Crohn's and Colitis UK** website provides useful information for patients with IBD, including medical therapy: http://www.crohnsandcolitis.org.uk/

European evidence-based consensus on the management of ulcerative colitis: current management. Travis, S. P. L., Stange, E. F., Lémann, M., Øresland, T., Bemelman, W. A., Chowers, Y., Colombel, J. F., D'Haens, G., Ghosh, S., Marteau, P., Kruis, W., Mortensen, N. J. McC., Penninckx, F. and Gassull, M. for the European Crohn's and Colitis Organisation (ECCO) (2008) *Journal of Crohn's and Colitis*, **2**, 24–62. https://www.ecco-ibd.eu/documents/UC_current_management.pdf

European evidence-based consensus on the management of ulcerative colitis: special situations. Biancone, L., Michetti, P., Travis, S., Escher, J. C., Moser, G., Forbes, A., Hoffmann, J. C., Dignass, A., Gionchetti, P., Jantschek, G., Kiesslich, R., Kolacek, S., Mitchell, R., Panes, J., Soderholm, J., Vucelic, B. and Stange, E. for the European Crohn's and Colitis Organisation (ECCO). (2008) *Journal of Crohn's and Colitis*, **2**, 63–92. https://www.ecco-ibd.eu/documents/UC_special_situations.pdf

European evidence based consensus on the diagnosis and management of Crohn's disease: current management. Travis, S. P. L., Stange, E. F., Lemann, M., Oeresland, T., Chowers, Y., Forbes, A., D'Haens, G., Kitis, G., Cortot, A., Prantera, C., Marteau,

P., Colombel, J.-F., Gionchetti, P., Bouhnik, Y., Tiret, E., Kroesen, A., Starlinger, M. and Mortensen, N. J. McM. for the European Crohn's and Colitis Organisation (ECCO) (2006). *Gut*, **55**(suppl. 1), i16–i35. http://gut.bmj.com/content/55/suppl_1/i16.abstract **European evidence based consensus on the diagnosis and management of Crohn's disease: special situations**. Caprilli, R., Gassull, M. A., Escher, J. C., Moser, G., Munkholm, P., Forbes, A., Hommes, D. W., Lochs, H., Angelucci, E., Cocco, A., Vucelic, B., Hildebrand, H., Kolacek, S., Riis, L., Lukas, M., de Franchis, R., Hamilton, M., Jantschek, G., Michetti, P., O'Morain, C., Anwar, M. M., Freitas, J. L., Mouzas, I. A., Baert, F., Mitchell, R., Hawkey, C. J. for the European Crohn's and Colitis Organisation (ECCO) (2006) *Gut*, **55**(suppl. 1), i36–i58. http://gut.bmj.com/content/55/suppl_1/i36 **European evidence-based consensus on the prevention, diagnosis and management of opportunistic infections in inflammatory bowel disease**. Rahier, J. F., Ben-Horin, S., Chowers, Y., Conlon, C., De Munter, P., D'Haens, G., Domènech, E., Eliakim, R., Eser, A., Frater, J., Gassull, M., Giladi, M., Kaser, A., Lémann, M., Moreels, T., Moschen, A., Pollok, R., Reinisch, W., Schunter, M., Stange, E. F., Tilg, H., Van Assche, G., Viget, N., Vucelic, B., Walsh, A., Weiss, G., Yazdanpanah, Y., Zabana, Y., Travis, S. P. L., Colombel, J. F. on behalf of the European Crohn's and Colitis Organisation (ECCO) (2009). *Journal of Crohn's and Colitis* 3, 47–91. https://www.ecco-ibd.eu/documents/ECCOconsensusOI.pdf

British National Formulary, 58, September 2009; http://www.bnf.org/.

CHAPTER 7

Management of the patient with more complex IBD

Jeremy Sanderson and Melissa Smith

Introduction

Despite the rather skewed impression that our patients may get from searching Crohn's disease and ulcerative colitis on the web, it is fair to say that most patients with IBD gain an effective remission on standard therapy and suffer few disease complications. Likewise, most are able to achieve their desired domestic, occupational and education goals, albeit with some interruptions along the way. However, for some, perhaps 5–10% of individuals, the disease proves much more complicated, leading to a much greater burden of illness and reduced quality of life. For children, adolescents and young adults this can be particularly threatening to individual expectations. For example, growth failure in children with complex IBD can be significant and permanent. Likewise, the lost educational and occupational opportunities for young adolescents and young adults can be irreversible (Boonen et al. 2002; Heuschkel et al., 2008).

Effective treatment decisions in this group of patients are therefore critically important. Such decisions are difficult because the patient with complex IBD has often already exhausted the conventional armamentarium available to IBD physicians. Nonetheless, effective treatment decisions can and should be made such that these patients can gain the kind of remission and quality of life gained more easily by those with less complicated IBD.

Who develops more complex IBD?

There are two main ways by which a patient comes to develop more complex IBD, each with factors of relevance to their subsequent treatment.

Firstly, it is clear that some individuals are predestined to run a more complicated course. In both CD and UC, it is most likely that genetic factors determine this difference (Canto *et al.*, 2007). Environmental factors are also important, particularly in CD where smoking, for example, more than doubles the risk of disease flares and relapse after surgery (Cosnes *et al.*, 1996; Yamamoto and Keighley, 2000).

Secondly, some individuals arrive at more complicated disease because of a lack of optimal therapy earlier in the course of their disease. For example, individuals who receive prolonged courses of steroids without early recourse to effective use of steroid sparing immunosuppression are more likely to have a greater burden of disease, progress to surgery and complications from the disease (e.g. progress to penetrating disease with fistulae and abscesses) or from treatment (e.g. osteoporosis, surgical complications) (Ezzat and Hamdy, 2010; Subramanian *et al.*, 2008).

What defines more complex IBD?

There is obviously no set definition of complex IBD and, to some extent, the cases debated each week in multidisciplinary IBD meetings across the globe are all complex cases. However, for the purpose of this chapter we have defined complex IBD as follows.

For CD, the definition would include:

- Cases unresponsive to all conventional drug therapy, including two biologicals
- Those with penetrating disease causing complicated fistulae, including perianal disease not responding to first-line treatment measures
- Those with multiple site involvement, particularly upper GI and oral disease
- Patients with ongoing active disease but who have undergone multiple resections previously
- Those with difficult extra-intestinal manifestations such as pyoderma gangrenosum

For UC, the definition would include:

- Steroid-dependent or refractory cases who are unresponsive to immunosuppression with a thiopurine
- Acute severe colitis failing to respond to intensive intravenous corticosteroids
- Patients with difficult extra-intestinal manifestations

Managing the patient with complex Crohn's disease

Some general principles are discussed below.

Case study

A 22-year-old female university student seeks your opinion regarding her Crohn's disease, which was diagnosed five years ago when she was 17 years old. She presented initially with abdominal pain and diarrhoea and was found to have an inflamed, ulcerated 25 cm segment of terminal ileum on colonoscopy and small bowel barium studies. The remaining small bowel and colon appeared unaffected. She received prednisolone 40 mg daily tapering over two months with good effect. However, her symptoms returned on steroid withdrawal and prednisolone was reinstated. She was started on azathioprine, 2 mg/kg daily which permitted successful steroid withdrawal and a relatively symptom free remission. She smokes between 5 and 10 cigarettes daily.

Two years later, she developed perianal pain, swelling and fever and required emergency surgery to drain a large perianal abscess. She also complained of recurrent lower lip swelling and painful oral ulceration. Examination under anaesthetic showed an anorectal stenosis which was dilated and active Crohn's proctitis. Oral examination revealed a firm swelling of the lower lip with surrounding erythema on the perioral skin, linear ulceration in the left buccal sulcus and nodular left buccal mucosa. She received further steroids and azathioprine was increased to 2.5 mg/ kg. She was improved on steroid therapy, but continued to have chronic drainage of pus from a perianal fistula. Six months later, her liver function tests were noted to be abnormal and azathioprine was stopped. The LFTs improved. Methotrexate was started at a dose of 15 mg once weekly, initially subcutaneously, then orally.

One year later, she comes to see you for an opinion. She has continued to have chronic perianal discharge. She suffers abdominal pain one hour after eating with borborygmi and distension and her weight has fallen significantly. She is tired and her university studies are being affected. Her mother comes with her, having read a lot about treatment for Crohn's disease on the Internet, and would like her to receive antibiotics aimed at treating *Mycobacterium paratuberculosis* infection. She has heard bad reports of reactions to biologic therapy for Crohn's disease. On examination, she is pale, thin and has erythema ab igne on the lower abdomen. There is a mildly tender mass in the right lower quadrant. Per rectum there are two tags, a chronic draining fistulous opening and a moderately tight anal stenosis.

How would you manage this patient?

What are the specific clinical issues in a particular patient?

This is a very important first question to answer because treatment choices stem directly and specifically from these considerations. In the patient with complex disease, there is always more than one issue, such that numerous management decisions need to be made. Hence in our case study the following management issues arise:

1. The history suggests that her ileal disease has evolved at least to stenotic disease with obstructive symptoms. This requires evaluation by appropriate imaging, but immediately raises the question of surgery as optimal management.
2. There is ongoing perianal disease requiring evaluation and management separately from the rest of her disease.
3. Regardless of the possible need for surgery, optimal medical therapy to control an active inflammatory component is needed. Biological therapy appears a likely option, but the reasons for failure of previous therapy and her own preferences and concerns need to be considered.
4. The involvement of the oral cavity requires separate specialist attention.
5. Her overall nutritional state is a concern.

What are the goals of therapy?

Before deciding on the appropriate plan of action for each of the clinical issues raised, it is important to be clear to yourself and the patient/family regarding the goals of therapy. This is important, particularly as it brings into debate the pros and cons of stronger immunosuppression or biological therapy as a means of inducing mucosal healing rather than merely symptomatic remission. Over recent years, goals of therapy in Crohn's disease have changed away from symptom improvement and more towards mucosal healing, prevention of complications and avoidance of surgery (Hyams and Markowitz, 2005; Lowenberg *et al.*, 2006). Importantly, evidence is now emerging that earlier use of both thiopurines and biologic agents leads not only to mucosal healing but also to reduced rates of surgical resection (Allez *et al.*, 2002; Colombel *et al.*, 2010; Froslie *et al.*, 2007; de Pineton *et al.*, 2010; Ramadas *et al.*, 2010; Schnitzler *et al.*, 2009; Van Assche *et al.*, 2010). Relapse of disease is known to be related to a failure to achieve long-term mucosal healing (Baert *et al.*, 2010). For the patient and family, however, this means that greater emphasis is put on the use of stronger immunosuppression and the risks and benefits of this need careful discussion. So, armed with clear therapeutic goals, how would we manage the five issues highlighted by the case of complex CD above? We deal with each in turn.

I. Evolution to fibrostenotic disease

Our patient has symptoms very suggestive of intermittent small bowel obstruction and, for this aspect, surgery is immediately brought into the equation as a highly likely outcome. Indeed, not to consider this would not be acting in their best interests. Evolution of Crohn's behaviour over time is common, from an inflammatory phenotype to that of fibrostenotic, to penetrating (fistulae/abscess), or both (Peyrin-Biroulet *et al.*, 2010). In our patient, the presence of a right lower quadrant mass is also predictive of a need for surgery (Gapasin *et al.*, 2010). Management of this aspect requires accurate imaging of small intestine in order to

- document the length and nature of the suspected stricture
- look for dilatation above the stricture (prestenotic dilatation) indicative of physiological obstruction
- determine, if possible, the balance between fibrosis and active inflammation within a stenotic segment of bowel
- rule out more proximal segments of disease

Whilst not available in all centres, MR enterography is the best means of achieving all of this information whilst avoiding the radiation exposure of more traditional barium contrast imaging. In addition, colonoscopy determines the presence of colonic disease requiring management separate to the stricturing ileal disease. In our patient, the MR enterography shows a 25 cm segment of distal ileal Crohn's disease with three tight strictures and dilatation of the small bowel above. There is no proximal disease, but there looks to be a fistulous tract running through to the mid sigmoid colon, confirmed on colonoscopy where a short segment of disease is seen in this region with suspicion of a fistulous opening. There is also significant Crohn's proctitis with an anorectal stenosis (see Step 2 below). The management of the ileal disease in this case is surgical. Very occasionally, a short (up to approximately 4 cm) fibrotic (Koltun, 2007) stricture can be dilated endoscopically and medical therapy employed, but in most cases surgery in this setting is inevitable. This is sometimes met with upset and disappointment by patients (and relatives), but it is important to make this a positive decision, emphasising both the inevitability and the restoration of good health, which far outweigh the risks and obvious downsides of surgery. In this particular case, there is a high chance that a temporary stoma will be required at surgery because of penetrating disease, nutritional deficit (Dionigi *et al.*, 2008) and smoking, all increasing the risk of anastomotic leak (Guo and Dipietro, 2010), and it is good practice for the physician to indicate this possibility (and the reasons why) to the patient rather than the surgeon, who can then concentrate more on the positive

121

aspects. This type of patient should always be discussed in a multidisciplinary IBD meeting to review clinical features and imaging and agree the plan for surgery with the IBD surgeon. With this management plan initiated, we can move to the second important issue raised. There is also the issue of optimising the patient's condition in the run-up to surgery, which is addressed in Step 5 below.

2. Management of the perianal disease
Our patient clearly has active perianal disease requiring management independent of the plan to operate on the ileal disease. Accurate assessment of this, whilst unfortunately meaning yet more investigations for the patient, is crucial to proper effective treatment. The goal of this assessment is to determine:

- the component of anorectal stenosis
- the presence and severity of associated active rectal inflammation
- the nature and complexity of fistulous tracks
- the presence of any drainable sepsis or collections

Consequently, pelvic MRI (fistula protocol), an examination under anaesthetic (EUA) and colonoscopy (or flexible sigmoidoscopy if more proximal endoscopy not needed) should each be undertaken. Endoanal ultrasound is also used in some centres. Multidisciplinary meeting discussion should ideally occur following endoscopy and MRI. The surgeon can then undertake an EUA with a view to drainage of sepsis, laying open of low fistulae and/or placing of seton sutures where appropriate, and dilatation of any significant anorectal stenosis. As soon as satisfactory drainage has been achieved, medical therapy should be initiated to control the active penetrating anorectal Crohn's disease, the driving force behind fistulation. At colonoscopy in our patient there was active Crohn's proctitis. We have agreed in Step 1 above that surgery is need for the stenosing ileal disease, but effective medical therapy is needed for the proctitis and perianal fistulation and, indeed, for post-operative relapse prevention.

3. Optimising medical therapy
Whilst there are reasons in our patient why thiopurines should be considered again (see below), the presence of penetrating rectal disease is an important indicator of a severe disease course (Thia *et al.*, 2010) and effective mucosal healing therapy must be instituted in this setting. Hence biologicals should be started (even if the patient is naïve to immunosuppression) because waiting for four months for the onset of action of a thiopurine and the lower efficacy in this setting are both unacceptable options for this type of disease.

The patient should receive either infliximab or adalimumab with a standard induction followed by initial maintenance (5 mg/kg 8 weekly or 40 mg every other week respectively). Most IBD specialists would agree that initial treatment with a biological should be for a year to give long enough for effective healing therapy. At one year, re-evaluation should occur, in this case, by pelvic MRI, colonoscopy and EUA, if deemed necessary, for accurate information on which to base decisions. If a seton was placed prior to initiation of therapy, there is debate as to whether this can be removed during induction or left until a one-year assessment. If there is good evidence of mucosal healing and fistula closure or quiescence with seton-*in-situ*, then a trial without biological should be considered.

Our patient had concerns regarding biologicals having read about treatment options on the Internet and was interested in alternative options. It is important in this situation to help the patient (and relatives) understand the critical balance between risks and benefits in Crohn's therapy – yes, biologicals carry an increased risk of allergic reaction, infection and rarer complications including malignancy, all of which need discussing, but these are outweighed satisfactorily by the benefits in terms of chances of fistula closure, mucosal healing and the knock-on benefits in terms of reduced complications and improved quality of life (D'Haens *et al.*, 2008). Getting this balance right is sometimes difficult, but alternative options here, such as second or third line immunosuppression or anti-mycobacterial antibiotic therapy, have a far inferior risk–benefit ratio. In other settings (i.e. away from penetrating rectal disease) this balance may be different, and hence the discussion might favour a defined trial of another therapy.

Having chosen to start a biological (see previous chapter for standard approach to initiation), it is still important to consider concomitant immunosuppression. There are two main reasons for this – firstly, there is no doubt that optimal efficacy, reduced loss of response and infusion reaction occur with combined therapy (Colombel *et al.*, 2010; Sokol *et al.*, 2010; Vermeire *et al.*, 2007) and secondly, there is the possibility of withdrawal of the biologic at, say, one year, with the aim that remission will be maintained on immunosuppression alone. This latter point is difficult because many patients (in the UK in particular) arrive at biologicals having failed on two or more immunosuppressive drugs. However, in my experience, a look back at previous immunosuppression often reveals opportunities for optimal or alternative use of immunosuppression, particularly thiopurines. Our patient is a good example of this. She developed abnormal liver function tests (LFTs) on azathioprine which resolved on stopping the drug. There are a number of reasons for abnormal LFTs on azathioprine, but the most frequent is the over-production of methylated metabolites compared to thioguanine nucleotides (TGN) (Dubinsky *et al.*, 2002), the metabolic end-product of thiopurines metabolism, considered responsible for the immunosuppressive effect of the drug (see Figure 7.1). Testing thiopurine methyltransferase (TPMT) activity prior to treatment predicts not only risk of myelosuppression due to TPMT deficiency (see previous chapter) but also reduced response due to hypermethylation (Ansari *et al.*, 2008a; Sparrow *et al.*, 2007). This can also be detected once established on treatment by measuring TGN levels. In most laboratories, checking TGN levels provides a measure of both TGN and methylated metabolites (6-MMP) allowing effective decision making according to results. For example, absent or very low levels of both indicates non-adherence, a problem in up to 10% of cases (Smith *et al.*, 2008). Sub-therapeutic levels indicate a need for simple dose escalation whilst high levels allow dose reduction to within the therapeutic range whilst maintaining response. My prediction is that, in our patient, the TGN was sub-therapeutic but the 6-MMP was very high, resulting in poor response and hepatotoxicity. Importantly, this can be circumvented by the combined use of allopurinol and low dose azathioprine (Ansari *et al.*, 2008b; Sparrow *et al.*, 2007), traditionally contra-indicated as concomitant therapy because of a high risk of myelotoxicity. However, by blocking xanthine oxidase and giving a low dose of azathioprine (25% of target), the kinetics of methylation are altered favourably such that therapeutic levels of TGN can be achieved without toxic level of methylated metabolites. In most cases this successfully circumvents the problem of abnormal LFTs.

If, however, the same problem occurs, then alternative immunosuppression is needed. The choices in our patient would be between methotrexate (MTX), tacrolimus, mycophenolate mofetil or perhaps thioguanine.

■ **Methotrexate** is the 'routine' choice, particularly as it is really the only other immunosuppressive agent for which reasonably strong randomised controlled data on efficacy exists (Feagan *et al.*, 1995). It is much better tolerated in IBD than in psoriasis, where liver toxicity concerns remain. Abnormal LFTs on azathioprine, as in our patient, do not predict hepatotoxicity on MTX. Optimal use is considered to be with 15–25 mg subcutaneously weekly, then switching to oral dosing with doses of folic acid (proven to diminish some toxicity related to folate antagonism) given for 1–3 days avoiding the days around the MTX (Patel *et al.*, 2009). Perhaps the most limiting aspect to starting MTX is the foetal toxicity (MTX, a folate analogue, was originally developed as an abortifacient), meaning that women (and theoretically men) of childbearing age must avoid conception. Thorough counselling regarding the risks and benefits should occur prior to initiation of treatment.

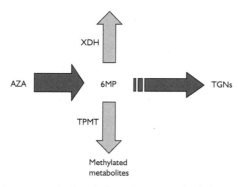

Figure 7.1 The basic metabolism of azathioprine (AZA) after ingestion. AZA is rapidly converted to 6-mercaptopurine (6MP) in the gut wall and liver mainly. 6MP then enters a three-way competitive metabolism, the balance of which determines how much is converted to 6-thioguanine nucleotides (TGNs), considered the active metabolites of the parent drug. 6-thiouric acid is formed by the action of the enzyme xanthine dehydrogenase (XDH), which can be inhibited by the drug allopurinol. Methylated metabolites, mainly 6-methyl mercaptopurine, are formed by the action of the enzyme thiopurine methyl transferase (TPMT). Unlike XDH, the activity of TPMT varies according to genetic polymorphism, leading to important inter-individual differences in the metabolism of AZA and 6MP.

- **Tacrolimus**, a potent macrolide, is an alternative option or, perhaps, third line immunosuppressant, particularly for refractory perianal disease (Taxonera *et al.*, 2009), given orally or, in some cases, topically as an adjunct for cutaneous aspects of perianal disease.
- **Mycophenolate mofetil** (MMF), an inhibitor of inosine monophosphate dehydrogenase (an enzyme in the same pathway affected by thiopurines) has become first line therapy in the prevention of transplant rejection. MMF, usually at a target dose of 1 g twice daily, has data to support efficacy in steroid dependent Crohn's disease (Neurath *et al.*, 1999), but its use is limited by gastrointestinal toxicity (diarrhoea and nausea mainly), which, not surprisingly, seems to be a much greater problem when used for IBD, for obvious reasons.
- Finally, **thioguanine** (6-tioguanine, 6-TG) is a logical choice of drug where there is thiopurine toxicity related to its parent drugs, azathioprine or 6-mercaptopurine. 6-TG bypasses most of the metabolism of thiopurines (see Figure 7.1), requiring only a single conversion step to 6-TGN. Used at doses

of 20–40 mg daily, there is uncontrolled data to support efficacy (Dubinsky *et al.*, 2001; Dubinsky *et al.*, 2003a) but its use has been limited by concerns regarding the development of nodular regenerative hyperplasia (NRH) in the liver (Dubinsky *et al.*, 2003b). 6-TG has been used mainly in the treatment of childhood acute lymphoblastic leukaemia (ALL), but was associated with significant levels of veno-occlusive disease, part of the spectrum into which NRH falls. In fact, concerns regarding NRH borne out of the original description of the use of 6-TG in thiopurine-intolerant IBD, have not been matched by reports from use in European centres (Ansari *et al.*, 2008c; Gilissen *et al.*, 2007) and, provided there is appropriate monitoring, including a close eye on the platelet count (a falling count heralds the presentation of significant NRH) and regular (yearly) hepatic MR scanning, 6-TG can have an important place in the management of refractory IBD.

Top-down versus step-up therapy

The concept of top-down versus step-up therapy is an important debate in the management of Crohn's disease, and indeed in many aspects of medicine. For moderate to severe Crohn's disease, the key question is whether it is better to use the most rapidly effective disease mucosal healing therapy (i.e. biologics) right at the start, aiming to withdraw to immunosuppression alone later, or whether the same goal can be achieved by a more conventional approach of steroid-induced remission sustained by the use of immunosuppression. In fact, it is a close call, and in studies looking at this, the main benefit of a top-down approach is the reduced exposure to corticosteroid (D'Haens *et al.*, 2008). In clinical practice, particularly in the UK, most patients arrive at the decision to use biologics from failure on immunosuppression (as in our case above), so the argument is not relevant. However, in the appropriate patient (moderate to severe Crohn's naïve to treatment) it is important to debate the option of top down therapy. The two main factors involved in the decision are as follows. Firstly, to what extent do you feel that corticosteroids will induce an effective *clinical* remission (to be maintained, with the aim of mucosal healing, by a thiopurine, and how 'acceptable' would corticosteroids be in the patient in question (for example, what is the bone density, is there a history of steroid adverse effects or non-response)? Secondly, what is the disease phenotype? Disease being simply severe may well respond very well to corticosteroids and thiopurines, but some patterns of disease, particularly penetrating disease, clearly do less well, and a strong argument can be made for using the most effective therapy available in this setting (i.e. biologics). I often talk to patients about 'saving biologics for a rainy day', which is a good concept, particularly as there is a slow but definite law of diminishing returns once these are started. However, if the cap fits, so to speak, don't hold back.

Managing the risks associated with immunosuppression

Over the next few years, it is hoped that further progress in the application of pharmacogenetics to guide drug choice before treatment starts, and translation of other measures to optimise therapy, like those mentioned above, will create a genuine era of individualised or personalised medicine. However, whilst responses to therapy will improve and unnecessary toxicity will be avoided, it is important also to realise that other types of toxicity may also increase. In particular, more profound immunosuppression will inevitably lead to a greater frequency of opportunistic infection and increase the known increase in risk of malignancy (particularly lymphoma). In recent years these risks have been defined more clearly in patients receiving immunosuppression for IBD. Thiopurines, for example, result in an approximately 3-fold increase in the chances of opportunistic infection (Toruner *et al.*, 2008) and around a 4-fold increase in relative risk of lymphoma (Kandiel *et al.*, 2005). There is also a less marked increase in risk of other malignancy, with skin cancer perhaps being the most pertinent to consider (Smith *et al.*, 2010). What action should we take and what should we tell our patients about these risks? It is clearly important to discuss these risks and put them into context. All patients going on to a thiopurine, for example, should have the possible short and long term risks explained and this should be documented in the clinical notes and/or in a letter following this consultation. It is important in this discussion to point out that, for lymphoma in particular, that the absolute risk is low (1 excess case per 300–1,300 years of treatment) and that a consensus of doctors treating IBD consider the benefits of treatment to far outweigh these risks (Smith *et al.*, 2010). In terms of taking action, there are definitely measures that can be taken. Firstly, screening for viral infections such as HIV, Hepatitis B, C and exposure to varicella zoster virus (VZV) should be routine prior to starting treatment, as proposed in the recent ECCO guidance (Rahier *et al.*, 2009). Also, it is good practice to have any live vaccines likely to be needed (for example yellow fever vaccine in young adults likely to travel to at-risk areas) prior to starting therapy (i.e. think ahead at diagnosis rather than waiting until treatment is already starting). Likewise, VZV and human papilloma virus (HPV) vaccine should be given to those who are non-immune prior to treatment where possible and appropriate. In terms of malignancy, patients should be encouraged to adhere to standard screening protocols for cancer and be advised of the importance of using standard protection measures against UV radiation from the Sun.

4. Managing oral Crohn's disease

Another aspect of our patient's condition is the involvement of the oral cavity. This is uncommon in Crohn's disease but can be very debilitating when present. It is common for patients to complain of recurrent mouth ulcers (aphthous stomatitis) particularly at times of disease flares. However, this is not true of oral Crohn's and, whilst haematinic deficiency may also be a factor, simple topical therapy and treatment of the underlying IBD lead to resolution. True oral Crohn's presents most frequently as firm lip swelling, with or without erythema spreading on to the face, and Crohn's-like ulceration and inflammation within the mouth, particularly affecting the buccal mucosa and buccal sulcus. Linear ulceration in the buccal sulcus is highly characteristic (Figure 7.2). Oro-facial granulomatosis (OFG) is an overlap term used to encompass oral Crohn's but also similar granulomatous chronic inflammation in the oral cavity presenting in isolation. These conditions are often indistinguishable, with perhaps only buccal sulcal involvement being truly indicative of intestinal Crohn's disease. The importance of OFG and oral Crohn's is that there appear to be separate factors driving the condition. Atopy rates are remarkably high in this group and much interest has focused on the role of dietary triggers. In particular, cinnamon and benzoate compounds (used as flavouring and preservatives) have been implicated, and there is good evidence of clinical benefit on a cinnamon- and benzoate-free diet (White *et al.*, 2006). Hence, in our patient, the involvement of the oral cavity should receive separate specialist attention to consider a cinnamon- and benzoate-free diet, in addition to the likely benefit from systemic therapy aimed at the intestinal and perianal Crohn's disease. In my experience, diet works well as an adjunct in this setting. At the same time, the presence of buccal sulcal ulceration is also a sign of likely need for systemic therapy, and of a good response to this treatment. There are currently very few clinics specialising in the management of oral Crohn's and patients often see a range of specialists, including dentists, oral surgeons and dermatologists, with variable outcomes. For disease not responding to initial approaches, referral to a specialist multidisciplinary clinic (including dietitian support) is recommended (such as the oral medicine/gastroenterology clinic at Guy's & St Thomas' Hospital).

5. Nutritional concerns

With lots of time being spent considering all the differing treatment options in our patient, it is easy to forget about their nutritional status and, indeed, whether, exclusive nutritional therapy may play a role, particularly in achieving improved overall health prior to surgery. In adults, despite the documented benefits of exclusive enteral nutrition (elemental or polymeric) in active small bowel Crohn's

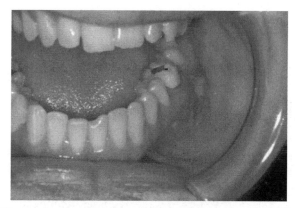

Figure 7.2 Photo of oral cavity showing linear ulceration and erythema in the left buccal sulcus characteristic of true oral Crohn's disease.

disease, patient (and physician) preferences often mean that this approach is little used. In children this is quite the opposite, driven appropriately by the importance of preventing growth retardation and avoiding steroids. In our patient, a good argument could be made for the use of enteral nutrition both as support and as therapy as a means of optimising nutritional health prior to surgery. In patients facing small bowel resection who have lost significant weight, a good plan is to admit the person for two weeks prior to surgery, deliver enteral nutrition (via an NG tube if necessary), optimise other nutritional aspects such as vitamin and mineral deficiency and attempt to withdraw all steroids (including budesonide) prior to operation. The benefit of this approach is significant in terms of improved outcome post-surgery. Care needs to be taken in those with significant obstruction (with upstream pre-stenotic dilatation), as enteral nutrition may simply fill up a dilated small intestine – hence parenteral nutrition with a small amount of enteral may be optimal in this group.

What if everything fails?
Anti-mycobacterial antibiotic therapy (rifabutin and clarithromycin) should also be considered if it has not been tried before. Other options would be an alternative biologic (for example, Nataluzimab, or entering the patient into a current local or national ongoing clinical trial). Many patients currently ask about Naltrexone, but on available data this seems unlikely to gain a significant remission in such severe Crohn's disease. There are also options such as leucophoresis or photophoresis,

available in certain centres. Finally, an autologous stem cell transplant (ASCT) could be considered.

In all units treating IBD, particularly tertiary referral units, there are a small number of patients in whom, unfortunately, all conventional treatment options are failing. It is even more important in these individuals to carefully evaluate exactly which areas of involvement are causing which symptoms and any contribution from factors unrelated to the Crohn's disease itself. Perhaps the most frequent scenario is the patient who still has predominant inflammatory disease in whom, with surgery considered inappropriate, a search is on for a medical therapy which might work. In general, my approach would be to first consider whether a diverting ileostomy (or colostomy) might be a way of restoring health whilst future options are considered. This option tends to be backed away from by physicians but, in my experience, can absolutely revolutionise the health of an individual, however young, who is highly symptomatic, failing education or a career and has minimal quality of life.

In terms of options for medical therapy in this situation, I suspect a poll of IBD physicians (and surgeons) would come up with 20 different preferences, which is fair because local experience influences the choice and suitability of any specific approach. My own approach would be as follows. I would certainly consider a trial of antimycobacterial antibiotics, as despite the lack of positive data from one randomised controlled trial, a small number of patients can clearly get a remarkable and sustained response (Gui *et al.*, 1997; Selby *et al.*, 2007). The standard approach is to use rifabutin 300–450 mg daily and Clarithromycin 750 mg daily in divided doses. Rifabutin can be poorly tolerated due to arthralgia and myalgia in particular and can cause uveitis requiring temporary withdrawal and steroid eye medication. Response can be fast, but a trial of three months in the first instance is appropriate, with therapy for two years (or longer) if there is a good response. Other options depend on local or regional availability and expertise. Natalizumab (Sandborn *et al.*, 2005), the alpha 4 integrin antibody, is available on a named patient basis in some centres and is worth considering as an alternative biologic, or there may be availability to enrol a patient in to a clinical trial locally. Leucophoresis (Maiden *et al.*, 2008) or, more recently, photophoresis (Tripodi *et al.*, 2007), have been used with some success but are only available in a limited number of units. Finally, some consideration should be given to referral for autologous stem cell transplantation (ASCT) (Marti *et al.*, 2001; Musso *et al.*, 2000). This rather dramatic option is currently under evaluation in the UK in a clinical trial, but results from the USA and some limited European experience are encouraging. In particular, in a group of patients generally severely affected by Crohn's disease, there is a suggestion that ASCT results in a resetting of the immune system such that responsiveness to conventional therapy (immunosuppression, biologics) is restored. The morbidity of this approach is high, but mortality is low (because less aggressive ablation is required) as has to be the case in the treatment of a disease itself only associated with a slight increase in mortality.

Application to ulcerative colitis

Clearly, much of the above management refers to Crohn's disease, which is the type of IBD more commonly taxing us regarding difficult management decisions. In refractory ulcerative colitis, many of the above options remain entirely relevant, particularly those concerning optimising immunosuppression. However, there are some important differences. The most important one concerns the role of surgery. Physicians, in particular, tend to view surgery as a last resort, but also tend to forget that the albeit imperfect cure gained by colectomy usually near normalises a patient's quality of life. Surgery will generally put a patient's life back on track, one that has been put on hold for many years because of chronic active UC and the knock-on effects on all aspects of life. Hence surgery *must* come into discussions with the patient with refractory UC early in a consultation, rather than being kept back as a bombshell to be dropped right at the end.

The other important difference concerns choice of second line immuno-suppression. There is an ongoing debate regarding the role of biologicals in UC and most would agree that the data from trials indicates a level of response significantly lower than that seen in CD (Rutgeerts *et al.*, 2005). Nonetheless, internationally, infliximab has become a routine second line option where thiopurines have failed in chronic active UC. In the UK, infliximab has not met the NICE threshold for cost-effectiveness and is therefore only available under an exceptional circumstances application. The choice of second line immunosuppression is therefore between ciclosporin A, for which there is reasonable data (D'Haens *et al.*, 2001; Lichtiger *et al.*, 1994; Van Assche *et al.*, 2003) but more potential toxicity than others, methotrexate (little data but less toxicity) or mycophenolate (even less data!).

In the acute severe situation things are a little different. If a standard intensive steroid regime has failed at day 3 or 5 of treatment and the situation is not fulminant or complicated (i.e. surgery is mandatory) then infliximab is considered an acceptable alternative to intravenous or oral ciclosporin (Jarnerot *et al.*, 2005). Further studies will hopefully inform us soon as to which option carries the best risk–benefit balance in this situation, but at present it is a matter of personal choice and local experience. Once again, in the acute severe UC setting surgery should be debated daily and attention paid to determinants such as height of CRP at presentation and, at day 3, albumin levels and complications (including an awareness of the masking effect of steroids). It would be ideal to have a marker of 'salvagability' in this setting to determine between a colonic mucosa that may recover with powerful immunosuppression and one that is irreversibly affected (for example with large areas of underlying muscularis visible at limited sigmoidoscopy). Where the latter has occurred, the adage 'save lives not colons' remains entirely valid today and surgery is the only option.

The role of the CNS in complex IBD management

For obvious reasons, decision-making in complex disease management tends to focus much more around the opinion and experience of a specialist IBD physician. However, there is also an argument that the CNS role is even more important in these types of cases than in patients with straightforward disease. Decisions on optimal management require input from the entire team (doctor, CNS, dietitian, pharmacist), the patient and their family. The IBD CNS plays a pivotal role in facilitating this process and ensuring all aspects of the patient's problem are considered. Moreover, the CNS is often critically important in conveying options to the patient and their family, explaining (or reiterating) risks and benefits of treatment approaches, and ensuring that important factors have not been missed. Finally, because the treatment option chosen may be both complex or, in some cases, unconventional, the CNS can be an important educational and explanatory bridge between the IBD team and other secondary care teams, primary care and, of course, family and friends.

Conclusion

Overall, it is clear that there are multiple aspects to consider when attempting to optimise the treatment of a patient with complex or more difficult IBD. Some aspects are supportive or deal with making sure an eye is kept on the broader complications of the disease; some involve the appropriate use of specialist surgery for each component of the disease; and finally, some aspects involve the optimal use of immunosuppressive drug therapy to control the chronic inflammation driving the disease. With optimal therapy, however, comes increased risk, which we have perhaps not seen previously because of therapy traditionally being less aggressive, geared to symptom control rather than mucosal healing. Nonetheless, the benefits of careful but aggressive therapy still far outweigh the risks but discussing this balance with patients and their family is now of much greater importance. Less aggressive therapy may seem attractive to many practitioners treating IBD, wary of causing harm, but there are no prizes later on for allowing a patient to suffer more complications, more surgery and a greater reduction in quality of life, education and career prospects.

Successful treatment involves balancing risks and benefits – the known risks of each treatment should be discussed, but always balance this with information regarding the expected level of benefit

---

Patient translation summary

- It is important in the management of complex IBD to break each of the patient's presenting problems down into separate issues and evaluate them thoroughly.
- Optimising drug treatment also involves careful appraisal of why previous or existing therapies might have failed with the hope of finding a means of getting a letter response to proven safe treatment rather than necessarily opting for stronger treatment.
- Always discuss the role of surgery with your patient – this should never be considered the last resort.

References

Allez, M., Lemann, M., Bonnet, J., Cattan, P., Jian, R. and Modigliani, R. (2002) Long term outcome of patients with active Crohn's disease exhibiting extensive and deep ulcerations at colonoscopy. *Am. J. Gastroenterol.*, **97**(4), 947–53.

Ansari, A., Arenas, M., Greenfield, S. M., Morris, D., Lindsay, J., Gilshenan, K., Smith, M., Lewis, C., Marinaki, A., Duley, J. and Sanderson, J. (2008a) Prospective evaluation of the pharmacogenetics of azathioprine in the treatment of inflammatory bowel disease. *Aliment. Pharmacol. Ther.*, **28**(8), 973–83.

Ansari, A., Elliott, T., Baburajan, B., Mayhead, P., O'Donohue, J., Chocair, P., Sanderson, J. and Duley, J. (2008b) Long term outcome of using allopurinol co-therapy as a strategy for overcoming thiopurine hepatotoxicity in treating inflammatory bowel disease. *Aliment. Pharmacol. Ther.*, **28**(6), 734–41.

Ansari, A., Elliott, T., Fong, F., Renas-Hernandez, M., Rottenberg, G., Portmann, B., Lucas, S., Marinaki, A. and Sanderson, J. (2008c) Further experience with the use of 6-thioguanine in patients with Crohn's disease. *Inflamm. Bowel. Dis.*, **14**(10), 1399–405.

Baert, F., Moortgat, L., Van, A. G., Caenepeel, P., Vergauwe, P., De, V. M., Stokkers, P., Hommes, D., Rutgeerts, P., Vermeire, S. and D'Haens, G. (2010) Mucosal healing predicts sustained clinical remission in patients with early-stage Crohn's disease. *Gastro-*

enterology, **138**(2), 463–8.

Boonen, A., Dagnelie, P. C., Feleus, A., Hesselink, M. A., Muris, J. W., Stockbrugger, R. W. and Russel, M. G. (2002) The impact of inflammatory bowel disease on labor force participation: results of a population sampled case-control study. *Inflamm. Bowel. Dis.*, **8**(6), 382–9.

Canto, E., Ricart, E., Busquets, D., Monfort, D., Garcia-Planella, E., Gonzalez, D., Balanzo, J., Rodriguez-Sanchez, J. L. and Vidal, S. (2007) Influence of a nucleotide oligomerization domain 1 (NOD1) polymorphism and NOD2 mutant alleles on Crohn's disease phenotype. *World J. Gastroenterol.*, **13**(41), 5446–53.

Colombel, J. F., Sandborn, W. J., Reinisch, W., Mantzaris, G. J., Kornbluth, A., Rachmilewitz, D., Lichtiger, S., D'Haens, G., Diamond, R. H., Broussard, D. L., Tang, K. L., van der Woude, C. J. and Rutgeerts, P. (2010) Infliximab, azathioprine, or combination therapy for Crohn's disease. *N. Engl. J. Med.*, **362**(15), 1383–95.

Cosnes, J., Carbonnel, F., Beaugerie, L., Le, Q. Y. and Gendre, J. P. (1996) Effects of cigarette smoking on the long-term course of Crohn's disease. *Gastroenterology*, **110**(2), 424–31.

D'Haens, G., Lemmens, L., Geboes, K., Vandeputte, L., Van, A. F., Mortelmans, L., Peeters, M., Vermeire, S., Penninckx, F., Nevens, F., Hiele, M. and Rutgeerts, P. (2001) Intravenous cyclosporine versus intravenous corticosteroids as single therapy for severe attacks of ulcerative colitis. *Gastroenterology*, **120**(6), 1323–9.

D'Haens, G., Baert, F., Van Assche, G., Caenepeel, P., Vergauwe, P., Tuynman, H., De, V. M., van, D. S., Stitt, L., Donner, A., Vermeire, S., Van de Mierop, F. J., Coche, J. C., van der, W. J., Ochsenkuhn, T., van Bodegraven, A. A., Van Hootegem, P. P., Lambrecht, G. L., Mana, F., Rutgeerts, P., Feagan, B. G. and Hommes, D. (2008) Early combined immunosuppression or conventional management in patients with newly diagnosed Crohn's disease: an open randomised trial. *Lancet*, **371**(9613), 660–7.

Dionigi, G., Dionigi, R., Rovera, F., Boni, L., Padalino, P., Minoja, G., Cuffari, S. and Carrafiello, G. (2008) Treatment of high output entero-cutaneous fistulae associated with large abdominal wall defects: single center experience. *Int. J. Surg.*, **6**(1), 51–6.

Dubinsky, M. C., Hassard, P. V., Seidman, E. G., Kam, L. Y., Abreu, M. T., Targan, S. R. and Vasiliauskas, E. A. (2001) An open-label pilot study using thioguanine as a therapeutic alternative in Crohn's disease patients resistant to 6-mercaptopurine therapy. *Inflamm. Bowel. Dis.*, **7**(3), 181–9.

Dubinsky, M. C., Yang, H., Hassard, P. V., Seidman, E. G., Kam, L. Y., Abreu, M. T., Targan, S. R. and Vasiliauskas, E. A. (2002) 6-MP metabolite profiles provide a biochemical explanation for 6-MP resistance in patients with inflammatory bowel disease. *Gastroenterology*, **122**(4), 904–15.

Dubinsky, M. C., Feldman, E. J., Abreu, M. T., Targan, S. R. and Vasiliauskas, E. A. (2003a)

Thioguanine: a potential alternate thiopurine for IBD patients allergic to 6-mercaptopurine or azathioprine. *Am. J. Gastroenterol.*, **98**(5), 1058–63.

Dubinsky, M. C., Vasiliauskas, E. A., Singh, H., Abreu, M. T., Papadakis, K. A., Tran, T., Martin, P., Vierling, J. M., Geller, S. A., Targan, S. R. and Poordad, F. F. (2003b) 6-thioguanine can cause serious liver injury in inflammatory bowel disease patients. *Gastroenterology*, **125**(2), 298–303.

Ezzat, Y. and Hamdy, K. (2010) The frequency of low bone mineral density and its associated risk factors in patients with inflammatory bowel diseases. *Int. J. Rheum. Dis.*, **13**(3), 259–65.

Feagan, B. G., Rochon, J., Fedorak, R. N., Irvine, E. J., Wild, G., Sutherland, L., Steinhart, A. H., Greenberg, G. R., Gillies, R. and Hopkins, M. (1995) Methotrexate for the treatment of Crohn's disease. The North American Crohn's Study Group Investigators. *N. Engl. J. Med.*, **332**(5), 292–7.

Froslie, K. F., Jahnsen, J., Moum, B. A. and Vatn, M. H. (2007) Mucosal healing in inflammatory bowel disease: results from a Norwegian population-based cohort. *Gastroenterology*, **133**(2), 412–22.

Gapasin, J., Van Langenberg, D. R., Holtmann, G., Hetzel, D. J. and Andrews, J. M. (2010) Potentially avoidable surgery in IBD: what proportion of patients come to resection without optimal preoperative therapy? A guidelines-based audit. *Intern. Med. J.* (in press).

Gilissen, L. P., Derijks, L. J., Driessen, A., Bos, L. P., Hooymans, P. M., Stockbrugger, R. W. and Engels, L. G. (2007) Toxicity of 6-thioguanine: no hepatotoxicity in a series of IBD patients treated with long-term, low dose 6-thioguanine Some evidence for dose or metabolite level dependent effects? *Dig. Liver Dis.*, **39**(2), 156–9.

Gui, G. P., Thomas, P. R., Tizard, M. L., Lake, J., Sanderson, J. D. and Hermon-Taylor, J. (1997) Two-year-outcomes analysis of Crohn's disease treated with rifabutin and macrolide antibiotics. *J. Antimicrob. Chemother.*, **39**(3), 393–400.

Guo, S. and Dipietro, L. A. (2010) Factors affecting wound healing. *J. Dent. Res.*, **89**(3), 219–29.

Heuschkel, R., Salvestrini, C., Beattie, R. M., Hildebrand, H., Walters, T. and Griffiths, A. (2008) Guidelines for the management of growth failure in childhood inflammatory bowel disease. *Inflamm. Bowel. Dis.*, **14**(6), 839–49.

Hyams, J. S. and Markowitz, J. F. (2005) Can we alter the natural history of Crohn's disease in children? *J. Pediatr. Gastroenterol. Nutr.*, **40**(3), 262–72.

Jarnerot, G., Hertervig, E., Friis-Liby, I., Blomquist, L., Karlen, P., Granno, C., Vilien, M., Strom, M., Danielsson, A., Verbaan, H., Hellstrom, P. M., Magnuson, A. and Curman, B. (2005) Infliximab as rescue therapy in severe to moderately severe ulcerative colitis: a randomized, placebo-controlled study. *Gastroenterology*, **128**(7), 1805–11.

Kandiel, A., Fraser, A. G., Korelitz, B. I., Brensinger, C. and Lewis, J. D. (2005) Increased risk of lymphoma among inflammatory bowel disease patients treated with azathioprine and 6-mercaptopurine. *Gut*, **54**(8), 1121–5.

Koltun, W. A. (2007) Dangers associated with endoscopic management of strictures in IBD. *Inflamm. Bowel. Dis.*, **13**(3), 359–61.

Lichtiger, S., Present, D. H., Kornbluth, A., Gelernt, I., Bauer, J., Galler, G., Michelassi, F. and Hanauer, S. (1994) Cyclosporine in severe ulcerative colitis refractory to steroid therapy. *N. Engl. J. Med.*, **330**(26), 1841–5.

Lowenberg, M., Peppelenbosch, M. and Hommes, D. (2006) Biological therapy in the management of recent-onset Crohn's disease: why, when and how? *Drugs*, **66**(11), 1431–9.

Maiden, L., Takeuchi, K., Baur, R., Bjarnason, I., O'Donohue, J., Forgacs, I., Chung-Faye, G., Sanderson, J. and Bjarnason, I. (2008) Selective white cell apheresis reduces relapse rates in patients with IBD at significant risk of clinical relapse. *Inflamm. Bowel. Dis.*, **14**(10), 1413–18.

Marti, J. L., Mayordomo, J. I., Isla, M. D., Saenz, A., Escudero, P. and Tres, A. (2001) PBSC autotransplant for inflammatory bowel disease (IBD): a case of ulcerative colitis. *Bone Marrow Transplant.*, **28**(1), 109–10.

Musso, M., Porretto, F., Crescimanno, A., Bondi, F., Polizzi, V. and Scalone, R. (2000) Crohn's disease complicated by relapsed extranodal Hodgkin's lymphoma: prolonged complete remission after unmanipulated PBPC autotransplant. *Bone Marrow Transplant.*, **26**(8), 921–3.

Neurath, M. F., Wanitschke, R., Peters, M., Krummenauer, F., Meyer Zum Buschenfelde, K. H. and Schlaak, J. F. (1999) Randomised trial of mycophenolate mofetil versus azathioprine for treatment of chronic active Crohn's disease. *Gut*, **44**(5), 625–8.

Patel, V., Macdonald, J. K., McDonald, J. W. and Chande, N. (2009) Methotrexate for maintenance of remission in Crohn's disease. *Cochrane Database Syst. Rev.*, 4, CD006884.

Peyrin-Biroulet, L., Loftus, E. V., Jr, Colombel, J. F. and Sandborn, W. J. (2010) The natural history of adult Crohn's disease in population-based cohorts. *Am. J. Gastroenterol.*, **105**(2), 289–97.

de Pineton, C. G., Peyrin-Biroulet, L., Lemann, M. and Colombel, J. F. (2010) Clinical implications of mucosal healing for the management of IBD. *Nat. Rev. Gastroenterol. Hepatol.*, **7**(1), 15–29.

Rahier, J., Ben-Horin, S., Chowers, Y., Conlon, C., De Munter, P., D'Haens, G., Domenech, E., Eliakim, R., Eser, A., Frater, J., Gassull, M. A., Giladi, M., Kaser, A., Lemann, M., Moreels, T., Moschen, A., Pollok, R., Reinisch, W., Schunter, M., Stange, E. F., Tilig, H., Van Assche, Viget, N., Vucelic, B., Walsh, A. M., Weiss, G., Yazdanpanph, Y., Zabana, Y., Travis, S. and Colombel, J. F. (2009) European evidence-based consensus on the prevention, diagnosis and management of opportunistic infections in inflammatory bowel disease. *Journal of Crohn's and Colitis*, **3**, 47–91.

Ramadas, A. V., Gunesh, S., Thomas, G. A., Williams, G. T. and Hawthorne, A. B. (2010) Natural history of Crohn's disease in a population-based cohort from Cardiff (1986–2003): a study of changes in medical treatment and surgical resection rates. *Gut*, **59**(9), 1200–6.

Rutgeerts, P., Sandborn, W. J., Feagan, B. G., Reinisch, W., Olson, A., Johanns, J., Travers, S., Rachmilewitz, D., Hanauer, S. B., Lichtenstein, G. R., de Villiers, W. J., Present, D., Sands, B. E. and Colombel, J. F. (2005) Infliximab for induction and maintenance therapy for ulcerative colitis. *N. Engl. J. Med.*, **353**(23), 2462–76.

Sandborn, W. J., Colombel, J. F., Enns, R., Feagan, B. G., Hanauer, S. B., Lawrance, I. C., Panaccione, R., Sanders, M., Schreiber, S., Targan, S., van, D. S., Goldblum, R., Despain, D., Hogge, G. S. and Rutgeerts, P. (2005) Natalizumab induction and maintenance therapy for Crohn's disease. *N. Engl. J. Med.*, **353**(18), 1912–25.

Schnitzler, F., Fidder, H., Ferrante, M., Noman, M., Arijs, I., Van, A. G., Hoffman, I., Van, S. K., Vermeire, S. and Rutgeerts, P. (2009) Mucosal healing predicts long-term outcome of maintenance therapy with infliximab in Crohn's disease. *Inflamm. Bowel. Dis.*, **15**(9), 1295–301.

Selby, W., Pavli, P., Crotty, B., Florin, T., Radford-Smith, G., Gibson, P., Mitchell, B., Connell, W., Read, R., Merrett, M., Ee, H. and Hetzel, D. (2007) Two-year combination antibiotic therapy with clarithromycin, rifabutin, and clofazimine for Crohn's disease. *Gastroenterology*, **132**(7), 2313–19.

Smith, M. A., Marinaki, A., Arenas, M., Escuredo, E. and Sanderson, J. (2008) The impact of introducing thioguanine nucleotide monitoring into clinical practice. *Gut*, **57**(suppl. 1), A387.

Smith, M. A., Irving, P. M., Marinaki, A. M. and Sanderson, J. D. (2010) Review article: malignancy on thiopurine treatment with special reference to inflammatory bowel disease. *Aliment. Pharmacol. Ther.*, **32**(2), 119–30.

Sokol, H., Seksik, P., Carrat, F., Nion-Larmurier, I., Vienne, A., Beaugerie, L. and Cosnes, J. (2010) Usefulness of co-treatment with immunomodulators in patients with inflammatory bowel disease treated with scheduled infliximab maintenance therapy. *Gut*, **59**(10), 1363–8.

Sparrow, M. P., Hande, S. A., Friedman, S., Cao, D. and Hanauer, S. B. (2007) Effect of allopurinol on clinical outcomes in inflammatory bowel disease nonresponders to azathioprine or 6-mercaptopurine. *Clin. Gastroenterol. Hepatol.*, **5**(2), 209–14.

Subramanian, V., Saxena, S., Kang, J. Y. and Pollok, R. C. (2008) Preoperative steroid use and risk of postoperative complications in patients with inflammatory bowel disease undergoing abdominal surgery. *Am. J. Gastroenterol.*, **103**(9), 2373–81.

Taxonera, C., Schwartz, D. A. and Garcia-Olmo, D. (2009) Emerging treatments for complex perianal fistula in Crohn's disease. *World J. Gastroenterol.*, **15**(34), 4263–72.

Thia, K. T., Sandborn, W. J., Harmsen, W. S., Zinsmeister, A. R. and Loftus, E. V., Jr (2010) Risk factors associated with progression to intestinal complications of Crohn's disease in a population-based cohort. *Gastroenterology* (in press).

Toruner, M., Loftus, E. V., Jr, Harmsen, W. S., Zinsmeister, A. R., Orenstein, R., Sandborn, W. J., Colombel, J. F. and Egan, L. J. (2008) Risk factors for opportunistic infections in patients with inflammatory bowel disease. *Gastroenterology*, **134**(4), 929–36.

Tripodi, G., Risso, M., Tenerini, L., Gandullia, P., Castellano, E. and Rivabella, L. (2007) Drug-resistant bullous pemphigoid and inflammatory bowel disease in a pediatric case successfully treated by plasma exchange and extracorporeal photochemotherapy. *J. Clin. Apher.*, **22**(1), 26–30.

Van Assche, G., D'Haens, G., Noman, M., Vermeire, S., Hiele, M., Asnong, K., Arts, J., D'Hoore, A., Penninckx, F. and Rutgeerts, P. (2003) Randomized, double-blind comparison of 4 mg/kg versus 2 mg/kg intravenous cyclosporine in severe ulcerative colitis. *Gastroenterology*, **125**(4), 1025–31.

Van, A. G., Vermeire, S. and Rutgeerts, P. (2010) The potential for disease modification in Crohn's disease. *Nat. Rev. Gastroenterol. Hepatol.*, **7**(2), 79–85.

Vermeire, S., Noman, M., Van, A. G., Baert, F., D'Haens, G. and Rutgeerts, P. J. (2007) The effectiveness of concomitant immunosuppressive therapy to suppress formation of antibodies to infliximab in Crohn's disease, *Gut*, **56**, 1226–31.

White, A., Nunes, C., Escudier, M., Lomer, M. C., Barnard, K., Shirlaw, P., Challacombe, S. J. and Sanderson, J. D. (2006) Improvement in orofacial granulomatosis on a cinnamon- and benzoate-free diet. *Inflamm. Bowel. Dis.*, **12**(6), 508–14.

Yamamoto, T. and Keighley, M. R. (2000) Smoking and disease recurrence after operation for Crohn's disease. *Br. J. Surg.*, **87**(4), 398–404.

CHAPTER 8

Dietary considerations in IBD

Miranda Lomer

Case study

Miss Y was diagnosed with ileocaecal Crohn's disease following an ileo-colonoscopy. She weighed 47 kg (BMI 18.2) having lost 9% of her body weight over the previous 6 months. She had loose watery stools, no blood or mucus and her bowels were opening with urgency 6–8 times per day. She was prescribed a reducing course of prednisolone but wanted to know if she could avoid taking steroids. Miss Y saw the dietitian, who provided some general dietary advice for newly diagnosed Crohn's disease and information for weight gain using nutritional supplements. The dietitian also discussed using enteral nutrition as a primary treatment for Crohn's disease and Miss Y decided to try this instead of the steroids. She was advised on a liquid polymeric feed as her only source of nutrition, which her GP prescribed. After 8 weeks Miss Y's weight had increased to 49 kg and she was feeling asymptomatic with more energy and keen to start eating. She began reintroducing food gradually using a modified exclusion diet.

Six months later Miss Y had intermittent episodes of abdominal pain associated with nausea and sometimes vomiting suggestive of obstructive symptoms. Her appetite was poor and this limited her food intake. Her weight had dropped to 45 kg. She had an MRI scan which confirmed an ileal stricture, inflammatory in nature, approximately 8 cm long. She was given dietary advice for stricturing disease and restarted nutritional supplements to meet her nutritional requirements. After several months Miss Y had an ileocaecal resection as she was still symptomatic. Within a few weeks of surgery her appetite was good and her weight increased to 52 kg (BMI 20). A diet history indicated she was managing a wide variety of foods and she was asymptomatic.

Box 8.1 Dietary considerations

■ Newly diagnosed patients may be concerned that their dietary habits have brought on their disease. Relatives may also have concerns about their risk of developing disease (see Diet as a cause of IBD).

■ Weight loss and nutritional deficiencies are common in IBD (see Nutritional issues in IBD).

■ Enteral nutrition can be used to treat active Crohn's disease and may be appropriate for some patients (see Dietary treatment of active Crohn's disease).

■ Dietary advice for stricturing disease depends on various factors (see Stricturing Crohn's disease).

Introduction

Access to appropriate dietary assessment and advice is of paramount importance to patients with IBD. However, often in clinical practice patients do not see a dietitian (UK IBD Audit Steering Group, 2006; UK IBD Audit Steering Group, 2008). New service standards recommend that the multidisciplinary healthcare team should include a dietitian with a special interest in gastroenterology and all patients should have access (IBD Standards Working Group, 2009). Specialist dietetic input for interpretation of symptoms, dietary assessment and therapeutic advice are invaluable to achieve comprehensive nutritional management for each patient. This chapter aims to address dietary and nutritional considerations in IBD.

Diet as a cause of IBD

At diagnosis, patients often think that diet has contributed to the cause of their disease. The highly processed modern Western diet is an appealing concept as an environmental risk factor. However, epidemiological evidence supporting dietary contribution to the development of IBD is lacking, despite a rising incidence in countries which are becoming more westernised. There is increasing interest in how the diet contributes to the gastrointestinal microbiota although the role is not yet clearly defined.

A high intake of refined carbohydrate in the pre-illness diet, especially sugar, has been described on numerous occasions in case-control studies (Porro and Panza, 1985; Reif *et al.*, 1997; Sakamoto *et al.*, 2005; Thornton *et al.*, 1979; Tragnone *et al.*, 1995), but dietary recall is difficult when carried out retrospectively and leads to inaccurate measurement of dietary intake. Dietary changes may occur soon after symptoms develop, but a confirmed diagnosis of IBD may take much longer. An increased likelihood of relapse in ulcerative colitis has been observed in patients with a high alcohol or high meat intake. Sulphur-containing compounds in these foods may be important substrates for sulphide-producing colonic bacteria and have been targeted as possibly being involved in the inflammatory process leading to disease relapse (Jowett *et al.*, 2004).

Fats, particularly polyunsaturated, have immunomodulatory effects; n-6 fats are considered to have pro-inflammatory properties and n-3 fats are anti-inflammatory. The ratio of n-6 to n-3 in the diet is important, with a healthy range from 1:1 to 4:1. A Japanese case control study has suggested that a high n-6 to n-3 ratio may contribute to the development of Crohn's disease (Shoda *et al.*, 1996). A prospective cohort study in over 260,000 European adults identified 139 incident cases of ulcerative colitis. Although no clear dietary associations were identified with the onset of disease, there was an association for an increased percentage of energy from total polyunsaturated fatty acids in the incident ulcerative colitis cases, but it did not quite reach significance ($p = 0.07$) (Hart *et al.*, 2008).

Exposure to *Mycobacterium avium paratuberculosis* (MAP) in milk, particularly unpasteurised milk, has been linked to the development of Crohn's disease due to MAP being present in cows and some milk, but results are conflicting and clinical interpretation is limited (Bernstein *et al.*, 2006; Danese *et al.*, 2004).

Despite the obesity epidemic, no association between obesity rates and the increasing incidence of IBD has yet been found. Obesity may be a risk factor for the development of Crohn's disease in the older person (Chapman-Kiddell *et al.*, 2010) but research is limited.

In summary, there is currently no conclusive evidence that diet is involved in the pathogenesis of IBD. However, the immunomodulatory role of fats in the cause of disease is an appealing mechanistic concept and further large prospective studies are needed. Relatives of patients with IBD should be encouraged to follow public health recommendations regarding general healthy eating and lifestyle.

Nutritional issues in IBD

Nutritional problems are common in IBD and develop from a multitude of causes (Table 8.1). They can occur very early on in the disease process, so access to appropriate dietary advice is essential soon after diagnosis. Changes in appetite and energy expenditure contribute to malnutrition and may be affected by chronic malabsorption and increased circulating pro-inflammatory cytokines (Bannerman *et al.*, 2001; Gassull and Cabre, 2001).

141

Inflammatory bowel disease nursing

Table 8.1 Nutritional considerations in IBD.

Nutritional problem	Possible causes
Reduced nutrient intake and anorexia	Nausea, vomiting, abdominal pain, intestinal obstruction (fibrotic scar tissue or active inflammation), upper gastrointestinal disease, enteric fistula, dietary exclusion, fear of eating, reduced appetite, fasting for investigations
Increasing energy expenditure and metabolism	Pro-inflammatory cytokines, surgery, pyrexia, infection
Anaemia	Blood loss, anaemia of chronic disease, poor dietary intake
Nutrient malabsorption	Inflamed mucosa, extensive small bowel disease, multiple resections, short bowel syndrome, bile salt malabsorption, secondary lactose malabsorption, bacterial overgrowth
Increased gastrointestinal losses	Diarrhoea, vomiting, fistulae, blood, protein, fluid, electrolytes
Dyspepsia	Upper gastrointestinal disease, drug side-effects (e.g. 5-ASA, metronidazole, corticosteroids)
Osteopenia and osteoporosis	Corticosteroids, poor calcium intake, calcium malabsorption, vitamin D deficiency

Loose bowel motions and chronic diarrhoea are common in IBD and can lead to electrolyte imbalance and micronutrient deficiencies. Diarrhoea may be due to a multitude of problems, and underlying mechanisms relate to the site, extent and severity of inflammation, and may be exacerbated by altered gastrointestinal microbiota, fermentation and malabsorption, altered motility and iatrogenic, causes such as infection, medication and diet.

Malnutrition occurs in up to 85% of patients with IBD; it is particularly high in active Crohn's disease (Gassull and Cabre, 2001) and often continues into disease remission (Geerling et al., 1998; Krok and Lichtenstein, 2003). Patients with malnutrition have higher mortality rates and spend significantly longer in hospital compared to those without malnutrition, thus increasing the burden on healthcare costs (Nguyen et al., 2008; Pirlich et al., 2003).

Weight loss is common and affects up to 80% of patients with Crohn's disease and 18–62% of patients with ulcerative colitis (Geerling et al., 1999). A single measurement of BMI is not a good indicator of lean body mass or nutritional status, and patients with a healthy BMI and/or in disease remission may have poor

Table 8.2 Prevalence of weight loss and nutritional deficiencies in IBD.

Nutritional problem or deficiency	Crohn's disease % of patients (reference)	Ulcerative colitis % of patients (reference)
Weight loss	80	18–62
Anaemia	6–74	9–67
Iron	36–90	81
Folate	3–54	6–36
Vitamin B$_{12}$	15–48	1–5
Calcium	13	*
Vitamin D	18–70	17–79
Magnesium	14–33	18–24
Zinc	3–5	6

Data are adapted from various sources (Geerling *et al*., 1999; Kulnigg and Gasche, 2006; O'Sullivan and O'Morain 2006; Vagianos *et al*., 2007; Valentini *et al*., 2008; Wilson *et al*., 2004) and summarise weight loss and suboptimal values for biochemical measurements of nutritional status.
*present but percentage of patients unknown

muscle function and micronutrient deficiencies (Vagianos *et al*., 2007; Valentini *et al*., 2008). Although a patient's BMI may be in the healthy range or even indicate overweight or obesity (Vagianos *et al*., 2007), a sudden or even gradual change in weight is important when considering nutritional status. Patients with IBD should routinely have their weight and body mass index (BMI) measured for long-term monitoring. All patients admitted to hospital should have their nutritional needs assessed (IBD Standards Working Group, 2009).

Nutritional deficiencies are prevalent in IBD (Table 8.2) and the two most relevant are those related to anaemia and osteoporosis. Magnesium and zinc deficiencies may be of specific concern in Crohn's disease. Magnesium deficiency may be due to increased intestinal losses, malabsorption, small bowel bacterial overgrowth or an ileal resection and zinc deficiency due to increased intestinal losses or high output fistulae.

Anaemia
Anaemia is frequent in IBD, with iron deficiency and/or anaemia of chronic disease being the most common causes (Gasche *et al*., 2004). Low dietary iron intakes have been reported (Lomer *et al*., 2004), and although assessment of dietary intake is important, poor intakes are unlikely to be the sole cause of anaemia in IBD. Rich

143

dietary sources of iron (red meat, fortified breakfast cereals) are often avoided due to food aversions or intolerances, so a dietary assessment will help to identify if poor oral intake is a contributing factor.

Diagnostic criteria and management

Assessment of iron deficiency in IBD is complex due to numerous contributing factors, e.g. inflammation and anaemia of chronic disease. Appropriate diagnostic criteria for iron deficiency in patients where inflammation is absent are serum ferritin $\leq$ 30 µg/l or transferrin saturation < 16%. Where there is evidence of inflammation, 100 µg/l is the lower limit of serum ferritin that is consistent with normal iron stores. In the presence of anaemia and inflammation, the diagnostic criteria for anaemia of chronic disease are serum ferritin > 100 µg/l and transferrin saturation < 16%. If the serum ferritin is 30–100 µg/l then iron deficiency and anaemia of chronic disease coexist (Gasche *et al.*, 2007). Haemoglobin levels may be abnormal due to other nutritional deficiencies, e.g. folate or vitamin B_{12}, or anaemia of chronic disease; however, microcytic anaemia (MCV $\leq$ 80 fl) is consistent with iron deficiency.

Oral iron supplementation is generally unhelpful in patients with IBD and iron deficiency due to gastrointestinal side-effects. When iron deficiency coexists with anaemia intravenous iron may be warranted (Gasche *et al.*, 2007).

Folate deficiency has often been described and may be due to inhibition of folate absorption in long-term use of sulphasalazine, although routine clinical use of sulphasalazine is far less common since the advent of mesalazine.

Vitamin B_{12} is a particular problem for patients with a diseased ileum or ileal resection. Vitamin B_{12} deficiency is not often seen in ulcerative colitis (Geerling *et al.*, 1999). Folate and vitamin B_{12} deficiencies may occur concurrently and could be due to poor dietary intake or malabsorption due to mucosal inflammation. Regular monitoring and oral supplementation (folate) or intravenous injection (vitamin B_{12}) may be required.

Osteoporosis

Bone mineral density is a growing concern for the IBD population and the prevalences of osteoporosis in Crohn's disease and ulcerative colitis are 3–58% and 4–50%, respectively (Tilg *et al.*, 2008). The cause of osteoporosis in IBD is multifactorial and includes age, malnutrition and malabsorption, vitamin D and calcium status, corticosteroid use and inflammation. Minimising the use of corticosteroids and ensuring an adequate intake of calcium and vitamin D are vital in osteoporosis prevention. Some patients limit their dairy food intake due to concerns over lactose intolerance, and dietary assessment is important to ensure that calcium intake is not limited.

Diagnostic criteria and management

Bone mineral density can be measured using dual energy X-ray absorptiometry (DEXA) and should be assessed for patients with IBD who are at high risk of osteoporosis. It is difficult to identify who may be at high risk and, in the absence of firm evidence, the British Society of Gastroenterology Guidelines propose that patients with IBD should have at least two of the following (Lewis and Scott, 2007):

- Continuing active disease
- Weight loss > 10%
- BMI < 20
- Age > 70

The recommended intake for calcium in IBD is 1000 mg/day (Lewis and Scott, 2007) and supplements (often in combination with vitamin D supplementation) may be required where dietary intake is low (e.g. lactose intolerance) or when corticosteroids are required.

Dietary treatment of active Crohn's disease

In Crohn's disease, nutrition can be used as a primary treatment for active disease, particularly in children and adolescents. Several decades ago 'bowel rest' was considered important and nutrition was provided as intravenous glucose. However, patients developed protein-energy malnutrition. Parenteral nutrition was introduced and, for a while, solved this nutritional dilemma, but total bowel rest led to gut atrophy and parenteral nutrition carried serious risks (Driscoll Jr and Rosenberg, 1978; Ostro et al., 1985). Since then a number of studies have assessed the clinical effectiveness of enteral nutrition and a Cochrane review has confirmed that enteral nutrition is not as effective as corticosteroids (Zachos et al., 2007). However, enteral nutrition is more effective than placebo and, in compliant patients, is as effective as corticosteroids. In paediatrics, enteral nutrition is often used as primary treatment as it avoids the use of corticosteroids which can impair growth. In adults, enteral nutrition can be considered in patients where other primary treatment is not possible or where it is used as an adjunctive therapy, particularly to address malnutrition.

The early enteral diets were chemically defined liquid 'elemental' diets, similar to those used by astronauts. Elemental diets are comprised of protein as free amino acids, carbohydrate as glucose or short chain maltodextrins, a small amount of fat as short chain triglycerides, and vitamins and minerals. The diets provided bowel rest, reducing faecal output and limiting gut atrophy. The mechanism of action was unknown but it was proposed that the diet lowered the antigenic load of the luminal contents, potentially reducing the inflammatory response.

By the 1970s elemental diets were being used to provide nutritional support in malnourished patients and, pre-operatively, their use improved surgical outcome (Rocchio *et al.*, 1974; Voitk *et al.*, 1973). In recent years, more palatable, peptide and whole protein diets were introduced and have been shown to be as efficacious in reducing remission as elemental diets (Zachos *et al.*, 2007). However, the therapeutic mechanisms remain unclear. Inorganic dietary microparticles have been proposed to contribute to intestinal inflammation, but their removal from the diet of patients with active Crohn's disease does not assist disease remission (Lomer *et al.*, 2005). Nutrients are important to the gastrointestinal environment, particularly the microbiota and their effect as inflammatory mediators. Studies comparing fat composition of enteral diets and immunomodulatory effects on remission induction have shown no difference in clinical effectiveness (Zachos *et al.*, 2007). Enteral nutrition may correct suboptimal micronutrient levels, improving mucosal defence mechanisms and, in paediatrics, growth (Bannerjee *et al.*, 2004; Gassull, 2004).

For enteral nutrition to be effective, and to aid compliance, patients need significant support from their multidisciplinary team, particularly the dietitian. Major barriers to successful enteral nutrition are poor palatability, particularly with elemental diets, and high volumes required to meet nutritional requirements (usually 1500–2500 ml per day). Starter regimens are useful to improve initial tolerance of the liquid diet, gradually building up the target volume over several days. Compliance can be improved by using flavours (which can be prescribed) and ensuring that the liquid is cold and taken from a closed beaker using a straw. An enteral feeding tube improves compliance (Rodrigues *et al.*, 2007) and is often used in paediatrics and may also be appropriate for some adult patients. Some patients will pass a nasogastric feeding tube every evening before bed for overnight nutrition while others have a gastrostomy feeding tube fitted.

Enteral nutrition is usually prescribed from two to eight weeks. At two weeks there should be a clinical response and patients may even go into remission, but continuation for up to eight weeks can achieve mucosal healing (Fell *et al.*, 2000). Enteral nutrition is considered to be most effective in patients with ileal disease, although there is insufficient evidence to support this (Zachos *et al.*, 2007).

Maintenance of Crohn's disease remission

Following a course of enteral nutrition, gradual food reintroduction is helpful. Firstly, this approach provides patients with a planned structure to introduce a nutritionally complete diet as quickly as possible, and secondly, it helps them to identify potentially problematic foods. The most widely used reintroduction diet is the LOFFLEX diet (Low Fat, Fibre Limited EXclusion diet) and achieves remission maintenance of 56% at two years (Woolner *et al.*, 1998).

Supplementary enteral nutrition providing 35–50% of energy requirements from an elemental or polymeric diet for up to 12 months may help with remission maintenance in 42–65% of cases, although data to support this is limited (Akobeng and Thomas 2007).

Other dietary considerations during the disease process

Stricturing Crohn's disease

Patients with an intestinal stricture should be advised to follow a diet that is limited in foods that may cause a mechanical obstruction in the gastrointestinal tract, which includes avoiding fibrous fruit and vegetables, nuts and seeds (Table 8.3) (Ballegaard *et al.*, 1997). Patients should be encouraged to chew food thoroughly and take time over meals to help limit obstructive-type symptoms as much as possible. The strictness of dietary avoidance of fibrous foods is dependent on the nature and extent of the stricture; some patients may only manage liquids (Raouf *et al.*, 1991) while others may manage a significantly wider variety of foods. Dietary advice should therefore be tailored to the individual's specific needs and nutritional supplements may be necessary to meet requirements.

Food aversions and intolerances

Patients often avoid high-fibre foods during a flare-up of disease, reducing the amount of residue passing through the gastrointestinal tract and thus alleviating symptoms. Patients may also have a fear of eating because of increased gastrointestinal symptoms and avoid specific trigger foods. Any food avoidance may limit the nutritional value of their diet (Ballegaard *et al.*, 1997; Lomer *et al.*, 2004; Sousa *et al.*, 2007) and long-term exclusion is not recommended; the nutritional adequacy of the diet should be monitored by a dietitian. Common food intolerances are to cow's milk, wheat and onion (Ballegaard *et al.*, 1997; Riordan *et al.*, 1993).

Symptoms in relation to cow's milk may be due to lactose malabsorption, which can result from chronic inflammation and occurs in up to 42% of patients

Table 8.3 Dietary considerations for gastrointestinal strictures.

General dietary advice	Chew food thoroughly and eat slowly as poorly digested food residue can cause blockages
	Eat small meals at regular intervals
	Introduce new foods one at a time to help identify what might trigger symptoms
Meat and fish	Avoid gristle and fat, tough skin, small edible bones (e.g. sardines)
	Include fish, lean meat
Fruit and vegetables	Avoid fibrous (woody) or stringy fruit and vegetables, e.g. broccoli and cauliflower stalks, celery, coconut, leeks, okra, orange pith, pineapple, runner beans
	Avoid fruit and vegetable skins and seeds, e.g. beans and pulses, berries, dried fruit, peppers, sweetcorn, tomato
	Avoid raw vegetables, e.g. carrots
	Include soft tinned fruit or ripe fresh fruit without skins or seeds, e.g. banana, melon, peach
	Include small amounts of fruit juice without pulp or fruit smoothie
	Include peeled cooked root vegetables, e.g. carrots, parsnip, potato, swede, sweet potato, turnip
Cereals and grains	Avoid wholegrains and wholewheat products, e.g. digestive biscuits, granary bread, popcorn, seeded bread, wholemeal bread
	Include corn flakes, crumpets, pancakes, plain bagels, plain biscuits, plain chapatti, plain crackers, plain muffins, plain naan, white pitta bread, plain scones, rice krispies, white bread, white pasta, white rice
Nuts and seeds	Avoid all nuts and seeds unless as a smooth nut butter
Milk and milk products	Include milk, yoghurt, cheese*

* If lactose intolerance present then choose calcium supplemented milk free alternatives – seek further advice from a dietitian

with Crohn's disease (Barrett *et al.*, 2009). Interestingly, the same study reported that 40% of patients with ulcerative colitis had lactose malabsorption which cannot be accounted for by chronic inflammation. It may be more likely that primary lactose intolerance is more common in patients with ulcerative colitis.

Intolerance to wheat and onion may be due to the fructan content. Fructans are polymers of fructose of varying length. They are poorly absorbed in the gastrointestinal tract and are available for rapid fermentation by the gastrointestinal microbiota (Gibson and Shepherd, 2005). Fructans and other poorly absorbed carbohydrates, such as fructose, galactans, lactose and polyols, may be responsible for functional gastrointestinal symptoms often associated with IBD (Simren *et al.*, 2002). Interestingly, fructose malabsorption occurs in up to 61% of patients with Crohn's disease and 42% of patients with ulcerative colitis (Barrett *et al.*, 2009). A diet low in fermentable oligo-, di- and monosaccharides and polyols (FODMAPs) may be helpful in combating functional gastrointestinal symptoms in IBD (Gearry *et al.*, 2009). Although this concept is of great interest, the low FODMAP diet, which was initially developed in Australia, requires careful adaptation for use in other countries before implementation can be successful. This would take into consideration local food supply, ingredient usage and suitable alternative 'free-from' foods to achieve dietary compliance and nutritional adequacy.

Diet, stomas and extensive small bowel resections

Patients with a colostomy or ileostomy may be concerned about their stoma output (e.g. volume, gas production) and request practical advice on how they can alter their diet to alleviate these problems (Table 8.4). Not all patients will have concerns about dietary effects on their stoma output and many will not need to change their diet at all. Patients who are likely to need specialist dietary advice are those with a high-output ileostomy or who have had an extensive small bowel resection with less than 150 cm of small bowel remaining (Table 8.5).

Probiotics and prebiotics

Much interest has been developing over the last decade regarding the role of probiotics and prebiotics in IBD. Definitions are shown in Table 8.6; they are called synbiotics when they are both added to the same product. Probiotics are available as single strains or combinations, and dose and preparation are important considerations. A huge increase in the availability of products commercially provides a plethora of choices, resulting in confusion over what may or may not be helpful.

Evidence indicates clinical effectiveness for probiotics in ulcerative colitis and pouchitis, but as yet their use in Crohn's disease is not convincing (Hedin *et al.*, 2007; Isaacs and Herfarth, 2008). Trials using single-strain probiotics, combinations and synbiotics have shown prevention of pouchitis, maintenance of remission and fewer relapses and treatment for ulcerative colitis. However,

Table 8.4 Dietary considerations for stomas.

Cause loose output	Alcohol, citrus fruit, dried fruit, fried foods, green leafy vegetables, hot drinks, pickles, raw vegetables, spices, strong tea and coffee, very hot or cold food
Thicken output	Bananas, boiled rice, dry toast, marshmallows, smooth peanut butter, yoghurt
Alleviate constipation	Fresh fruit and vegetables Ensure adequate fluid intake
Increase bulk	Brown rice, dried fruit, nuts and seeds, sweetcorn, wholemeal bread and pasta
Stoma blockages	Chew food thoroughly and eat slowly – poorly digested food residue can cause blockages Take extra caution with beans and pulses, celery, coconut, fruit and vegetable skins (e.g. tomato), mushrooms, nuts and seeds, orange pith, pineapple, sweetcorn and any other fibrous 'woody' fruit or vegetables
Cause flatus and gas	Carbonated drinks, alcohol (particularly lager and beer) Beans and pulses, broccoli, cabbage, cauliflower, mushrooms, spinach, onions, garlic, turnips, nuts
Cause odour	Asparagus, baked beans, Brussels sprouts, cabbage, eggs, fish, garlic, onion
Alleviate odour	Orange juice, parsley, tomato juice, yoghurt
Affect colour	Beetroot, blackberries, blueberries, liquorice, strawberries Iron tablets
Hydration	Ensure adequate fluid intake (at least 1500 ml/day). Some patients will require replacement water and salt For high-output stomas dehydration may be a problem and oral rehydration solution will be required

NB: Patients vary in their response to food and many will be unaffected by foods listed here.

not all studies have been positive. Prebiotics are often used in combination with probiotics, so it is difficult to assess their effects in isolation. The gastrointestinal microbiota, immune dysregulation, disease phenotype and disease severity may all impact their effectiveness and are key to better understanding the role that probiotics and prebiotics may have in the management of IBD.

Table 8.5 Dietary considerations for extensive small bowel resection (short bowel syndrome).

Length of resection	Nutritional concerns
Small bowel resection > 100 cm	Uncommon, possibly IV fluids and oral supplements may be required especially in patients where residual bowel is inflamed
Residual jejunum < 100 cm	IV fluids and electrolytes
Residual jejunum < 75 cm	IV fluids, electrolytes and parenteral nutrition
Residual jejunum < 50 cm + colon	IV fluids, electrolytes and parenteral nutrition

Table 8.6 Definitions and examples of probiotics and prebiotics

Definition	Examples
Probiotics are live micro-organisms, which, when administered in adequate amounts, confer a beneficial health effect on the host (de Vrese and Schrezenmeir 2008)	■ Bifidobacteria (*infantis, breve, longum, bifidum*) ■ Lactobacillus (*bulgaricus, casei, rhamnosus GG, reuteri, plantarum*) ■ *Streptococcus thermophilus* and the yeast *Saccharomyces boulardi*
Prebiotics are selectively fermented ingredients that allow specific changes, both in the composition and/or activity in the gastrointestinal microflora, that confer benefits upon the well-being and health of the host (de Vrese and Schrezenmeir 2008)	■ Fructo-oligosaccharide ■ Galacto-oligosaccharides ■ Inulin

Future research

The effect of diet on the gastrointestinal luminal contents and environment in IBD is fascinating and is of major interest to clinicians and patients alike. However, it is still unclear what role diet plays in both the cause and management of disease. Despite a huge number of case control studies looking at the pre-illness diet, further epidemiological evidence is necessary before associations between the diet and the aetiopathogenesis of IBD can be confirmed. Understanding how the gut environment, especially the microbiota, influences disease progression may help to unlock answers as to why (i) enteral nutrition can treat active Crohn's disease and (ii) probiotics and prebiotics are effective in the management of ulcerative colitis and pouchitis. Improvement in the palatability of enteral diets is necessary to improve patient compliance in patients that may benefit, particularly to treat malnutrition in IBD or for treatment for active Crohn's disease. Limiting fermentable substrates from the diet that are presented to the gastrointestinal tract (e.g. a diet low in FODMAPs) is a novel innovative dietary approach to help manage gastrointestinal symptoms that are functional in nature.

Key points

- New service standards recommend that all patients should have access to a dietitian for assessment and specialist advice.
- Newly diagnosed patients may be concerned that their disease has been triggered by diet. Patients should be informed that there is no strong evidence to link diet to the development of IBD. Relatives of people with IBD should be encouraged to follow public health recommendations regarding general healthy eating.
- Well patients with IBD should be encouraged to eat as wide a variety of foods as possible and should follow healthy eating guidelines. Foods should only be avoided if known to aggravate symptoms.
- Eating habits may be compromised for a number of reasons, delivering a suboptimal level of micronutrients. Nutritional supplements which can be prescribed may be helpful for malnourished patients and those with a restricted diet or a poor appetite. Loose bowel motions or diarrhoea can lead to fluid and electrolyte imbalances alongside poor calcium, magnesium and zinc status, all of which may need routine monitoring. Multivitamin/mineral supplementation may be necessary whether or not disease is active.
- In-patients with IBD should have a nutritional risk assessment carried out as standard according to local policy.
- Risk of osteoporosis: ensure patients have an adequate calcium intake (1000 mg/day). Calcium and vitamin D supplements may be required and should be prescribed if patient is taking corticosteroids.
- Enteral nutrition can be considered as a primary or adjunctive treatment for active Crohn's disease in patients who will comply.
- Use of probiotics and prebiotics may be helpful in ulcerative colitis and pouchitis and should be discussed with the clinical team.
- Recommend that patients join a support group, e.g. Crohn's and Colitis UK.

Patient translation: practical tips on healthy living related to diet and IBD

- At present, there is no good evidence to link diet to the cause of IBD.
- There is no standard correct diet for people with IBD, and individual symptoms will determine what can be eaten. Ask your healthcare team about seeing a dietitian.
- Eat as wide a variety of foods as possible to ensure your diet is nutritionally complete. Keep well hydrated, chew food thoroughly and take time over meals.
- Monitor your weight and inform your healthcare team if you are concerned that you are losing weight. If your appetite is poor eat small frequent meals and aim to have three small meals and three snacks per day.
- Commercially available food allergy and intolerance tests are not reliable for identifying problem foods in relation to gut symptoms. Avoidance of foods or food groups could limit nutritional adequacy. Seek professional advice from a dietitian before excluding foods thought to provoke symptoms.
- A liquid diet can be used to treat active Crohn's disease in some patients. Discuss your treatment options with your healthcare team.
- Probiotics and prebiotics may be helpful in the management of ulcerative colitis or pouchitis. Discuss further with your healthcare team.

References

Akobeng, A. K. and Thomas, A. G. (2007) Enteral nutrition for maintenance of remission in Crohn's disease (Review). *Cochrane Database Syst. Rev.*, **3**.

Ballegaard, M., Bjergstrom, A., Brondum, S., Hylander, E., Jensen, L. and Ladefoged, K. (1997) Self-reported food intolerance in chronic inflammatory bowel disease. *Scand. J. Gastroenterol.*, **32**, 569–71.

Bannerjee, K., Camacho-Hubner, C., Babinska, K., Dryhurst, K. M., Edwards, R., Savage, M. O., Sanderson, I. R. and Croft, N. M. (2004) Anti-inflammatory and growth-stimulating effects precede nutritional restitution during enteral feeding in Crohn's disease. *J. Pediatr. Gastroenterol. Nutr.*, **38**, 270–5.

Bannerman, E., Davidson, I., Conway, C., Culley, D., Aldhous, M. C. and Ghosh, S. (2001) Altered subjective appetite parameters in Crohn's disease patients. *Clin. Nutr.*, **20**, 399–405.

Barrett, J. S., Irving, P. M., Shepherd, S. J., Muir, J. G. and Gibson, P. R. (2009) Comparison of the prevalence of fructose and lactose malabsorption across chronic intestinal disorders. *Aliment. Pharmacol. Ther.*, **30**, 165–74.

Bernstein, C. N., Rawsthorne, P., Cheang, M. and Blanchard, J. F. (2006) A population-based case control study of potential risk factors for IBD. *Am. J. Gastroenterol.*, **101**, 993–1002.

Chapman-Kiddell, C. A., Davies, P. S., Gillen, L. and Radford-Smith, G. L. (2010) Role of diet in the development of inflammatory bowel disease. *Inflamm. Bowel Dis.*, **16**, 137–51.

Danese, S., Sans, M. and Fiocchi, C. (2004) Inflammatory bowel disease: the role of environmental factors. *Autoimmun. Rev.*, **3**, 394–400.

de Vrese, M and Schrezenmeir, J. (2008) Probiotics, prebiotics, and synbiotics. *Adv. Biochem. Eng. Biotechnol.*, **111**, 1–66.

Driscoll, R. H., Jr and Rosenberg, I. H. (1978) Total parenteral nutrition in inflammatory bowel disease. *Med. Clin. North Am.*, **62**, 185–201.

Fell, J. M., Paintin, M., Arnaud-Battandier, F., Beattie, R. M., Hollis, A., Kitching, P., Donnet-Hughes, A., MacDonald, T. T. and Walker-Smith, J. A. (2000) Mucosal healing and a fall in mucosal pro-inflammatory cytokine mRNA induced by a specific oral polymeric diet in paediatric Crohn's disease. *Aliment. Pharmacol. Ther.*, **14**, 281–9.

Gasche, C., Lomer, M. C., Cavill, I. and Weiss, G. (2004) Iron, anaemia, and inflammatory bowel diseases. *Gut*, **53**, 1190–7.

Gasche, C., Berstad, A., Befrits, R., Beglinger, C., Dignass, A., Erichsen, K., Gomollon, F., Hjortswang, H., Koutroubakis, I., Kulnigg, S., Oldenburg, B., Rampton, D., Schroeder, O., Stein, J., Travis, S. and Van, A. G. (2007) Guidelines on the diagnosis and management of iron deficiency and anemia in inflammatory bowel diseases. *Inflamm. Bowel Dis.*, **13**, 1545–53.

Gassull, M. A. (2004) Review article: the role of nutrition in the treatment of inflammatory bowel disease. *Aliment. Pharmacol. Ther.*, **20**(suppl. 4), 79–83.

Gassull, M. A. and Cabre, E. (2001) Nutrition in inflammatory bowel disease. *Curr. Opin. Clin. Nutr. Metab. Care*, **4**, 561–9.

Gearry, R. B., Irving, P. M., Barrett, J. S., Nathan, D. M., Shepherd, S. J. and Gibson, P. R. (2009) Reduction of dietary poorly absorbed short-chain carbohydrates (FODMAPs) improves abdominal symptoms in patients with inflammatory bowel disease. *J. Crohn's and Colitis*, **3**, 8–14.

Geerling, B. J., Badart-Smook, A., Stockbrugger, R. W. and Brummer, R. J. (1998) Comprehensive nutritional status in patients with long-standing Crohn's disease currently in remission. *Am. J. Clin. Nutr.*, **67**, 919–26.

Geerling, B. J., Stockbrugger, R. W. and Brummer, R. J. (1999) Nutrition and inflammatory bowel disease: an update. *Scand. J. Gastroenterol.,* **Suppl**. 230, 95–105.

Gibson, P. R. and Shepherd, S. J. (2005) Personal view: food for thought – western lifestyle and susceptibility to Crohn's disease. The FODMAP hypothesis. *Aliment. Pharmacol. Ther.*, **21**, 1399–409.

Hart, A. R., Luben, R., Olsen, A., Tjonneland, A., Linseisen, J., Nagel, G., Berglund, G., Lindgren, S., Grip, O., Key, T., Appleby, P., Bergmann, M. M., Boeing, H., Hallmans, G., Danielsson, A., Palmqvist, R., Sjodin, H., Hagglund, G., Overvad, K., Palli, D., Masala, G., Riboli, E., Kennedy, H., Welch, A., Khaw, K. T., Day, N. and Bingham, S. (2008) Diet in the aetiology of ulcerative colitis: a European prospective cohort study. *Digestion*, **77**, 57–64.

Hedin, C., Whelan, K. and Lindsay, J. O. (2007) Evidence for the use of probiotics and prebiotics in inflammatory bowel disease: a review of clinical trials. *Proc. Nutr. Soc.*, **66**, 307–15.

IBD Standards Working Group (2009) *Quality Care: Service Standards for the Healthcare of People Who Have Inflammatory Bowel Disease (IBD)*. http://www.ibdstandards.org.uk/uploaded_files/IBDstandards.pdf.

Isaacs, K. and Herfarth, H. (2008) Role of probiotic therapy in IBD. *Inflamm. Bowel Dis.*, **14**, 1597–605.

Jowett, S. L., Seal, C. J., Pearce, M. S., Phillips, E., Gregory, W., Barton, J. R. and Welfare, M. R. (2004) Influence of dietary factors on the clinical course of ulcerative colitis: a prospective cohort study. *Gut*, **53**, 1479–84.

Krok, K. L. and Lichtenstein, G. R. (2003) Nutrition in Crohn's disease. *Curr. Opin. Gastroenterol.*, **19**, 148–53.

Kulnigg, S. and Gasche, C. (2006) Systematic review: managing anaemia in Crohn's disease. *Aliment. Pharmacol. Ther.*, **24**, 1507–23.

Lewis, N. R. and Scott, B. B. (2010) *Guidelines for Osteoporosis in Inflammatory Bowel Disease and Coeliac Disease.* http://www.bsg.org.uk/clinical-guidelines/ibd/guidelines-for-osteoporosis-in-inflammatory-bowel-disease-and-coeliac-disease.html14-1-2010.

Lomer, M. C., Kodjabashia, K., Hutchinson, C., Greenfield, S. M., Thompson, R. P. and Powell, J. J. (2004) Intake of dietary iron is low in patients with Crohn's disease: a case-control study. *Br. J. Nutr.*, **91**, 141–8.

Lomer, M. C., Grainger, S. L., Ede, R., Catterall, A. P., Greenfield, S. M., Cowan, R. E., Vicary, F. R., Jenkins, A. P., Fidler, H., Harvey, R. S., Ellis, R., McNair, A., Ainley, C. C., Thompson, R. P. and Powell, J. J. (2005) Lack of efficacy of a reduced microparticle diet in a multi-centred trial of patients with active Crohn's disease. *Eur. J. Gastroenterol. Hepatol.*, **17**, 377–84.

Nguyen, G. C., Munsell, M. and Harris, M. L. (2008) Nationwide prevalence and prognostic significance of clinically diagnosable protein-calorie malnutrition in hospitalized inflammatory bowel disease patients. *Inflamm. Bowel Dis.*, **14**, 1105–11.

O'Sullivan, M. and O'Morain, C. (2006) Nutrition in inflammatory bowel disease. *Best. Pract. Res. Clin. Gastroenterol.*, **20**, 561–73.

Ostro, M. J., Greenberg, G. R. and Jeejeebhoy, K. N. (1985) Total parenteral nutrition and complete bowel rest in the management of Crohn's disease. *J. Parenter. Enteral Nutr.*, **9**, 280–7.

Pirlich, M., Schutz, T,, Kemps, M., Luhman, N., Burmester, G. R., Baumann, G., Plauth, M., Lubke, H. J. and Lochs, H. (2003) Prevalence of malnutrition in hospitalized medical patients: impact of underlying disease. *Dig. Dis.*, **21**, 245–51.

Porro, G. B. and Panza, E. (1985) Smoking, sugar, and inflammatory bowel disease. *Br. Med. J. (Clinical Research Edition)*, **291**, 971–2.

Raouf, A. H., Hildrey, V., Daniel, J., Walker, R. J., Krasner, N., Elias, E. and Rhodes, J. M. (1991) Enteral feeding as sole treatment for Crohn's disease: controlled trial of whole protein v amino acid based feed and a case study of dietary challenge. *Gut*, **32**, 702–7.

Reif, S., Klein, I., Lubin, F., Farbstein, M., Hallak, A. and Gilat, T. (1997) Pre-illness dietary factors in inflammatory bowel disease. *Gut*, **40**, 754–60.

Riordan, A. M., Hunter, J. O., Cowan, R. E., Crampton, J. R., Davidson, A. R., Dickinson, R. J., Dronfield, M. W., Fellows, I. W., Hishon, S. and Kerrigan, G. N. (1993) Treatment of active Crohn's disease by exclusion diet: East Anglian multicentre controlled trial. *Lancet*, **342**, 1131–4.

Rocchio, M. A., Cha, C. J., Haas, K. F. and Randall, H. T. (1974) Use of chemically defined diets in the management of patients with acute inflammatory bowel disease. *Am. J. Surg.*, **127**, 469–75.

Rodrigues, A. F., Johnson, T., Davies, P. and Murphy, M. S. (2007) Does polymeric formula improve adherence to liquid diet therapy in children with active Crohn's disease? *Arch. Dis. Child*, **92**, 767–70.

Sakamoto, N., Kono, S., Wakai, K., Fukuda, Y., Satomi, M., Shimoyama, T., Inaba, Y., Miyake, Y., Sasaki, S., Okamoto, K., Kobashi, G., Washio, M., Yokoyama, T., Date, C. and Tanaka, H. (2005) Dietary risk factors for inflammatory bowel disease: a multicenter case-control study in Japan. *Inflamm. Bowel Dis.*, **11**, 154–63.

Shoda, R., Matsueda, K., Yamato, S. and Umeda, N. (1996) Epidemiologic analysis of Crohn disease in Japan: increased dietary intake of n-6 polyunsaturated fatty acids and animal protein relates to the increased incidence of Crohn's disease in Japan. *Am. J. Clin. Nutr.*, **63**, 741–5.

Simren, M., Axelsson, J., Gillberg, R., Abrahamsson, H., Svedlund, J. and Bjornsson, E. S. (2002) Quality of life in inflammatory bowel disease in remission: the impact of IBS-like symptoms and associated psychological factors. *Am. J. Gastroenterol.*, **97**, 389–96.

Sousa, G. C., Cravo, M., Costa, A. R., Miranda, A., Tavares, L., Moura-Santos, P., Marquesvidal, P. and Nobre, L. C. (2007) A comprehensive approach to evaluate nutritional status in Crohn's patients in the era of biologic therapy: a case-control study. *Am. J. Gastroenterol.*, **102**, 2551–6.

Thornton, J. R., Emmett, P. M. and Heaton, K. W. (1979) Diet and Crohn's disease: characteristics of the pre-illness diet. *Br. Med. J.*, **2**, 762–4.

Tilg, H., Moschen, A.R., Kaser, A., Pines, A. and Dotan, I. (2008) Gut, inflammation and osteoporosis: basic and clinical concepts. *Gut*, **57**, 684–94.

Tragnone, A., Valpiani, D., Miglio, F., Elmi, G., Bazzocchi, G., Pipitone, E. and Lanfranchi, G. A. (1995) Dietary habits as risk factors for inflammatory bowel disease. *Eur. J. Gastroenterol. Hepatol.*, **7**, 47–51.

UK IBD Audit Steering Group. *IBD Audit 2006: National Results for the Organisation and Process of IBD Care in the UK.* http://www.rcplondon.ac.uk/clinical-standards/ceeu/Current-work/Documents/ceeu_uk_ibd_audit_2006.pdf14-1-2010.

UK IBD Audit Steering Group. *IBD Audit 2008: National Results for the Organisation and Process of IBD Care in the UK.* http://www.rcplondon.ac.uk/clinical-standards/ceeu/Current-work/Documents/UK-IBD-Audit-2nd-Round-Full-National-Report-Appendices.pdf14-1-2010.

Vagianos, K., Bector, S., McConnell, J. and Bernstein, C. N. (2007) Nutrition assessment of patients with inflammatory bowel disease. *J. Parenter. Enteral Nutr.*, **31**, 311–19.

Valentini, L., Schaper, L., Buning, C., Hengstermann, S., Koernicke, T., Tillinger, W., Guglielmi, F. W., Norman, K., Buhner, S., Ockenga, J., Pirlich, M. and Lochs, H. (2008) Malnutrition and impaired muscle strength in patients with Crohn's disease and ulcerative colitis in remission. *Nutrition*, **24**, 694–702.

Voitk, A. J., Echave, V., Feller, J. H., Brown, R. A., Gurd, F. N. (1973) Experience with elemental diet in the treatment of inflammatory bowel disease. Is this primary therapy? *Arch. Surg.*, **107**, 329–33.

Wilson, A., Reyes, E. and Ofman, J. (2004) Prevalence and outcomes of anemia in inflammatory bowel disease: a systematic review of the literature. *Am. J. Med.*, **116**(suppl. 7A), 44S–49S.

Woolner, J. T., Parker, T. J., Kirby, G. A. and Hunter, J. O. (1998) The development and evaluation of a diet for maintaining remission in Crohn's disease. *J. Hum. Nutr. Dietetics*, **11**, 1–11.

Zachos, M., Tondeur, M. and Griffiths, A. M. (2007) Enteral nutrition therapy for induction of remission in Crohn's disease (Review). *Cochrane Database of Systematic Reviews*, **1**.

CHAPTER 9

Surgical management

Sue Clark

Introduction

The surgical management of inflammatory bowel disease encompasses a variety of operations performed in elective and emergency settings for two similar, overlapping, but at times quite different diseases. Overall the principles of surgery are to remove the diseased area of bowel, minimise complications, retain gastrointestinal continuity if possible and achieve the best functional outcome for the patient.

Ulcerative colitis

Overall about 30% of patients with ulcerative colitis eventually come to surgery. For many of these, emergency surgery is required for acute colitis. In ulcerative colitis, surgery to remove the large bowel can cure the disease, as the entire affected area can be removed.

Emergency surgery for ulcerative colitis

Indications

The advent of intravenous steroids, and more recently ciclosporin and infliximab, has greatly improved the outlook in acute severe colitis. However, in some patients

> ### Case study (part 1)
> A 21-year-old woman presented with rapid onset of malaise and diarrhoea. She was referred to a gastroenterologist who diagnosed ulcerative colitis and treated her with oral steroids. Her symptoms rapidly resolved. She was started on mesalazine and weaned off her steroids.

> Six months later the symptoms recurred; she continued to deteriorate despite re-starting oral steroids. She was admitted to hospital for intravenous steroids. Stool cultures were negative and there was no evidence of CMV on biopsies from flexible sigmoidoscopy. She continued to worsen and after three days was started on intravenous ciclosporin. She continued to open her bowels 15 times per 24 hours, and her inflammatory markers remained raised. Plain abdominal X-ray showed a transverse colon dilated to 8 cm with thickened mucosa. At that point the decision was made by the team that she needed surgery, and a subtotal colectomy with formation of end ileostomy was performed.

these treatments fail and surgery is required. Surgery is indicated in the following circumstances:

1. Toxic megacolon
By definition, this is present in any patient with evidence of systemic sepsis (tachycardia, pyrexia, hypotension, raised white cell count) and a colon dilated beyond 5.5 cm.

2. Non-response to medical therapy
Prior to the introduction of ciclosporin it was accepted that surgery should be undertaken if there was no improvement in acute colitis after 3–5 days of intravenous steroids. Now ciclosporin is generally added at that point, and patients on this treatment pathway need to be very closely monitored and surgery undertaken if they fail to respond.

3. Incomplete response to medical therapy
A number of patients respond to some extent to intravenous steroids and/or ciclosporin, but do not improve sufficiently to be able to leave hospital. Whilst surgery in this group is less urgent, it is often required.

Inpatients being treated for acute colitis should be managed by a multidisciplinary team including a consultant gastroenterologist, consultant colorectal surgeon and specialist nurses. Clinical monitoring of vital signs and fluid balance, and regular imaging of the large bowel to assess for dilatation, are essential. High-dose intravenous steroids can mask the signs of systemic deterioration and peritonitis. Assessment of whether medical treatment is succeeding or not can be difficult and contentious, meaning that the decision-making around timing of surgery is complex.

It is important that clear plans are made and discussed with the patient and that medical therapy is not carried on too for long if it is not working. Early involvement of the entire team and good communication with the patient and family give time for the patient to become mentally and emotionally prepared for the possibility of surgery and ensure that they can be fully counselled.

Pre-operative preparation

Any patient in hospital with acute severe colitis should be prepared for the possibility of surgery. Fluid and electrolyte balance should be carefully maintained with particular attention to potassium and magnesium levels, which often fall because of high losses in diarrhoea. Some patients become anaemic because of loss of blood in the faeces and should be adequately transfused prior to surgery. These patients are also at increased risk of thromboembolic disease and should have prophylactic low molecular weight heparin and graduated compression stockings. The fact that there is significant blood loss in the faeces is not a contra-indication to prophylactic heparin, as the risk of thromboembolism is considerably raised in active IBD and outweighs the increase in bleeding caused by this level of anticoagulation.

Most patients having emergency surgery for ulcerative colitis will require a temporary ileostomy. Early referral to a stoma nurse for counselling ensures that they have adequate time to absorb information about this potentially distressing facet of the surgery. An optimum site for the ileostomy should be marked.

Bowel preparation is not required, and in the context of severe acute colitis may be harmful and should not be given.

Surgery

The standard operative procedure under the circumstances of acute severe colitis is a subtotal colectomy. This is usually performed through a midline incision but increasingly now is being performed laparoscopically. The benefit of a laparoscopic approach is that small 'port site' wounds replace the long midline wound needed for open surgery. This reduces the physiological trauma experienced, and decreases analgesic requirements, speeding up recovery. In the longer term the lack of a substantial wound reduces the future risk of incisional hernia and wound-related adhesions. The drawback is that this is a technically challenging procedure and requires an experienced laparoscopic colorectal surgeon to perform it, together with substantially longer theatre time than an open procedure. Suitable facilities and expertise are by no means universally available in the UK, particularly in an emergency setting.

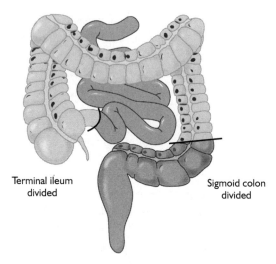

Terminal ileum divided

Sigmoid colon divided

Figure 9.1 Subtotal colectomy and ileostomy.

The operation is illustrated in Figure 9.1 The terminal ileum is divided just before it joins the caecum, and the entire large bowel down to the distal part of the sigmoid colon is removed. The end of the terminal ileum is brought out to form an end ileostomy, usually in the right iliac fossa. The divided distal end of the bowel can be managed in several ways (Figure 9.2). The simplest is to close it off using staples or sutures or a combination of the two. Some surgeons simply leave the closed-off end of the bowel in the abdomen. Others fix this piece of the bowel underneath the midline incision so that its location is known and if the staple

(a) Closed off in abdomen

(b) Closed and fixed deep to abdominal wound

(c) Mucus fistula

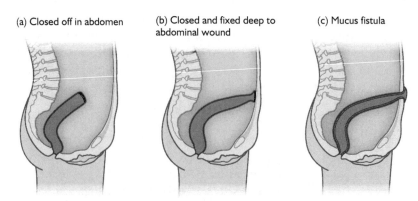

Figure 9.2 Management of the rectum after subtotal colectomy.

162

line breaks down any discharge will pass out through the wound rather than into the abdomen. If this part of the bowel is very diseased, with a high likelihood of 'stump blow out', a mucus fistula can be formed, sited in the left iliac fossa or the lower end of the wound itself. This is effectively a small colostomy, which allows rectum and distal sigmoid colon to vent out via the abdominal wall.

Complications

Complications related to abdominal surgery are listed in Table 9.1 and are subdivided into those that occur early or late. Specific complications related to subtotal colectomy are discussed below. Patients are often debilitated by their disease and immunosuppressed by medical therapy, increasing these risks.

Table 9.1 Complications of abdominal surgery.

Early complications	Thromboembolism
	Chest infection
	Urinary tract infection
	Wound infection
	Prolonged ileus
Late complications	Incisional hernia
	Adhesion obstruction

Specific complications of subtotal colectomy
- *Rectal stump blow out*
  So called 'rectal stump blow out' is a specific early complication that occurs when a combination of build-up of secretions within the retained sigmoid colon and rectum and inflammation of the sealed-off end results in this perforating and the contents of the rectum passing into the abdominal cavity. This results in severe acute sepsis. It can be avoided by either placing a drain in the rectum to allow the secretions to escape or forming a mucus fistula at the operation.
- *Proctitis*
  Later, proctitis in the remaining rectosigmoid segment can be a troublesome problem. Ulcerative colitis is a disease that affects the large bowel continuously from the rectum proximally. Therefore the remaining large bowel after a subtotal colectomy is still affected by the disease. In addition much of the nutrition of the lining of the bowel comes from material in the faeces. Following subtotal colectomy with a formation of ileostomy, faeces

no longer pass through the rectum, which may become inflamed as a result (diversion proctitis). A combination of ongoing ulcerative colitis in the rectum (ulcerative proctitis) and diversion proctitis can result in some patients passing bloody mucus or pus and even having a generalised systemic illness as a result. This can be treated with 5-amino-salicylate suppositories or steroid suppositories, often with some success. Sometimes, however, the symptoms are severe enough that the rectum eventually needs to be removed.

■ *Dysplasia and cancer*
There is an increased incidence of cancer in the colon and rectum in ulcerative colitis, probably due to chronic inflammation. This risk remains in the rectum even though the colon has been removed. It is therefore important either to remove the rectum or monitor it very carefully using endoscopy. This can prove difficult, as ongoing proctitis means that patients frequently pass blood and do not notice any new symptoms, and when an endoscope is inserted into the rectum good views often cannot be obtained.

■ *Ileostomy-related complications*
Later the ileostomy can prolapse, retract or become associated with a parastomal hernia.

Post-operative care

Patients should be aware that on return to the ward they will have an intravenous infusion and a urinary catheter. Many will have an epidural for pain relief for the first for 48 hours or so. Sometimes a nasogastric tube and abdominal drain may also be used. There will be a newly fashioned ileostomy.

The rate of recovery is really determined by the speed of return of gut function. It is now known that allowing oral intake can stimulate this and therefore drinks and then food should be reintroduced as quickly as possible. However, some patients may have a prolonged ileus, particularly if they have been unwell, and the speed of introduction of oral intake needs to be assessed on a case-by-case basis. Patients should be mobilised as soon as possible.

Most will have been on intravenous steroids and will require this to be continued in the immediate post-operative period. Such patients will then need to be discharged on a decreasing dose to wean them off the steroids altogether. If steroids are stopped suddenly or reduced too quickly, the combination of the stress of surgery and adrenal suppression can result in an Addisonian crisis.

Input from the stoma nurses (as outlined in Chapter 11) will be required from the beginning to familiarise the patient with their ileostomy and how to care for it. Some may have a high stoma output initially and need Loperamide or codeine phosphate to help thicken up the effluent. Most patients remain in hospital for around seven days following this type of surgery.

The longer term

Many of these patients, once recovered will go on to have their rectum removed and an ileoanal pouch formed (as described below) to allow them to be rid of their ileostomy. Before this operation was available some patients underwent an ileorectal anastomosis once recovered, in which the ileum is joined onto the distal sigmoid colon or proximal rectum. This has considerable disadvantages, in that the rectum often develops worsening inflammation, resulting in poor function. In addition, the rectum remains at risk of cancer. In some circumstances, however, this operation is occasionally still done, but it is something of a compromise.

Some patients have little in the way of symptoms from their rectum and are content to remain as they are. So long as the rectum can be adequately examined by flexible sigmoidoscopy so that the risk of developing cancer is minimised, there is no reason that they should not be able to remain as they are with no further surgery.

Elective surgery for ulcerative colitis

Indications

Patients with ulcerative colitis require elective surgery under three circumstances: failure of medical treatment, development of dysplasia or cancer, or to remove the remaining rectum after emergency subtotal colectomy.

Failed medical therapy

Some patients are managed as an outpatient but go through the whole range of drug treatment for ulcerative colitis without achieving satisfactory control. Others may have their disease controlled by steroids, but despite the use of other immunosuppressants relapse whenever steroids are withdrawn. Long-term high-dose steroids cause significant complications, including osteoporosis, hypertension, peptic ulceration, weight gain, diabetes, skin thinning, cataracts, immunosuppression and adrenal suppression. Both of these groups of patients eventually come to surgery. There is great individual variation with regard to how long patients go on, on various medical therapies, before this point is reached.

Dysplasia or cancer

Long-standing ulcerative colitis results in an increased risk of dysplasia (precancerous change) and cancer in the colon and rectum. This risk starts to rise from

165

about ten years after the diagnosis of disease. It is for this reason that patients with long-standing ulcerative colitis undergo regular colonic surveillance. If an area of dysplasia or cancer is found there is a very high risk of abnormality elsewhere and it is therefore important that the entire colon and rectum are removed.

Case study (part 2)

The woman presented earlier in the chapter made an excellent recovery from her surgery, and at follow-up three months post-operatively was off all medication, and had just got engaged. She was experiencing troublesome discharge of bloody mucous from the anus, and rigid sigmoidoscopy showed that her rectum was inflamed. She had a long discussion with her nurse specialist and surgeon about further surgery to remove her rectum and restore intestinal continuity with an ileoanal pouch. She was started on mesalazine suppositories.

Two months later she returned to the clinic, her anal discharge much improved. She had decided to defer further surgery until she had completed her family, because of concerns about the effect of pelvic surgery on her fertility. She was followed up annually, and six years later (having had two children) underwent restorative proctectomy with formation of an ileoanal pouch.

Surgical options

Removal of the entire colon and rectum cures ulcerative colitis. Even if only the distal part of the colon is affected, when a patient reaches a point where surgery is required the entire large bowel should be removed, as there is good evidence that if any is left behind it is very likely to develop ulcerative colitis later. In the case of cancer or dysplasia, there is a high risk of any remaining large bowel becoming affected in future, so generally it is recommended that the entire large bowel is removed under these circumstances too. Increasingly this surgery is being performed laparoscopically.

Total proctocolectomy

In this procedure the entire colon, rectum and anus are removed. The skin is closed at the site where the anus has been excised, leaving a scar. A permanent end ileostomy is formed. Prior to the advent of the ileoanal pouch in the late 1970s this was the 'gold standard' procedure for ulcerative colitis. The advantage is that all the diseased (or potentially diseased) bowel is removed. There are no surgical anastomoses, so that there is no risk associated with anastomotic leak. The major drawback is that a permanent ileostomy is formed.

Total colectomy and ileorectal anastomosis

This procedure is rarely now performed. The colon is removed but the rectum remains. The small bowel is joined directly onto the rectum. Ongoing inflammation can result in poor function in many patients and a risk of rectal cancer remains.

Kock continent ileostomy (Kock pouch)

Before the advent of the ileoanal pouch (see below) there was considerable interest in this procedure, which used small bowel as a faecal reservoir just inside the ileostomy, with a special configuration which has a valve effect, so that the ileostomy is continent (Figure 9.3). The faeces are emptied on a regular basis by

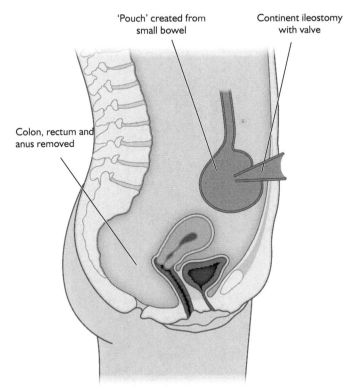

'Pouch' created from
small bowel

Continent ileostomy
with valve

Colon, rectum and
anus removed

Figure 9.3 Kock pouch.

the patient using a soft catheter to intubate the ileostomy. This improves lifestyle for many patients, as they do not need to wear a standard stoma appliance, and they can control where and when they evacuate, but the procedure is fraught with complications and often requires revision. It is now rarely performed.

Restorative proctocolectomy (ileoanal pouch)

This is now the 'gold standard' procedure for ulcerative colitis. The whole of the colon and rectum is removed and a new faecal reservoir formed of small bowel, which is anastomosed to the anus (Figure 9.4). Ultimately this has the advantages

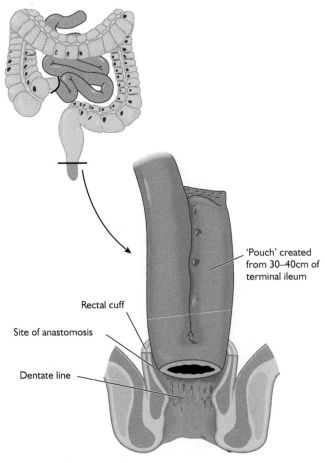

'Pouch' created from 30–40cm of terminal ileum

Rectal cuff

Site of anastomosis

Dentate line

Figure 9.4 Restorative proctocolectomy.

of removing almost the entire large bowel and also resulting in intestinal continuity. The procedure can be performed in one, two or three stages.

■ *One-stage procedure*
The colon and rectum are removed. The ileoanal pouch is formed and attached inside the anus. A drain is usually placed within it to reduce the risk of anastomotic leakage.

■ *Two-stage procedure*
Because formation of the ileoanal pouch results in creation of quite long suture lines, and any resulting leakage can cause severe pelvic sepsis and ultimately poor pouch function, the majority of surgeons defunction the newly created pouch for a period of approximately three months to allow all of the joins to heal before the pouch is put into use. In the two-stage procedure the first stage of the operation comprises removal of the colon and rectum, formation of the ileoanal pouch and attachment of this to the anus and then formation of a defunctioning loop ileostomy proximal to the pouch. The second stage of the procedure is closure of the ileostomy.

■ *Three-stage procedure*
Many patients who have ileoanal pouch formation have already undergone an emergency subtotal colectomy as described above under emergency surgery. This is the first of the three stages. In the second stage the remaining rectum is removed and the ileoanal pouch formed and attached to the anus. A defunctioning loop ileostomy is formed to protect the pouch and pouch anal anastomosis. The third stage of the procedure is closure of the ileostomy. This is a much more straightforward procedure which does not require the abdomen to be opened. A cut is simply made around the ileostomy to free it up and the bowel is joined and placed back inside the abdomen. The small resulting wound is closed.

Some patients who have not had emergency surgery undergo a three-stage procedure. Reasons for this approach might be a patient who is on high-dose oral steroids where there is concern about healing. A subtotal colectomy can be performed and then the patient weaned off steroids prior to completion proctectomy (removal of the remaining rectum) and formation of the ileoanal pouch. In some patients it is not entirely clear whether they have Crohn's colitis or ulcerative colitis. Removal of the colon allows the pathologist to have a very large specimen to study, which may clarify the diagnosis. For further information on pouch care, refer to Chapter 10.

Pre-operative preparation

In the elective setting it is important that all of the surgical options are fully discussed with the patient so that they can make an informed decision about what surgery they would like to have. Ideally this should also include contact with a patient support group, such as the Red Lion Group (see list of support groups on p. 185) and specialist nurses who can often put the patient in touch with others who have been through the same illness.

It is important that the patients understand that the medical part of the surgery is removal of the large bowel. The formation of an ileoanal pouch has no medical purpose. Its only advantage is to avoid a permanent ileostomy. Whilst ileoanal pouch function can be extremely good, on average one would expect the patient to open their bowels about five times a day and once at night and have some occasional slight soiling. Some patients may have problems with pouchitis and in a few pelvic sepsis is a major complication. Ultimately about 10–15% of pouches will have failed after 15 years for a variety of reasons, resulting in a permanent end ileostomy. Many patients in whom this happens will have been through a period of quite severe ill health as a result.

Many patients are happy to accept the possibility of pouch failure and potentially poor function in an attempt to avoid an ileostomy, but for others an ileostomy is acceptable and they would prefer not to expose themselves to the more complex procedure of pouch surgery. All of these issues need to be thoroughly discussed and the patient comfortable with their decision before surgery goes ahead.

In many units patients undergo a pre-admission visit for the pre-operative blood samples to be taken and are admitted either the day before or on the morning of surgery itself. It is important that an ileostomy site is marked. If a patient has already had a subtotal colectomy, and has an end ileostomy, usually the same site can be used. Pre-operative thrombo prophylaxis should be given. There is no need for formal bowel preparation, although in those with an intact colon and rectum many surgeons use a phosphate enema.

Complications

General complications of surgery and ileostomies have already been described in the section on emergency surgery.

Removal of the rectum (proctectomy) carries additional specific risks. The nerve supply to the bladder and penis can be damaged during the dissection, resulting in erectile or ejaculatory dysfunction in 2–5% of men, and in impaired bladder function. In women fertility is approximately halved, probably due to formation of adhesions around the Fallopian tubes. Young women who have had subtotal colectomy may wish to postpone removal of the rectum and creation of an ileoanal pouch until after they have completed their family for this reason, though others are prepared to accept this risk in order to be rid of their ileostomy.

Any surgery involving the creation of joins between pieces of bowel (formation of Kock or ileoanal pouch, connection of ileal pouch to anus, ileorectal anastomosis, and closure of ileostomy) carries the risk of leakage, which can cause severe peritonitis if not detected promptly, and often requires further surgery.

Post-operative care

Patients need to be aware that after the operation they will have an intravenous infusion and a urinary catheter. Many will have an epidural for analgesia otherwise a patient controlled analgesia is usually used. There will be an ileostomy (unless a single stage procedure has been done) and there may be a drain in the pelvis or pouch.

The management for a subtotal colectomy has already been described under emergency surgery. If a total proctocolectomy has been performed the patient will have a perineal wound and should avoid prolonged sitting for the first week or so following surgery. All patients with a stoma will need to be seen by a stoma nurse. This is necessary even if the patient previously had an end ileostomy and now has a loop ileostomy defunctioning a pouch, as this will be in a different configuration and they may well need a different type of appliance.

The principles of enhanced recovery are increasingly being used, the rationale being that a combination of modifications to surgery and post-operative care will contribute to rapid recovery and shorter hospital stay. These include avoidance of bowel preparation and pelvic drainage, early introduction of oral intake and mobilisation, and minimising the use of intravenous fluids and analgesics (which are thought to delay the return of gut function).

Patients after ileostomy closure or who have had a one-stage pouch formed often find that they have urgency and even frank incontinence for the first few days once the pouch starts to work. Many find this very distressing indeed and require considerable support and reassurance that they will regain their adequate bowel function quickly.

Crohn's disease

In contrast to ulcerative colitis, the majority of patients (80%) require surgery at some point and many patients require repeated operations for Crohn's disease. Only about 10% of surgery for Crohn's disease is done as an emergency, the rest being elective.

Intestinal Crohn's disease

Small bowel Crohn's disease

Crohn's disease affects the bowel either by stricturing (narrowing) or by fistulation, where deep ulcers perforate the bowel resulting in intra-abdominal abscesses, sepsis and fistulation to the skin or other areas of bowel.

As with ulcerative colitis, medical therapies have become increasingly complex and successful in Crohn's disease. However, stricturing or fistulating disease, resulting in either obstructive symptoms or sepsis, usually requires surgical management. The surgical management of Crohn's disease aims to be conservative, meaning that as little bowel as possible is removed, given that Crohn's disease recurs at another site in the bowel over time after surgery.

Colonic Crohn's disease

Colonic Crohn's disease generally behaves in a similar way to ulcerative colitis but is often confined to one part only of the large bowel. It can be more extensive, however, and can result in acute colitis indistinguishable from ulcerative colitis. In these circumstances it is managed in exactly the same way with a subtotal colectomy.

Pre-operative preparation

Because of the 'skip lesions' in Crohn's disease, and the fact that it can affect any part of the bowel, it is important that the entire gastrointestinal tract is assessed prior to surgery. Usually this will involve a barium follow-through and a colonoscopy.

If at all possible the patient's nutritional status should be optimised. In some cases, particularly in patients with stricturing disease who are chronically malnourished, this may involve oral nutritional supplementation or even admission for intravenous nutrition for a few weeks prior to surgery. For fistulating disease it may be advantageous to drain any abscesses percutaneously to try to control sepsis prior to surgery.

As with ulcerative colitis these patients are at increased risk of thromboembolic disease and should have appropriate prophylaxis.

Preparation for the risks

One of the main risks in bowel surgery is that of anastomotic leakage. This is increased in patients who have been on steroids or who are malnourished or septic. Even if the intention is to remove a piece of diseased bowel and perform an anastomosis, patients should be warned that an ileostomy might be required and be counselled and marked appropriately.

No bowel preparation is required for small bowel surgery or right-sided colonic surgery, and in most cases an enema is sufficient for surgery involving the left side of the colon. There remain some circumstances in which bowel preparation might be required.

Surgery

Traditionally surgery was done through a midline laparotomy or transverse incision, but it is increasingly being performed laparoscopically to reduce surgical trauma and pain, speed up recovery and minimise wound-related complications.

The principle of surgery is to remove the diseased area and perform an anastomosis if this is considered safe. The commonest site of Crohn's disease is the terminal ileum, so the most common operation is removal of the terminal ileum and caecum (ileocaecectomy) with formation of an ileocolic anastomosis. Disease more proximally in the small bowel is managed by small bowel resection and anastomosis.

There is evidence that the time to recurrence of Crohn's and further surgery is increased if a side-to-side anastomosis is performed, presumably because the wide anastomosis takes much longer to re-stenose down compared with a narrower end-to-end anastomosis. This type of anastomosis is usually made with staples, although it can be performed hand sewn (Figure 9.5).

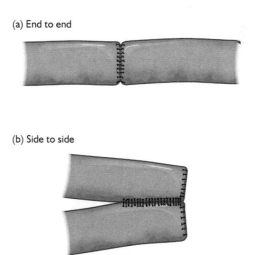

(a) End to end

(b) Side to side

Figure 9.5 Types of anastomosis.

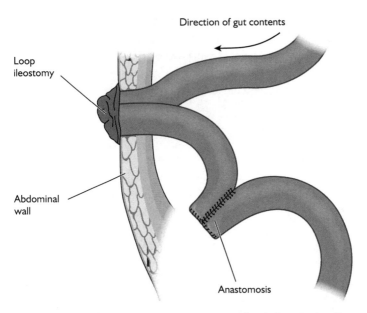

Figure 9.6 Anastomosis protected by defunctioning ileostomy.

If an anastomosis is not thought to be safe the options are to create an end ileostomy and close the distal end of the bowel (or create a mucous fistula) and perform an anastomosis at a later date, once the patient has recovered form sepsis and malnutrition, or to create an anastomosis, but protect it with an upstream defunctioning ileostomy (Figure 9.6).

Stricturoplasty
Repeated bowel resections can result in insufficient small bowel remaining leading to problems with nutrition, therefore rather than removing strictured bowel a stricturoplasty is sometimes performed instead. This is effectively a plastic surgical procedure in which narrowed areas are made wider.

Colonic Crohn's disease
In contrast to the situation in ulcerative colitis, if only a part of the large bowel is affected with Crohn's it is perfectly reasonable simply to remove this part (segmental colectomy). It may be that further Crohn's will develop in future, but this is not necessarily the case. The principle is similar to small bowel surgery in that the affected area is removed and an anastomosis performed if it is safe

to do so. If an anastomosis is considered unsafe either one can be formed and defunctioned with a temporary loop ileostomy or an end colostomy can be brought out and a further operation can be performed to rejoin the bowel at a future date if so desired.

Once the patient has recovered following a subtotal colectomy, an ileorectal anastomosis can produce a good result for the patient, provided the rectum is free of Crohn's disease.

Restorative proctocolectomy in Crohn's disease

In patients with Crohn's affecting the colon and rectum restorative proctocolectomy, as performed in ulcerative colitis, is in theory an attractive option. However, the pouch failure rate following this is very much higher, probably in excess of 50%. It is therefore very contentious whether it is ever justified to perform restorative proctocolectomy in Crohn's disease. It is important that if it is being contemplated an experienced pouch surgeon is involved and that the patient is fully aware of the very high chances of failure. This option should only be considered if there is no evidence of any small bowel Crohn's disease or perianal disease.

Complications

The complications of intestinal surgery in Crohn's disease are essentially the same as those for surgery in ulcerative colitis. There is the additional issue that these patients may face repeated surgery throughout their lifetime, in contrast to ulcerative colitis, where surgery effectively cures the disease.

Each subsequent operation is likely to be more difficult than the last because of adhesion formation and distorted anatomy, with an associated risk of accidental bowel injury and fistulation through the abdominal wound. Repeated small bowel resection can eventually leave insufficient bowel remaining, resulting in diarrhoea, dehydration and malnutrition (short bowel syndrome); refer to Chapter 12 on Intestinal failure.

Post-operative management

There is evidence that restarting medical therapy for Crohn's disease early can prevent or delay recurrence after surgery, so gastroenterologists should be involved in the immediate post-operative period. If the patient is a smoker they should be very strongly encouraged to give up and be offered help in doing so, as smoking is a potent risk factor for recurrent Crohn's disease.

Perianal Crohn's disease

A significant proportion of patients with Crohn's disease develop perianal sepsis and a fistula-in-ano. Some of these may have active Crohn's disease in the rectum immediately adjacent, but many do not. Most of them will actually have small bowel Crohn's disease.

The aetiology of perianal Crohn's disease is unclear. Patients commonly develop anal fissures, large oedematous anal skin tags and perianal abscesses, which form fistulae once they discharge out through the skin or are surgically drained

The principles of treatment

The first priority is to drain sepsis, by incision and drainage of abscesses. Next the underlying fistula needs to be controlled, to prevent recurrent abscess formation. This is usually done by insertion of a seton (Figure 9.7), which holds the fistula open, allowing drainage.

If Crohn's disease remains active fistulae are likely to recur and any attempts at definitive treatment are very likely to fail. The entire gastrointestinal tract needs to be assessed for the site and activity of Crohn's disease and appropriate treatment

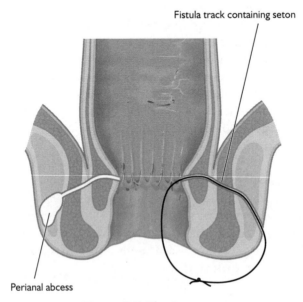

Fistula track containing seton

Perianal abcess

Figure 9.7 Fistula-in-ano.

given to control it. If medical treatment fails surgery may be necessary. Only then can definitive treatment be considered for the fistula.

Definitive treatment of fistulae

The main difficulty with treating anal fistulae is that laying them open whilst curing the fistula can cause impaired continence because it involves dividing the anal sphincter muscles to some extent (see Figure 9.7). Low fistulae can usually be treated with lay open with only a small risk of incontinence to flatus and slight mucus leakage. However, the higher a fistula is the more chance there is of jeopardising continence.

A range of surgical options exist to try to close fistulae, including advancement flaps (where the fistula is cored out and the internal opening closed using a full thickness rectal flap) and fistula plugs (which are fibrin-based plugs designed to close the fistula and encourage tissue ingrowth and healing). Unfortunately the success rates of the procedures are very variable, with probably in the region of 25–50% being realistic.

It has been shown that infliximab treatment can result in healing in conjunction with adequate surgical drainage. This option requires full involvement of the MDT.

In some cases of fistulae associated with severe proctitis, proctectomy and formation of permanent colostomy is needed if the disease cannot be controlled.

Conclusion

The relationship between medical and surgical management of inflammatory bowel disease is becoming increasingly complex. This is particularly the case in the situation of the acute colitic that is being medically treated but may require emergency surgery, and in the management of perianal Crohn's where surgical drainage and the use of new biological agents go hand in hand. It is essential that appropriately experienced specialists manage these patients in a multidisciplinary setting, and that the patients are well informed and have access to appropriate support.

Patient translation summary

Sometimes emergency surgery for IBD is unavoidable, and it is important for a surgeon to be involved closely in the care of inpatient with severe ulcerative colitis or Crohn's disease. An ileostomy is often required in large bowel surgery, but is usually temporary. There are a number of surgical options

> available, and it is crucial to consider carefully how each impacts on lifestyle factors important to the individual – such as body image, work and sports requirements, sexual functioning and family planning. The management of perianal Crohn's often involves a combination of surgery and drugs such as infliximab. It is important that a surgeon and gastroenterologist are both closely involved in delivering care.

Further reading and supporting evidence

Brown, S., Haboubi, N., Hampton. J. *et al.* (2008) The management of acute severe colitis: ACPGBI position statement. *Colorectal Dis.*, **10**(suppl. 3), 8–29.

Carter, M. J., Lobo, A. J., Travis, S. P.; IBD Section, British Society of Gastroenterology (2004) Guidelines for the management of inflammatory bowel disease in adults. *Gut*; **53**(suppl. V), v1–v6.

Cohen, J. L., Strong, S. A., Hyman, N. H. *et al.* (2005) Practice parameters for the surgical treatment of ulcerative colitis. *Dis. Colon Rectum*, **48**, 1997–2009.

Sandborn, W. J., Fazio, V. W., Feagan, B. G. and Hanauer, S. B. (American Gastroenterology Association Clinical Practice Committee) (2003) AGA technical review on perianal Crohn's disease. *Gastroenterology*, **125**, 1508–30.

Stange, E. F. and Travis, S. P. for the European Crohn's and Colitis Organisation (ECCO) (2008) European evidence-based consensus on the diagnosis and management of ulcerative colitis. *J. Crohn's Colitis*, **2**, 63–92.

Strong, S. A., Koltun, W. A., Hyman, N. H. *et al.* (2007) Practice parameters for the surgical treatment of Crohn's disease. *Dis. Colon Rectum*, **50**, 1735–46.

CHAPTER 10

Ileoanal pouch care

Zarah L. Perry-Woodford and Simon D. McLaughlin

Introduction

Ulcerative colitis (UC) is a chronic relapsing condition. The majority of patients respond to medical treatment; however, large studies performed in the 1980s and 1990s suggest that about one-third of patients will eventually require surgery (Langholz *et al.*, 1992; Hendriksen *et al.*, 1985). Whilst it is possible that increased use of immunosuppressant medication and novel drugs may have reduced the need for surgery, there is currently no good evidence that this is the case.

In the last 100 years there have been considerable advances in surgical treatment of ulcerative colitis. In 1913, Brown used a loop ileostomy to defunction the large bowel. However, this did not slow the disease spread and had a high mortality rate (Zelas and Jagleman, 1980). By 1920, ileorectal bypasses were introduced, but these still presented with a high mortality rate (Lacey, 1982). Miller and Canadian colleagues treated UC patients by resection of the colon with an ileostomy in the 1940s with no mortality noted in the 24 patients. However, complications with the stoma were disproportionate (Miller *et al.*, 1949). It was not until 1952 that Brooke used a conventional proctocolectomy and developed the everted spout ileostomy in order to manage some of the complications of the ileostomy (Brooke, 1952). Even though this was a successful procedure many surgeons and some patients did not like the idea of a permanent ileostomy. Kock (1969) reported the use of an ileal reservoir as a means of a continent ileostomy. The Kock pouch is rarely created now due to problematic valves resulting in long-term pouch dysfunction. During the period from 1970 to 1976 Sir Alan Parks combined the advantages of previous surgical developments to create the modern restorative proctocolectomy (RPC) and in 1978 Professor John Nicholls joined forces to perfect the RPC with the ileoanal pouch as we know it today, avoiding the need for a permanent ileostomy (Parks *et al.*, 1980).

RPC can offer patients an excellent quality of life while avoiding much of the physiological and psychological implications that permanent ileostomy may incur (Persson *et al.*, 2005). RPC is associated with an excellent functional outcome, but it does not provide normal bowel function. In addition there is a high morbidity from complications (Bengtsson *et al.*, 2007). In this chapter we aim to provide an overview of the ileoanal pouch operation, portraying normal pouch function and the methods involved in diagnosing and treating pouch dysfunction. The pre- and post-surgical nursing management which is vital for holistic patient care will be discussed. A case study has been used to integrate medical theory and nursing practice.

Case study

Mr Patel aged 43 is an accountant and works in a busy London firm. He lives with his wife, three young children and elderly father. Following failed medical treatment for UC he opted for an ileoanal pouch. He has adapted well to his pouch and his stool frequency is approximately six times in a 24 hour period, with one evacuation overnight. He can defer evacuation for up to an hour. He is a pescetarian (a vegetarian who consumes fish). In the last month he has felt tired and his pouch frequency has doubled. He has not noticed any blood in his stool, but he has increased urgency. There has been one episode of nocturnal leakage, which he had not previously experienced. He has increased stress at work and is undertaking more overtime, to which he attributes his erratic pouch function. He describes his symptoms as resembling those of UC. History taking and investigation with flexible pouchoscopy confirms the clinical diagnosis of pouchitis and he is treated with four weeks of antibiotic therapy and his pouch function returns to normal. He is followed up in the outpatient clinic.

RPC with ileo pouch anal anastomosis

RPC is an elective procedure. Depending on local surgical practice RPC may require one or two operations. Caution must be taken if performing a one-stage pouch, as a discrepancy between initial and final diagnosis may occur. Lucarotti *et al.* (1995) report that 3 of 19 patients had their diagnosis of UC revised to Crohn's disease following a one stage RPC. This data suggests that caution should be exercised in performing synchronous proctocolectomy with the formation of an ileoanal pouch.

RPC is most commonly performed in two stages. The first stage involves a total colectomy, formation of the ileoanal pouch and a defunctioning loop ileostomy. A gastrografin enema (an X-ray contrast study sometimes referred to as a pouchogram) may be organised to exclude an anastomotic leak before the stoma is closed. The patient then returns in approximately three months to close the ileostomy.

The ileoanal pouch is formed from 30–60 cm of terminal ileum, which usually absorbs bile acids and vitamin B_{12}. Most patients will have stores of vitamin B_{12} which can last up to 10 years. However, if pouch patients are found to have low vitamin B_{12} levels on annual blood screening, they should be referred to their GP for three-monthly supplementary injections (McLaughlin *et al.*, 2008). People with an ileoanal pouch open their bowels between 3 and 8 times a day, passing on average 600–800 g of stool. Acutely unwell patients require a conventional subtotal colectomy and temporary ileostomy primarily. RPC is then performed once corticosteroids or immunosuppressive medications have been withdrawn and the patient has recovered fully from the initial operation.

Laparoscopic surgery

RPC is performed laparoscopically in some surgical units. The technique was first described in the early 1990s and has grown in acceptance. Patients usually prefer the superior cosmetic result of a laparoscopic compared to an open surgical approach. The short-term advantages of laparoscopic RPC appear to be limited and the clinical significance arguable when compared to the open procedure (Ahmed *et al.*, 2009).

Patient selection

Indications

Indications for RPC include failure of medical treatment, growth failure in children and development of colonic dysplasia or carcinoma. Age is not an absolute contraindication. RPC has been successfully performed in patients from 3 years of age to over 80 years (Nicholls *et al.*, 1993). Some studies suggest that patients over the age of 55 may have an increased risk of anal leakage following pouch surgery due to deterioration of anal sphincter function, which is more common in women than in men. This is likely to be due to anal sphincter damage following childbirth (Schafer *et al.*, 1997).

Contraindications

Crohn's disease

Most surgeons agree that Crohn's disease is a contraindication for RPC because of the unacceptably high pouch failure rate of up to 60% (Tekkis *et al.*, 2005). Failure of RPC in Crohn's disease can occur due to fistulae, abscess formation or anastomotic breakdown resulting in eventual pouch excision.

Incompetent anal sphincter

Normal anal sphincter function is required in order to hold large volumes of semi-formed stool. Sphincter function can be assessed using a combination of clinical examination and anorectal physiology. Females who have undergone difficult or instrumental vaginal deliveries require careful assessment (Oberwalder *et al.*, 2003) before consideration of RPC.

Low rectal cancer

In those for whom the indication is carcinoma of the colon, it must be clear that there is an absence of low rectal cancer. RPC is a successful surgical approach for patients with coexisting colorectal cancer in UC providing there is evidence of good clearance margins (Remzi and Preen 2003).

Indeterminate colitis

Indeterminate colitis (IC) and primary sclerosing cholangitis (PSC) are not contraindications to RPC, but patients should be advised that both conditions are associated with an increase in complications and pouch failure rate. The term IC is often used interchangeably with IBD-unclassified (see Chapter 3). PSC is inflammation of the bile ducts and liver associated with extra-intestinal manifestations of UC and can be detected on a screening blood test. Patients with UC and PSC have a higher risk of developing colorectal dysplasia/carcinoma than UC patients without PSC (Broome and Bergquist, 2006). Following RPC, pouchitis rates increased in 39% patients with extra-intestinal manifestations of UC compared to 26% of those who had not. The same study reported that patients who develop extra-intestinal manifestations post-operatively had an incidence of pouchitis of 53% compared to 25% in the group of patients without extra-intestinal manifestations (Lohmuller *et al.*, 1990).

Pre- and post-operative counselling

Despite the ileoanal pouch operation becoming the surgical procedure of choice for some patients with ulcerative colitis, some aspects of the operation remain contentious. Great care must be taken to explain the advantages, disadvantages and alternatives to patients considering this surgery. It is important to advise patients that RPC does not result in normal bowel function and is mainly considered a lifestyle operation rather than a necessity. It is therefore offered as an elective procedure. Concordance is better achieved if the patient is fully informed about their condition and treatment options, which will allow them to become involved in the decisions as to which course of action to take. They will also be partially responsible for monitoring and reporting back to the medical and surgical teams.

Candidates for RPC should be given as much information and pre-operative counselling as possible. Most patients are provided with statistical evidence related to the complications of the operation. In order to obtain informed consent patients must be aware of the failure rate of the pouch, which is reported to be between 3.5% and 17% (Tekkis and Nicholls, 2008). Cumulative failure irrespective of diagnosis is approximately 5% at year 5, 10% at year 10 and 15% at year 15 (Tulchinsky *et al.*, 2003). Many patients experience some form of complication, with rates ranging from 20–60% (McLaughlin *et al.*, 2008). Patients should be made aware that even though RPC is considered curative for UC, extra-intestinal manifestations of the disease may still develop. These include skin, ophthalmic or enteropathic arthropathy conditions (Rayhorn and Rayhorn, 2002). The risk of developing carcinoma within the ileoanal pouch is rare. Nineteen cases have been reported in the literature, of which 13 were due to residual rectal mucosa following surgery (Naik *et al.*, 2008). In almost all of these patients dysplasia or invasive cancer in the large bowel was present before RPC (McLaughlin *et al.*, 2008). Current recommendations from our institution are that those with a history of dysplasia or carcinoma prior to RPC, those with PSC or those with chronic severe pouchitis undergo annual surveillance pouchoscopy. In all others surveillance is not recommended (Das *et al.*, 2007).

The British Society for Gastroenterology (BSG) recommend that patients requiring surgery for IBD are best managed under the joint care of a colorectal surgeon and gastroenterologist (Carter *et al.*, 2004). Only when the two specialist areas combine can the patient attempt to view surgery as an extension of their medical management and not as a last resort or medical failure. Patients that undergo RPC for UC with a history of recurrent relapse may accept surgery better than those who have experienced minimal inflammatory problems. This is

183

possibly because they have elected for surgery and have had time to achieve a better awareness of their illness (Perry-Woodford, 2008a).

Fertility and sexual function

Sexuality and sexual counselling is a vital part of pre- and post-operative information. This is not usually the easiest of subjects for healthcare professionals to discuss, but it is possibly the most vital to the patient. Sexual questioning should be direct but considerate and professional. This support is essential in helping patients to deal effectively with the consequences should they occur. Pouch patients are commonly young adults who are often still developing their own sexuality or personal relationships. A continent procedure is seen to improve the quality of sexual life in approximately 85% of both men and women (Nicholls *et al.*, 1993) . It is important to note that if a patient has unresolved problems with their pouch then their perception of quality of life is greatly reduced.

The effect of RPC on fertility and sexual function should be discussed in the early preoperative period in elective candidates. Fecundity measures the length of time in which a woman having unprotected sex will become pregnant (Cornish *et al.*, 2007). In patients with UC this showed a modest decrease when compared with the general population; however, following RPC fecundity decreases and infertility rates increase by up to 48% (Stein and Michelassi, 2008; Olsen *et al.*, 1999). This is mainly contributed to by anatomical changes within the pelvis, tubal obstruction or the adhering of fallopian tubes to the dorsal pelvic wall. If fecundity is over 12 months following RPC women should be referred for *in vitro* fertilisation (IVF). Young women should be advised to consider a subtotal colectomy and end ileostomy as a holding measure and defer RPC until they have completed their family. However, in our experience few young women wish to defer RPC.

Before considering RPC, men must be made aware of the potential risk of ejaculatory and erectile dysfunction due to pelvic nerve damage. Erectile dysfunction occurs in 1–2%, and failure of ejaculation in 3–4% (Colwell and Gray, 2001). Sperm banking is not usually necessary as RPC does not affect the manufacture of sperm unless the patient is scheduled for chemotherapy or radiotherapy.

After abdominal surgery, patients may complain of lack of libido, fear and anxiety of incontinence or discomfort during intercourse. Women may complain of vaginal dryness, which can be relieved with the use of water-based lubrication. It has been reported that following RPC dyspareunia increased, but sexual satisfaction was enhanced as fear of leakage during intercourse was reduced and general health following surgery improved (Tiainen and Matikainen, 1999). Intercourse can be resumed when the patient has recovered from the effects of surgery and feels ready to resume a sexual relationship. Patients should be advised pre-operatively that anal intercourse should be avoided to reduce damage to the pouch-anal anastomosis. Stricture formation is common at the stapled ileoanal anastomosis and this may prevent anal penetration. Overall, sexual function post-RPC remains stable. In one study it was reported that 67% of males and 78% of females reported unchanged or increased sexual activity following RPC (Curran and Hill, 1990).

Pouch compliance and urge resistance techniques

Pouch compliance and urge resistance techniques can be discussed with the patient even before the stoma is reversed. Once the stoma is closed the pouch will usually start to work within 2–3 days. Most patients will initially experience some urgency and frequency, which resolves quickly. The pouch needs to adapt to hold the effluent and gently expand to fulfil its new role. Patients can encourage this by extending the time from when they first feel the urge to defecate to when they empty the pouch. The time can start at just a few minutes and be increased within reasonable measures and within individual pain tolerance. The anal sphincter muscles which were defunctioned by the stoma will need to regain strength, and occasionally leakage may occur overnight when the patient is relaxed. This is normal and reassurance can be provided that these nocturnal episodes usually become less frequent over time. Some patients wear pads at night for peace of mind. Thin and discrete sanitary pads can be used by both sexes, as seepage is usually minimal. Pouch frequency can be as often as every 2–3 hours during the day; therefore barrier cream and good quality anal hygiene should be introduced as soon as the stoma is reversed and the pouch is active. Support in the community can be provided by the GP, the practice nurse, and the pouch or stoma clinician. Specialist pouch support groups or charities (Box 10.1) can offer non-medical lifestyle advice and information from members who have already undergone RPC.

Box 10.1 Support groups and charities

- Ileostomy and Internal Pouch Support Group: http://www.the-ia.org.uk/
- Crohn's and Colitis UK: http://www.nacc.org.uk/
- The Red Lion Group: http://www.redliongroup.org/
- Ostomy Lifestyle Careline: http://www.lifestylecareline.com/
- Bladder and Bowel Foundation: http://www.bladderandbowelfoundation.org/

With the absence of the terminal ileum and large bowel, pouch output is loose and often an irritant to perianal skin. If output is high (8 times or more in 24 hrs) excoriated skin is inevitable. Sometimes patients may complain of associated rectal burning or anal itch. This could arise from the effluent being in contact with the pouch–anal anastomosis. Frequency and leakage are the commonest cause of perianal soreness. Taking good care of the perianal skin can help stop these problems occurring. However, it is important to exclude an anal fissure. Anal fissures can be treated topically with either a steroid-based cream or glyceryl trinitrate ointment prescribed by a doctor. Pouch patients are advised to keep the perianal area clean by washing and drying after every motion or by using wet, unperfumed wipes. The perianal skin should be dry before applying barrier creams and thoroughly removed before reapplication. Loose cotton underwear should also be worn. About one-third of patients will require anti-diarrhoeal medication to obtain satisfactory pouch function (Tekkis *et al.*, 2009). Loperamide up to 32 mg is usually effective. In those where this is not effective codeine phosphate should be recommended.

Pouch absorption and diet

It is important to understand the effect of pouch formation on water, sodium and nutrient absorption in order to detect potential problems and provide dietary advice. Annual blood tests are performed to exclude anaemia and vitamin B_{12} and iron deficiencies. In addition, monitoring of liver function tests may aid in identifying the development of PSC. Osteopenia and osteoporosis are no more common in RPC patients than in the general IBD population and standard guidelines regarding the need for DEXA screening should be followed (McLaughlin *et al.*, 2010).

Commonly pouch patients will require supplementary vitamin B_{12} injections (McLaughlin *et al.*, 2008). Importantly, vitamin deficiency may not become apparent for many years, as some patients have up to 10 years of body stores. Iron deficiency is also common in RPC patients. The cause of this is not well understood, but may occur due to reduced absorption and increased loss from low grade pouch inflammation. Unfortunately, many patients have low tolerance to oral iron therapy and intravenous iron replacement is often required.

In the early post-operative period following closure of the ileostomy, a soft, light and low-fibre diet should be provided similar to ileostomy dietary advice. Food and drink can usually be increased to the patient's preferences within two to three weeks. Most pouch patients enjoy a healthy well-balanced diet. Over time, most patients realise the effects of certain foods on their pouch function; however, it appears that pouch function is not solely based on dietary intake (Coffey *et al.*, 2002).

A high-fibre diet may cause blockages within the pouch or pre-pouch ileum or increase frequency. Therefore patients should be advised to choose soluble rather than insoluble fibre. Vegetarians in particular should be advised of this. Fruit and vegetables should be peeled, cooked or chewed well. Some foods can increase anal itching or burning. Examples include coconut and citrus fruit and may be avoided or taken in moderation. Dietary obstruction is usually resolved by avoiding food for 24 hours and only drinking fluids. Activities such as walking, a warm bath or massaging the abdomen may help relieve a blockage. Patients need to be advised to seek medical advice if the pouch stops working and/or they start vomiting.

Pouch dysfunction and management of complications

In order to diagnose and manage pouch complications it is usually necessary to take a full history and perform a clinical examination, as most cases of pouch dysfunction present with similar symptoms. The importance of patient history can not be overestimated. The most useful initial test is a flexible pouchoscopy with biopsy (Figure 10.1). In addition, the clinician should arrange for stool testing to exclude gastrointestinal infections, including *Clostridium difficile*. The most common causes of pouch dysfunction are described below, and in addition an algorithm for the investigation of pouch dysfunction is illustrated (Figure 10.2).

Pouchitis

Pouchitis is the most common cause of pouch dysfunction and occurs in up to 50% of patients (Figure 10.3). About 39% of patients who develop pouchitis will have a single episode which is easily treated, while the remaining 61% will suffer at least one further episode (Lohmuller *et al.*, 1990) and about 5–19% of patients will develop chronic relapsing pouchitis (Mowschenson *et al.*, 2000; Hurst *et al.*, 1998; Madiba and Bartolo, 2001). Therefore in clinical practice pouchitis is rarely a significant problem. Patients with PSC are at increased risk of developing chronic pouchitis and should be counselled regarding this risk before RPC. Pouchitis usually presents with urgency and an increase in stool frequency and abdominal cramping. Rarely patients may complain of bleeding. Non-steroidal anti-inflammatory drugs (NSAIDs) can precipitate pouchitis (Shen *et al.*, 2007). The clinician should enquire about these medications, as withdrawal alone may be sufficient to induce remission. Diagnosis is usually made at flexible pouchoscopy; however stool for faecal calprotectin is also a reliable test (Johnson *et al.*, 2008) and may be requested by the clinician. Antibiotics remain the mainstay of treatment.

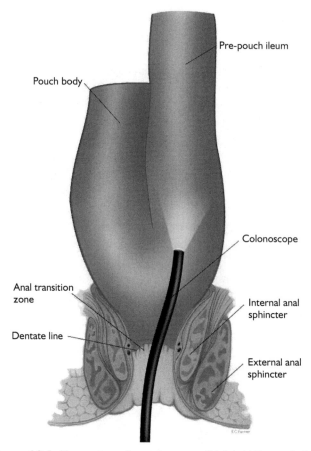

Pre-pouch ileum

Pouch body

Colonoscope

Anal transition zone

Internal anal sphincter

Dentate line

External anal sphincter

Figure 10.1 Illustration of pouchoscopy (McLaughlin *et al.*, 2009).

In patients with chronic pouchitis maintenance treatment with antibiotics or a probiotic such as VSL#3 may be required. Contradictory research remains on the effectiveness of VSL#3 in promoting remission in pouchitis. Mimura *et al.* (2004) state VSL#3 has no role in patients who have not first responded to antibiotic treatment for pouchitis. The treatment of pouchitis is summarised in Figure 10.4.

Pelvic sepsis

Pelvic sepsis occurs due to a leak at the pouch–anal anastomosis. It most commonly occurs soon after surgery; however, it can present many years later (Heuschen *et al.*, 2002). In the early post-operative period it may present with fever and/or pain. Delayed pelvic sepsis usually presents with poor function and/or pain. A pelvic

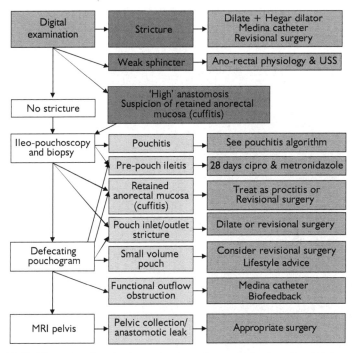

Figure 10.2 Algorithm for the investigation of pouch dysfunction (McLaughlin *et al.*, 2008).

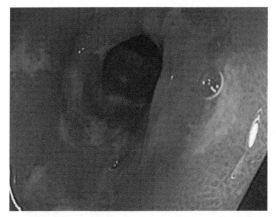

Figure 10.3 Endoscopic view of pouchitis.

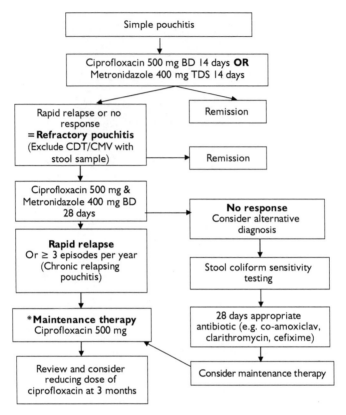

Figure 10.4 Algorithm for the treatment of pouchitis (McLaughlin *et al.*, 2008).

MRI scan is the usual diagnostic tool. Treatment includes antibiotics and in some cases surgery to de-function or excise the pouch.

Fistulation

Pouch–vaginal or pouch–perineal fistula may develop at any time following RPC. Most are associated with sepsis at the ileoanal anastomosis. Only a minority are due to undiagnosed Crohn's disease. Surgery (pouch advancement or an advancement flap) will result in closure in most cases, although this often requires several procedures and a temporary ileostomy (McLaughlin *et al.*, 2008).

Functional outflow obstruction

Functional outflow obstruction occurs where there is difficulty evacuating the pouch despite the absence of a stricture. Patients complain of stool frequency and difficulty evacuating the pouch. Diagnosis is made following a defecating pouchogram. Evacuation of the pouch using a Medina catheter (flexible soft plastic tube) is an effective treatment in those patients who cannot spontaneously evacuate. The clinician is fundamental in instigating treatment, which requires teaching intermittently catheterisation of the pouch using a Medina catheter (Perry-Woodford and McLaughlin, 2009).

Pouch failure

Pouch failure is defined as the need to remove the pouch or form a permanent ileostomy. The incidence of pouch failure increases over time; large studies report a failure rate of 5% at 5 years and 10–15% at 20 years. The majority of failures occur in the first year following surgery. The most common causes of failure are pelvic sepsis, poor pouch function and pouchitis (Tulchinsky *et al.*, 2003).

Retained rectal cuff (cuffitis)

Most surgeons now use a stapling device to join the pouch to the anal canal. This technique requires a 0.5–2 cm cuff of rectum to be left *in situ*. In about 5% of patients this can become sufficiently inflamed to cause symptoms similar to proctitis with anal pain, urgency, frequency and bleeding. Diagnosis is made at flexible pouchoscopy. Treatment is similar to proctitis using mesalazine or steroid suppositories (McLaughlin *et al.*, 2008).

Crohn's disease

About 2–3% of patients will be reclassified to Crohn's disease following pouch surgery (Hahnloser *et al.*, 2007). Some of these patients will have been diagnosed with IBD-unclassified, indeterminate colitis and some with UC prior to surgery. Patients may present with fistula, stricture or treatment resistant pouchitis (McLaughlin *et al.*, 2008).

Special considerations

Pregnancy

Pregnancy is safe following RPC, but women should be advised that pouch dysfunction is common, especially in the third trimester as the foetus enlarges. Expectant mothers commonly report increased stool frequency, urgency, perianal irritation and nocturnal incontinence as the foetus develops. Women should be reassured that normal function returns after delivery. Advice on anal skin care, diet and general reassurance can be helpful. Some women find it helpful to speak to others who have experienced pregnancy and childbirth with a pouch. The main controversy lies in the chosen method of delivery. Whilst vaginal delivery is usually safe, most colorectal surgeons recommend delivery by Caesarean section because of the potential risk of anal sphincter injury associated with vaginal delivery (Lepisto *et al.*, 2007).

Children

Children as young as five years of age have undergone RPC successfully. However, some paediatric surgeons may advocate alternate operations or wish to postpone surgery as long as safely possible. In a study by Rintala and Lindahi (2002), 29 children were followed up for eight years following RPC. The median age at operation was 13 years. Fifty-three per cent of the children had a complication, which is in line with adult complication rates. None of the pouches had to be removed. Supporting evidence state that RPC is the preferred technique for children suffering with UC and offer an excellent quality of life (Fonkalsrud *et al.*, 2001). For most children it is paramount to include the family in all aspects of care. Care of the temporary stoma, lifestyle and support information is necessary for the carers of the child. It may also be helpful for the clinician to liaise with the school, as the transition may be daunting for the patient and their family following bowel surgery.

Elderly

RPC is offered with care to patients over the age of 60, not because of the reduced success of RPC in the elderly, but mainly due to the increased co-morbidities that coincide with age. It is paramount that the anal sphincter is deemed effective before RPC in an elderly person. However, complication rates (such as for anal leakage) were comparable to that of a younger population following RPC (Tan *et al.*, 1997). Patient mobility and comprehension of the surgery need to be taken into account, as chronic, unremitting pouchitis is a possible disabling complication of pouch surgery in the elderly. There is, however, no evidence to suggest that the elderly population is more at risk of pouchitis than a younger group.

Quality of life (QOL)

Many studies have reported the QOL in patients with an ileoanal pouch as comparable with the general population (Coffey *et al.*, 2002). There is a strong association between functional outcome and QOL in patients after RPC (Carmon *et al.*, 2003). However, patient age at time of surgery seems to strongly influence both functional outcome and QOL with reduction in both with increased age. Much of the improvement in QOL may result from the reassurance that the diseased colon and the risk of colonic cancer are removed, although this perception can vary between patients. There is also no gold standard to measure QOL in patients after pelvic surgery, as all validated methods have advantages and disadvantages (Fazio *et al.*, 1999). This finding should be taken into consideration during pre-operative counselling. Others have compared the high long-term complication rate to the relatively small quality of life advantage associated with RPC and advise that patients be thoroughly counselled prior to surgery (Camilleri-Brennan *et al.*, 2003).

A multidisciplinary team (MDT) approach to follow-up

Nurse-led initiatives continue to identify areas of independent practice where they are able to initiate and deliver care to patients and incorporate certain aspects of clinical work previously carried out by medical staff (NMC, 2006). The traditional role of the medical team solely managing the needs of the pouch patient has drastically changed over the last decade, with more patients being cared for by the MDT and in outpatient settings. A specialist nursing interest in the management of pouch complications was observed in 1996 when the pouch nurse role was first established at St Mark's Hospital, caring exclusively for patients considering, or having undergone, pouch surgery. Other centres have set up pouch nurse-led clinics, which have started to show improvements in patient follow-up and overall satisfaction. Although the literature on pouch nurse-led clinics is sparse, Perrin (2005) states that 88% of patients were happy to have their internal examinations undertaken by a nurse specialist and 96% were happy to discuss their concerns or related issues with the nurse. Supporting evidence by Perry-Woodford (2008b) suggest that the nurse specialist is able to reduce clinic waiting times by adding patients on to their own lists and accessing problems without necessarily having a doctor present. Patients are now discharged into the care of their GP for routine follow-up and annual blood tests following pouch surgery unless they have chronic antibiotic dependent/resistant pouchitis or were found to have rectal carcinoma/dysplasia at colectomy. For this high-risk group, annual surveillance is recommended. Complications arising from RPC are best managed in specialist centres where appropriate follow-up and testing can be achieved. This follow-up procedure enhances the support that pouch patients receive post-operation, whilst providing a cost-effective service to an over-stretched NHS. Some inflammatory bowel disease nurse specialists at several centres have adapted the role of managing pouch patients following surgery. These nursing roles are supported by the medical teams should they need advice or assistance.

Telephone helplines and telephone clinics run by nurse specialists are also increasingly used in order to combat the problems associated with long waiting lists, wasted clinic appointments and cost restraints (Hennell *et al.*, 2006). Nurse specialists have become vital in the management of pouch patients' care. Medical teams are beginning to acknowledge the nurses' diverse knowledge and skills in other areas, such as providing psychological and practical support, referring to other members of the multidisciplinary team and continuation of patient care. This extended role for nurses has seen an increase in job satisfaction, confidence and accountability for assessing patient needs and developing and managing areas of research to improve the quality of care and outcomes of pouch patients (Campbell *et al.*, 1999).

Conclusion

One of the greatest advances in colorectal surgery over the last 30 years has been the development of RPC with ileo pouch anal anastomosis for patients suffering with UC. This operation can offer patients an acceptable quality of life while avoiding a permanent ileostomy. It has also allowed clinicians in gastroenterology to take their place alongside medical specialists and more importantly establish themselves as a principal carer in many diverse roles when dealing with the patient suffering with UC (Norton and Kamm, 2002). However, management of the post-operative complications and long-term dysfunction seen in some pouch patients warrants more research and randomised controlled trials in order to provide expert care to all patients with an ileoanal pouch.

Key points

- Effective pre-operative assessment and counselling will enhance patient experience, expectation and long-term satisfaction following RPC.
- Effective management of complications such as pouchitis is required in maintaining normal/acceptable pouch function. This is also with interaction from the MDT.
- The quality of life in patients with an ileoanal pouch is comparable with the general population.

Patient translation summary

RPC is an operation that can offer patients with UC an acceptable quality of life while avoiding some of the complications that permanent ileostomy may incur. RPC is an elective procedure and patient concordance is necessary for pouch success. It must be made clear that RPC with an ileoanal pouch does not allow normal defecation. However, the anal route is preserved and defecation can take place in an accustomed manner. The pros and cons of a pouch should be discussed in the pre-operative stage and risks discussed in order for the patient to make an informed choice. The possibility of differential diagnoses must be explored in order to exclude Crohn's disease, indeterminate colitis, PSC or a rectal cancer. If these conditions occur a patient must be aware of the increased failure rates of RPC should they continue with pouch surgery. Patient expectations and lifestyle are paramount in deciding if a pouch is a suitable surgical option for management of relapsing UC. Medical help lines or support groups are available to those considering RPC.

References

Ahmed, A. U., Keus, F., Heikens, J. T. *et al.* (2009) Open versus laparoscopic (assisted) ileo pouch anal anastomosis for ulcerative colitis and familial adenomatous polyposis. *Cochrane Database Syst. Rev.*, CD006267.

Bengtsson, J., Borjesson, L., Lundstam, U. and Oresland, T. (2007) Long-term function and manovolumetric characteristics after ileal pouch-anal anastomosis for ulcerative colitis. *Br. J. Surg.*, **94**, 327–32.

Brooke, B. (1952) The management of an ileostomy including its complications. *Lancet*, **2**, 102–4.

Broome, U. and Bergquist, A. (2006) Primary sclerosing cholangitis, inflammatory bowel disease, and colon cancer. *Semin. Liver Dis.*, **26**, 31–41.

Campbell, J., German, L. and Lane, C. (1999) Radiotherapy outpatient review: a nurse led clinic. *Nursing Standard*, **13**(22), 39–44.

Camilleri-Brennan, J., Munro, A. and Steele, R. J. (2003) Does an ileoanal pouch offer a better quality of life than a permanent ileostomy for patients with ulcerative colitis? *J. Gastrointest. Surg.*, **7**, 814–19.

Carmon, E., Keidar, A., Ravid, A., Goldman, G. and Rabau, M. (2003) The correlation between quality of life and functional outcome in ulcerative colitis patients after proctocolectomy ileal pouch anal anastomosis. *Colorectal Dis.*, **5**, 228–32.

Carter, M. J., Lobo, A. J. and Travis, S. P. (2004) Guidelines for the management of inflammatory bowel disease in adults. *Gut*, **53**(suppl. 5), V1–16.

Coffey, J. C., Winter, D. C., Neary, P., Murphy, A., Redmond, H. P. and Kirwan, W. O. (2002) Quality of life after ileal pouch-anal anastomosis: an evaluation of diet and other factors using the Cleveland Global Quality of Life instrument. *Dis.Colon Rectum*, **45**, 30–8.

Colwell, J. C. and Gray, M. (2001) What functional outcomes and complications should be taught to the patient with ulcerative colitis or familial adenomatous polyposis who undergoes ileal pouch anal anastomosis? *J. Wound Ostomy Continence Nurs.*, **28**, 184–9.

Cornish, J. A., Tan, E. and Teare, J. *et al.* (2007) The effect of RPC on sexual function, urinary function, fertility, pregnancy and delivery: a systematic review. *Dis. Colon Rectum*, **50**, 1128–38.

Curran, F. T. and Hill, G. L. (1990) Results of 50 ileoanal J pouch operations. *Aust. NZ J. Surg.*, **60**, 579–83.

Das, P., Johnson, M. W., Tekkis, P. P. and Nicholls, R. J. (2007) Risk of dysplasia and adenocarcinoma following RPC for ulcerative colitis. *Colorectal Dis.*, **9**, 15–27.

Fazio, V. W., O'Riordain, M. G., Lavery, I. C., Church, J. M., Lau, P., Strong, S. A. and Hull, T. (1999) Long-term functional outcome and quality of life after stapled restorative proctocolectomy. *Ann. Surg.*, **230**, 575–84.

Fonkalsrud, E. W., Thakur, A. and Beanes, S. (2001) Ileoanal pouch procedures in children. *J. Pediatr. Surg.*, **36**, 1689–92.

Hahnloser, D., Pemberton, J. H., Wolff, B. G., Larson, D. R., Crownhart, B. S. and Dozois, R. R. (2007) Results at up to 20 years after ileal pouch-anal anastomosis for chronic ulcerative colitis. *Br. J. Surg.*, **94**, 333–40.

Hendriksen, C., Kreiner, S. and Binder, V. (1985) Long term prognosis in ulcerative colitis – based on results from a regional patient group from the county of Copenhagen. *Gut*, **26**, 158–63.

Hennell, S., Spark, E., Wood, B. and George, E. (2006) An evaluation of nurse-led rheumatology telephone clinics. *Musculoskeletal Care*, **3**, 233–40.

Heuschen, U. A., Allemeyer, E. H., Hinz, U., Lucas, M., Herfarth, C. and Heuschen, G. (2002) Outcome after septic complications in J pouch procedures. *Br. J. Surg.*, **89**, 194–200.

Hurst, R. D., Chung, T. P., Rubin, M. and Michelassi, F. (1998) The implications of acute pouchitis on the long-term functional results after restorative proctocolectomy. *Inflamm. Bowel. Dis.*, **4**, 280–4.

Johnson, M. W., Maestranzi, S., Duffy, A. M. *et al.* (2008) Faecal calprotectin: a non-invasive diagnostic tool and marker of severity in pouchitis. *Eur. J. Gastroenterol. Hepatol.*, **20**, 174–9.

196

Kock, N. (1969) Intra abdominal 'reservoir' in patients with permanent ileostomy. *Arch. Surg.*, **99**, 223–31.

Lacey, J. (1982) Sir Arbuthnot Lane, Chronic intestinal stasis and autointoxication. *Ann. Int. Med.*, **96**, 365–9.

Langholz, E., Munkholm, P., Davidsen, M. and Binder, V. (1992) Colorectal cancer risk and mortality in patients with ulcerative colitis. *Gastroenterology*, **103**, 1444–51.

Lepisto, A., Sarna, S., Tiitinen, A. and Jarvinen, H. J. (2007) Female fertility and childbirth after ileal pouch-anal anastomosis for ulcerative colitis. *Br. J. Surg.*, **94**, 478–82.

Lohmuller, J. L., Pemberton, J. H., Dozois, R. R., Ilstrup, D. and van Heerden, J. (1990) Pouchitis and extraintestinal manifestations of inflammatory bowel disease after ileal pouch-anal anastomosis. *Ann. Surg.*, **211**, 622–7.

Lucarotti, M. E., Freeman, B. J., Warren, B. F. and Durdey, P. (1995) Synchronous procto-colectomy and ileoanal pouch formation and the risk of Crohn's disease. *Br. J. Surg.*, **82**, 755–6.

Madiba, T. E. and Bartolo, D. C. (2001) Pouchitis following restorative proctocolectomy for ulcerative colitis: incidence and therapeutic outcome. *J. R. Coll. Surg. Edinb.*, **46**, 334–7.

Miller, G., Gardener, C. and Ripstein, C. (1949) Primary resection of the colon in ulcerative colitis. *Can. Med. Assoc. J.*, **60**, 584–5.

Mimura, T., Rizzello, F., Helwig, U. *et al.* (2004) Once daily high dose probiotic therapy (VSL#3) for maintaining remission in recurrent or refractory pouchitis. *Gut*, **53**, 108–14.

McLaughlin, S. D., Clark, S. K., Tekkis, P. P., Ciclitira, P. J. and Nicholls, R. J. (2008) Review article: RPC, indications, management of complications and follow-up – a guide for gastroenterologists. *Aliment. Pharmacol. Ther.*, **27**, 895–909.

McLaughlin, S. D., Clark, S. K., Thomas-Gibson, S., Tekkis, P. P., Ciclitira, P. J. and Nicholls, R. J. (2009) *Inflamm. Bowel Dis.*, **15**(8), 1256–63.

McLaughlin, S. D., Perry-Woodford, Z. L., Clark, S. K. *et al.* (2010) Osteoporosis in patients over 50 years of age following RPC for ulcerative colitis: is DXA screening warranted? *Inflamm. Bowel. Dis.*, **16**, 250–5.

Mowschenson, P. M., Critchlow, J. F. and Peppercorn, M. A. (2000) Ileoanal pouch operation: long-term outcome with or without diverting ileostomy. *Arch. Surg.*, **135**, 463–5.

Naik, V. S., Patil, S. B., Scholefield, J. *et al.* (2008) Adenocarcinoma arising in a background of chronic atrophic pouchitis in an ileoanal pouch for ulcerative colitis. *Histopathology*, **53**, 354–8.

Nicholls, R. J., Bartolo, D. C. and Mortenson, N. J. (1993) *Restorative Proctocolectomy*. Oxford: Blackwell Scientific.

Nursing and Midwifery Council (2006) *Independent Practice*. http://www.nmc-uk.org/ (accessed 12 June 2006).

Norton, C. and Kamm, M. A. (2002) Specialist nurses in gastroenterology *J. R. Soc. Med.*, **95**, 331–5.

Oberwalder, M., Connor, J. and Wexner, S. D. (2003) Meta-analysis to determine the incidence of obstetric anal sphincter damage. *Br. J. Surg.*, **90**, 1333–7.

Olsen, K. O., Joelsson, M., Laurberg, S. and Oresland, T. (1999) Fertility after ileal pouch-anal anastomosis in women with ulcerative colitis. *Br. J. Surg.*, **86**, 493–5.

Parks, A., Nicholls, R. and Belliveau, P. (1980) Proctocolectomy with ileal reservoir and anal anastamosis. *Br. J. Surg.*, **67**, 533–8.

Perrin, A. (2005) Development of a nurse led ileo-anal pouch clinic. *Br. J. Nurs.*, **14**(16), S21–S24.

Persson, E., Gustavsson, B., Hellstrom, A. L., Lappas, G. and Hulten, L. (2005) Ostomy patients' perceptions of quality of care. *J. Adv. Nurs.*, **49**, 51–8.

Perry-Woodford, Z. L. (2008a) Intestinal pouches. In: *Stoma Care* (ed. J. Burch). London: Wiley Blackwell Publishing.

Perry-Woodford, Z. L. (2008b) A clinical audit of the ileo-anal pouch service at St Mark's Hospital. *Gastroint. Nurs.*, **6**(2), 36–9.

Perry-Woodford, Z. L. and McLaughlin, S. D. (2009) Ileoanal pouch dysfunction and the use of a Medina catheter following hospital discharge. *Br. J. Community Nurs.*, **14**, 502–6.

Rayhorn, N. and Rayhorn, D. J. (2002) Inflammatory bowel disease: symptoms in the bowel and beyond. *Nurse Pract.*, **27**, 13–27.

Remzi, F. H. and Preen, M. (2003) Rectal cancer and ulcerative colitis: does it change the therapeutic approach? *Colorectal Dis.*, **5**, 483–5.

Rintala, R. J. and Lindahl, H. G. (2002) Proctocolectomy and J-pouch ileo-anal anastomosis in children. *J. Pediatr. Surg.*, **37**, 66–70.

Schafer, R., Heyer, T., Gantke, B. *et al.* (1997) Anal endosonography and manometry: comparison in patients with defecation problems. *Dis. Colon Rectum*, **40**, 293–7.

Shen, B., Fazio, V. W., Remzi, F. H. *et al.* (2007) Effect of withdrawal of nonsteroidal anti-inflammatory drug use on ileal pouch disorders. *Dig. Dis. Sci.*, **52**, 3321–8.

Stein, S. L. and Michelassi, F. (2008) How can fecundity be preserved in patients undergoing pelvic surgery? *Nat. Clin. Pract. Gastroenterol. Hepatol.*, **5**, 308–9.

Tan, H. T., Connolly, A. B., Morton, D. and Keighley, M. R. (1997) Results of restorative proctocolectomy in the elderly. *Int. J. Colorectal Dis.*, **12**, 319–22.

Tekkis, P. P. and Nicholls, R. J. (2008) Ileal pouch dysfunction: diagnosis and management. *Gastroenterol. Clin. N. Am.*, **37**, 669–83.

Tekkis, P. P., Heriot, A. G., Smith, O., Smith, J. J., Windsor, A. C. and Nicholls, R. J. (2005) Long-term outcomes of RPC for Crohn's disease and indeterminate colitis. *Colorectal*

Dis., **7**, 218–23.

Tekkis, P. P., Lovegrove, R. E., Tilney, H. S. *et al.* (2009) Long-term failure and function after RPC – a multi-centre study of patients from the UK National Ileal Pouch Registry. *Colorectal Dis.*, **9**(S3), 1.

Tiainen, J. and Matikainen, M. (1999) Health-related quality of life after ileal J-pouch-anal anastomosis for ulcerative colitis: long-term results. *Scand. J. Gastroenterol.*, **34**, 601–5.

Tulchinsky, H., Hawley, P. R. and Nicholls, J. (2003) Long-term failure after RPC for ulcerative colitis. *Ann. Surg.*, **238**, 229–34.

Zelas, P. and Jagelman, D. (1980) Loop ileostomy in the management of Crohn's colitis in the debilitated patient. *Ann. Surg.*, **191**, 164–8.

CHAPTER 11

Caring for stomas and fistulae

Jennie Burch

Introduction

This chapter covers caring for stomas and fistulae in inflammatory bowel disease (IBD). People with inflammatory bowel disease may, during their lifetime, require a temporary or permanent stoma to treat their IBD, or experience a fistula resulting from their disease or treatment. The chapter will discuss the role of the stoma clinical nurse specialist (CNS) including the education and practical management techniques he or she may employ as well as the issues patients may encounter when living with a stoma and/or a fistula.

Case study

Sarah was in her mid-twenties; she had been diagnosed with ulcerative colitis three years before and had tried multiple oral medications. A recent disease flare had led to an emergency admission; Sarah's bowels were open in excess of a dozen times daily and intravenous steroids were commenced. Sarah was informed by the medical team that surgery was likely if the intravenous therapy was ineffective.

Sarah was introduced to the surgical team and the stoma CNS and given information. The stoma CNS explained the various surgical options. The initial operation (if medical therapy failed) would be a subtotal colectomy, removal of the inflamed colon, retaining of the rectum (as it is unsafe to remove this during periods of severe inflammation) and formation of a temporary end ileostomy. The subsequent options of an ileo-pouch anal anastomosis or a proctectomy (removal of the rectum) were briefly mentioned. The issue that concerned Sarah was whether she would still be able to have children in the future, and she was reassured that this would generally be possible.

Sarah did progress to surgery and was taught how to care for her stoma, becoming independent five days after her operation. She quickly learnt how to empty the drainable stoma appliance. Once she was home she needed to empty this about five times daily, and she changed the appliance every morning. Although Sarah and her partner were able to talk through the options of further surgery together, Sarah had not yet chosen how to proceed. However, her general condition improved rapidly after removal of her colon.

Stomas

There are three main types of stoma: the ileostomy, colostomy and urostomy. The faecal stomas are the colostomy and ileostomy, which are formed to pass faeces and flatus from the body and may be temporary or permanent. The urinary stoma is termed a urostomy. For the purpose of this chapter, urostomy will not be discussed in detail.

Ileostomy

The most commonly seen stoma for patients with inflammatory bowel disease is the ileostomy, which may be formed to treat either ulcerative colitis or Crohn's disease. An ileostomy is made from the small bowel or ileum, often the terminal ileum; however, patients with Crohn's disease may have a shortened small bowel if they have undergone a small bowel resection (see Chapter 12). The output from an ileostomy is flatus and loose faeces, often described as 'porridge like'; again, this will be looser in consistency if there has been a small bowel resection or if there is active small bowel Crohn's disease.

The stomal output is collected in a one-piece or two-piece drainable appliance, often with a Velcro-like fastening. Appliances will be explained later in the chapter. In general, an ileostomy appliance will be emptied three to six times each day into the toilet and the appliance will be replaced every one to three days.

In appearance an ileostomy is red or pink, wet, warm, and circular or egg shaped. The ideal ileostomy has a small spout of about 25 mm. The ileostomy spout helps to keep the faecal output away from the skin, reducing the risk of sore skin developing. Ileostomates (people with an ileostomy) with a spout shorter than 20 mm are more likely to experience appliance leaks than ileostomates with longer spouts (Persson *et al.*, 2009).

Colostomy

A colostomy is formed from the colon (usually the sigmoid or descending colon) and thus should pass flatus and soft, formed stool. Although a colostomy is most commonly formed for a rectal cancer, it is also formed for people with perianal Crohn's disease. The stomal output is generally collected in a closed bag, which can be either a one-piece or two-piece appliance. The stoma is usually active somewhere between once every three days to three times daily, depending upon the diet consumed or the segment of bowel used for the colostomy formation. Therefore the appliance needs to be replaced when a third to a half full, which is generally between three times daily and three times a week. In appearance the colostomy is red or pink, wet and warm. The size of a colostomy can vary widely, but an average size, once post-operative oedema has resolved, is about 35 mm in diameter (Burch, 2008) and the stoma is ideally minimally raised above the skin surface.

Urostomy

The urostomy, or ileal conduit, is the least commonly formed stoma and is not usually related to IBD. The most frequent reason to form a urostomy is to treat bladder cancer and involves the anastomosis of the two ureters to a small section of ileum. This segment of ileum is removed from the rest of the ileum, but the blood supply is maintained. One end of the ileal segment is over-sewn and the other is formed into a stoma, which has the appearance of an ileostomy. The output is urine, mixed with mucus from the bowel segment. The urostomy appliance used to collect the stomal output is drainable, with a tap or bung that is used to release the urine. The appliance is emptied about six times daily and usually changed every one or two days.

High-output stomas

There are also high-output faecal stomas that are generally defined as stomas with an output of more than one litre daily. Patients with Crohn's disease that have undergone extensive small bowel resections may have a stoma formed high in the ileum or even more rarely within the jejunum. People with a high-output ileostomy or jejunostomy have a high-volume, loose faecal output and may require a drainable appliance with a bung-type fastening that can be attached to a bag similar to a catheter bag at night. It is also possible that these patients will be on parenteral nutrition. This will be further elucidated in Chapter 12.

Mucous fistula

A mucous fistula is formed to release mucus from the body, but a person with a mucous fistula will therefore also have a faecal output stoma that will pass faeces.

203

A mucous fistula may be formed in the emergency situation for people with ulcerative colitis. For example, when the subtotal/total colectomy is performed the rectum might be brought to the skin surface to pass the mucus. The mucus is usually intermittent and can be quite malodorous. A small stoma cap is used to collect the mucus.

Rectal mucus

It is also possible that ostomates (people with a stoma) who have a retained rectum or ileo-pouch anal anastomosis will pass mucus anally. The mucus can be malodorous and jelly-like in consistency, or liquid with blood mixed in if the diseased rectum is still *in situ*. This mucus is usually passed under voluntary control, occurring intermittently to multiple times daily. However, some ostomates are not troubled with mucus, as the bowel reabsorbs it.

Role of the stoma clinical specialist nurse

The role of the stoma CNS varies slightly with each organisation and/or individual, but in general will include some or all of the following roles:

- Pre-operative care, including information provision such as advice on appliances, stomas, diet and stoma siting
- Post-operative training, including reinforcing information given preoperatively
- Follow-up care.

Pre-operation

The specific care of stomas falls under the remit of stoma CNSs, who are available in most hospitals in the UK. Once the decision to operate has been made by the surgical or multidisciplinary team, a referral is made to the stoma CNS, who will further discuss the operation and implications of this with the patient.

Stoma siting

The stoma CNS ideally sites or marks the patient's abdomen for the best position for the stoma to be formed for all planned operations. Siting is important to avoid skin creases and to enable good subsequent care of the stoma after surgery. Siting allows the patient to see where the stoma will be formed and also to have a role in choosing the position for the surgeons to use (Rust, 2009). A poorly sited stoma may result in post-operative problems, such as a leaking appliance, which can lead to sore skin and social isolation in some cases.

Surgery

Stoma-forming surgery in IBD is fully explored in Chapter 9; however, Table 11.1 lists the most common surgical procedures resulting in stoma formation.

Table 11.1 Surgical procedures in IBD leading to stoma formation.

Ulcerative colitis	Crohn's disease
Panproctocolectomy and permanent end ileostomy	Panproctocolectomy and permanent end ileostomy
Subtotal/total colectomy and temporary end ileostomy	Subtotal/total colectomy and temporary end ileostomy
Ileo-pouch anal anastomosis or ileoanal pouch and temporary loop ileostomy (IPAA)	Abdominoperineal resection of the rectum and permanent end colostomy (APER)
	Formation of a temporary loop colostomy

Management of stomas

There are many different types of appliance and various manufacturers are available to assist in stoma management. This provides variety but can also be confusing to the nurse and the ostomate.

Appliances

The function of a stoma appliance is to collect and contain the stomal output. The appliance therefore contains any odour from the faeces and helps to maintain healthy, intact peristomal skin (skin around the stoma). This is obviously necessary for ostomate comfort and to allow further appliances to securely adhere to the abdominal skin. A stoma appliance consists of the flange or base plate and the bag or pouch and can be defined as one-piece and two-piece appliances. Ostomates may have a personal preference, but in general either is suitable for the majority of ostomates. Worldwide, stoma care practice varies; in the UK one-piece products are generally preferred, whereas in America two-piece appliances are the product of choice. This is often related to cost, as two-piece appliances can be more cost-effective. In Germany it is common practice for ileostomates to use a convex ileostomy appliance (see below).

Appliances are available with a 'starter hole', which is a small aperture. The starter hole can then be enlarged and cut to the size and shape of the stoma (2–3 mm larger than the actual stoma, to allow for errors in placing or cutting). After about eight weeks the stoma will have 'shrunk' as the post-operative oedema resolves. Following this there are pre-cut stoma appliances available in a variety of sizes that suit most ostomates.

One-piece appliances
A one-piece appliance has the flange, which is the adhesive part of the appliance, joined to the bag. The adhesive part of the appliance adheres to the abdominal wall and these appliances are generally thin and flexible (Bradshaw and Collins, 2009).

Two-piece appliances
A two-piece appliance comes in two parts. These are initially separate but are joined together with a two plastic circles that 'click' together (McPhail, 2003); more recently, adhesive joins the two parts together (White and Berg, 2005).

Stoma accessories
There is a vast array of stoma accessories available. However, for ostomates with complications there may be the need for products such as:

- Convex appliances: these have a shaped flange which can be used for situations such as a non-spouted ileostomy to prevent appliance leakage.
- Skin protection accessories: these include wipes and sprays used to protect peristomal skin at risk of trauma from the stomal output, for example.
- Extra adhesion products: seals/washers and paste are used to reduce the risks of a leaking stoma appliance by increasing adhesion directly around the stoma.
- Skin cleansing accessories: these include adhesive remover, which is useful for ostomates who find it uncomfortable when removing their appliance.

Stoma accessories should be advised by a stoma CNS (Rudoni and Dennis, 2009) prior to use to enable a thorough assessment of the ostomate's requirements.

Stoma appliances in the UK community
When discharged home it is general practice to provide the ostomate with two weeks' supply of stoma appliances. Ongoing supplies are obtained on prescription from the family doctor and can be received via the chemist or a delivery company. The delivery company will often provide free cleaning wipes and disposal bags. It should be noted that anyone in the UK with a permanent stoma is currently exempt from prescription charges, but needs to complete the appropriate exemption paperwork; see http://www.nhs.uk/ for further information.

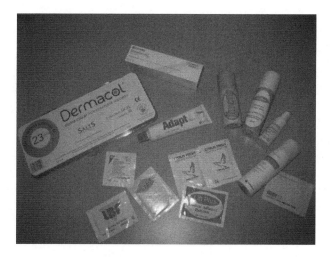

Figure 11.1 Appliances.

Colostomy irrigation

An alternative to a stoma appliance for colostomates (people with a colostomy) is to perform colostomy irrigation. This is undertaken to evacuate faeces and flatus from the distal colon and negates the need for a stoma appliance (Readding, 2006). The process involves instilling water into the colostomy, which will subsequently leave the stoma, evacuating the faeces and flatus. Specialist equipment is required, which the stoma CNS will be able to advise the colostomate on. Although this procedure allows the colostomate to be free from a colostomy appliance for one or two days, it is not a popular option in the UK and is potentially contraindicated for people with Crohn's disease because of concerns about a disease flare.

Nutrition

When considering diet ideally all ostomates can eat and drink anything. However, in practice this advice does not suit all ostomates, as everyone is individual. Diet will be considered for the colostomy and ileostomy separately.

Diet for colostomates

In general, colostomates can eat whatever foods they used to enjoy prior to their stoma-forming surgery. Adequate fluids and fibre help to prevent constipation and a balanced diet should be advised (Pearson, 2008). A balanced diet should of course consist of all the major food groups.

Diet for ileostomates

Ileostomates are not at risk of constipation (as the colon has been removed) and thus dietary fibre can be reduced, which many ostomates find to be beneficial. However, as the faeces are looser it is important to ensure that adequate fluids are taken (approximately two litres daily). Sodium is lost in the looser faeces, but most Western diets contain adequate sodium, so this loss is already compensated for without the need for an additional salt intake. Some foods, such as high-fibre or spicy foods, and alcoholic drinks can be less well tolerated and may cause loose stool. Problems such as a food bolus obstruction can occur if certain foods are not well chewed. These foods include fruit and vegetable skins, nuts, peas and sweetcorn; however, this list of potentially problematic foods is incomplete and may not be relevant to all ileostomates. A food bolus is most likely to occur in the first few weeks following surgery; thus some foods that are not initially tolerated may be suitable after the post-operative oedema has resolved.

Post-operation

During the hospital period the patient is trained by the stoma CNS to be independent with their stoma. This is a practical skill that in the majority of cases is mastered within a few days of the surgery by the ostomates. It should be noted that patients have only a short period in hospital in which to adapt and learn about their stoma and this period of time can be quite intense. Additionally, pre-operative information is reinforced to enable a safe discharge home.

Adjusting to life with a stoma

There are many issues that can psychologically affect ostomates, including changes to their body image (Borwell, 2009), grief at the loss of their body function or concerns about sexuality. Possible issues related to altered body image include the ostomate seeing the stoma as being disfiguring and embarrassing. Stoma formation is often an anxious and emotional time, with concerns for the changes that will and do occur. A few ostomates suffer with psychological problems that require referral for specialist therapy, although most, over time, do cope well. Nurses are in an ideal position to assist ostomates to cope with these concerns by listening, offering advice or arranging for ostomates to meet established ostomates.

In the initial post-operative period many individuals are preoccupied with learning to cope with their stoma appliance changes and often do not even consider other issues. These can manifest themselves weeks or months later, when recovery from the actual surgery has occurred. Wade (1990) reported on psychological adjustment at ten weeks and a year following surgery. Despite this work being 20 years old it has been confirmed by more recent studies by Pittman (2008), who found that there were a number of factors that can assist ostomates to cope, including a supportive partner. Wade's research suggests that follow-up at a year after surgery is beneficial to ostomates. Recent government legislation also supports yearly follow-up and although this is financially driven, it nonetheless should still be beneficial to ostomates.

Bathing and showering
Bathing and showering are safe and generally encouraged whilst still in the hospital. They can be undertaken with the appliance either on or off, depending on choice. However, there is a chance that the stoma will be active during this time, so most ostomates choose to wear an appliance. It should be noted that the appliance is easily and quickly dried if it is not to be replaced after bathing.

Discharge from hospital
Following discharge home, ostomates continue their adaptation to their stoma (Readding, 2005). There has been research on coping with a stoma, and when ostomates go home this can be a very difficult period. The problems that are reported relate to ostomates in general and are not specific to people with inflammatory bowel disease. Other issues of concern include the safety of resuming work or hobbies. However, in general after stoma-forming surgery it is possible to undertake almost any activity that was done prior to surgery. Patients with particular concerns regarding post-operative activities are encouraged to discuss them with the CNS and/or healthcare team.

Follow-up care
Usually there is follow-up by the surgeon and the stoma CNS, within a few weeks of discharge home. Currently in many areas there are few home visits performed either by the stoma CNS or the district nurse in the UK due to cost cuts. Follow-up in many hospitals by the stoma CNS is now performed in nurse-led stoma clinics. Follow-up care can vary widely, but will ideally include a post-operative review of the skin, stoma function, stoma appliance and stoma accessories. In the initial and longer term, it is important to ensure the ostomate is adjusting well, both physically and psychologically, to their stoma.

Written discharge information is important to reinforce oral information and to be used as a reminder. Education and knowledge that there is ongoing care, if required is essential. Many ostomates find local and/or national stoma support groups useful, but this is not appropriate for all. Details are given at the end of the chapter.

Common issues for ostomates

Work and hobbies

Within reason there is nothing that ostomates cannot do. However, it is important not to undertake heavy activities for a minimum of six weeks following the procedure, to allow healing to occur. This helps to reduce the risk of a parastomal hernia (herniation around the stoma), which is reported in up to three quarters of ostomates. Care is required if work or hobbies, such as contact sports, might inadvertently damage the stoma. To protect the stoma, a stoma shield and belt can be used. General advice following surgery would be not to return to work for at least two weeks. This will depend upon the age of the individual, the surgery undertaken and the level of recovery. Light duties or a shorter working week may be advisable when first returning to work, if possible.

Travel

Travel and a stoma are compatible. However, there are precautions that should be undertaken if flying. These include taking the stoma appliances as part of the hand luggage, in case of problems with luggage. It is also advisable to take twice as many supplies as are generally used. It can be useful to discuss extra hand luggage allowance with the airline prior to the flight. Some holiday insurance companies can be problematic for ostomates and in this instance the stoma support groups can be very useful. It should be noted that is not advisable to fly immediately after surgery in most cases.

Exercise

Although in the long term almost all exercises are possible for ostomates, it is advisable after any abdominal surgery not to undertake heavy lifting or strenuous exercise until the ostomate is fully recovered. As already mentioned, a parastomal hernia is common and wearing a support belt during exercise appears to reduce the risks of herniation (Thompson, 2008).

However, activities such as making a cup of tea/coffee and gentle housework are usually possible for most ostomates when first discharged home. This does not include more strenuous activities, such as vacuuming, for several weeks.

Many exercises are not suitable to be undertaken for several months after stoma-forming surgery, such as gym work or swimming. Swimming should not be undertaken until all wounds have healed, and should be deferred often for several months after surgery to allow healing to occur. Gentle exercise like walking is encouraged from the day following the operation. Early mobilisation helps to

prevent post-operative complications such as a chest infection or a DVT (deep vein thrombosis) and is beneficial in many other ways.

Driving is not advised for a period of time after the surgery. Usually a minimum of two weeks is advocated and only then if the person is physically able to undertake an emergency stop. Patients should be advised to check with their insurance company.

Clothing

Clothing requires consideration, but in general many ostomates can wear the clothes they wore prior to their stoma-forming surgery. There are several companies that produce specialist clothes for ostomates; these include underwear and swimming costumes with pockets that hold the stoma appliance; the stoma CNS can provide details of these products. Additionally some men choose to wear braces rather than belts as they find this more comfortable. High-waisted trousers may help to disguise the stoma appliance.

Quality of life

Work has been undertaken on the quality of life of ostomates, and although this was not specifically addressing people with IBD, the results indicated that the quality of life is more affected by issues other than the stoma itself (Pittman *et al.*, 2008). This includes the reason why the stoma was formed and whether it was curative, which for Crohn's disease it may not be. Nichols and Riemer (2008) surveyed ostomates, including people with IBD, and found that people with a supportive stable environment, such as married ostomates and those whose occupations remained the same after their stoma-forming surgery, reported a better quality of life.

Cultural and religious issues

There are a variety of cultural and religious issues that can affect the ostomate, such as language, food and clothing. Religious considerations are very individual and each member of particular faiths has different requirements. Muslims, for example, may use a 'clean' and 'dirty' hand and require cleansing before praying, which occurs five times daily. This may make changing the stoma appliance difficult, but can often be resolved by speaking to the religious leader (Black, 2009). Using a two-piece appliance in this situation, however, reduces the trauma to the peristomal skin caused by removing the stoma flange. Fasting and strict vegetarian diets can also cause problems with stoma function, and any issue raised should be individually addressed (Williams and Da Costa, 2006).

211

Sexual issues

Although many ostomates will not broach the subject of sex, it is important for the nurse to discuss this issue with patients. Patients following stoma-forming surgery are generally able to have sexual intercourse and children can usually be conceived. However, it is important to be realistic with ostomates and explain that in some cases problems can occur. Problems can include a possible reduction in fertility or erectile dysfunction, most commonly following pelvic surgery. However, the majority of ostomates can regain a fulfilling sex life. Some ostomates report that they have improved libidos following surgery, when the symptoms of IBD including lethargy are resolved.

Some practical tips on the subject include, prior to undertaking sexual relations, that the ostomate should ensure that the stoma appliance is securely intact and (in the case of ileostomates) that the appliance is emptied. This serves two purposes: there is less chance of appliance leakages and additionally the ostomate will have increased confidence and thus should be more relaxed.

Pregnancy for female ostomates may lead to potential problems with the appliance. As the abdomen grows during the pregnancy the stoma itself may increase in diameter, change shape or become shorter in length, and the appliance used prior to the pregnancy may no longer be the most appropriate appliance. The stoma CNS is the ideal person to assist the ostomate in this situation. It is advisable for the pregnant ostomate to see the stoma CNS for advice, as the stoma output may also become erratic in the later months of pregnancy.

Complications

In general, complications specific to stomas are best resolved by the stoma CNS. However, a basic knowledge is useful for all nurses. Two frequently encountered problems are appliance leakage and sore skin. The causes and treatment options are discussed below.

Appliance leakage

A common problem that can occur for ostomates in relation to their stoma is appliance leakage, which can be distressing; the stoma CNS should be contacted for advice. The cause may be, for example, a short-spouted ileostomy (Redmond *et al.*, 2009) and the appliance leakage can be resolved by using a convex stoma appliance and a belt. However, this needs to be assessed for suitability prior to being used, as convex appliances may not be appropriate in all situations, such as for patients with a parastomal hernia.

A change in weight, either a loss or gain, can change the shape of the abdomen and in particular the peristomal skin. This may result in skin creases or skin dips next to the stoma. These creases/dips can be 'levelled' by using a filler paste, strip paste or seals/washers to 'smooth' the skin surface prior to adhesion of the stoma appliance. This will more securely adhere the appliance to the skin and therefore stop the appliance from leaking.

Sore skin

Sore skin can occur quickly and is often the result of faeces touching the peristomal skin, caused by the appliance leaking. Sore skin can compromise the security of the stoma appliance and thus make it more likely that further leaks will occur. However, following assessment these are often easily resolved using specialist stoma accessories, as discussed earlier. The cause of the problem needs to be established by a careful nursing assessment of the ostomate. Sore skin might be the result of poor appliance changing technique, for example. This may include the skin being treated 'roughly' by the ostomate when removing the appliance or poor cleansing or drying of the peristomal skin. This problem can be resolved by re-training the ostomate or using adhesive remover. If the skin is wet and oozing it might be appropriate to use a sparse sprinkling of protective stoma powder, or a cool hairdryer can be used to dry the skin prior to the application of the stoma appliance.

Fistulae

A fistula is rare but potentially difficult to care for. Fistulae can occur for a number of reasons, but in relation to patients with IBD it is more common in people with Crohn's disease. A fistula can be described as an abnormal communication between two epithelial surfaces; more specifically, there can be joins between the bowel and the skin, known as enterocutaneous fistulae, which can be seen in Figure 11.2. There are many types of fistula; some of the most common are outlined in Table 11.2. This chapter will focus on the care of individuals with enterocutanous, rectovaginal, perianal and anorectal fistulae. The management of fistulae will require input from many members of the team, including gastroenterologists, surgeons and nurses, and most importantly the patients themselves.

Enterocutaneous fistulae

Post-operative enterocutaneous fistulae may be large or small in size. The fistulae will often pass through a weak area of skin, which may be the site of the operation,

Table 11.2 Types of fistula.

Type of fistula	Description
Rectovaginal	Connection between rectum and vagina
Perianal	Bowel to the perineum
Simple	Fistula track passing through the external sphincter muscles only
Complex	Can be multiple fistula tracks passing through the internal and external sphincter muscles
Enterocutaneous	Join between the bowel and the skin
Simple	Single bowel perforation without complications
Complex	Disruption of the bowel and seepage into the surrounding areas
High-output	Output that exceeds 500 ml daily
Low-output	Output below 500 ml daily
Post-operative	Possibly due to an anastomotic leak

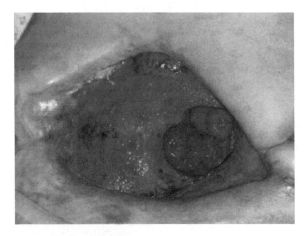

Figure 11.2 Enterocutaneous fistulae.

though an old surgical scar or drain site. Alternatively, there may be catastrophic complications following surgery and the abdominal wound may break down, resulting in a large open wound with faeces passing through it. This can be extremely distressing for the patient, as often the bowel is clearly visible in the wound bed and, even if the wound heals, there may be one or more areas of bowel left above the level of the abdominal wall. This in many cases can later be repaired surgically (Slater, 2009).

Case study

Carl was in his early thirties and had a long history Crohn's disease. At 21 Carl underwent a right hemi colectomy and was relatively well following this for several years. However, in the last two years Carl had multiple admissions to hospital and was diagnosed with strictures in his small bowel and a narrow anastomosis at the site of his previous resection. These led to obstructive symptoms, vomiting and abdominal pain. Carl was admitted to hospital and it was decided that surgery would be the best options: resection of the strictures.

The surgery was undertaken but Carl did not progress well, in the first few post-operative days his bowels did not open, his abdomen became distended and he began to have pain and vomiting. Other signs also worried the surgeons: Carl became pyrexial and his blood tests became deranged. Carl was taken back to theatre on the emergency list and was found to have a leakage from one of the joins of the small bowel. This was repaired and several drains were inserted. Unfortunately soon after surgery, bile-stained fluid passed from both drains and the wound dehisced. The wound size was in excess of 25 cm and there was disrupted bowel visible at the base of the wound. It was decided not to return to theatre but to manage the patient medically. Parenteral nutrition and intravenous antibiotics were commenced. Carl was initially instructed to be nil by mouth.

The stoma CNS assessed the fistula and advised the use of a wound manager, with seals/washers and paste to build up and smooth the surrounding skin. The wound manager was connected to a catheter bag and the 1500 ml output was recorded to ensure that appropriate volumes of fluid could be prescribed to replace losses. The wound manager took about one and a half hours to replace and was replaced every Tuesday and Friday. The surrounding skin occasionally became sore, but only rarely did the appliance leak. Six months after the last operation plans were made by the surgical team to re-operate. During this period Carl regained strength and continued on parenteral feed. Carl was allowed to gradually introduce a low-fibre diet and oral fluids and was discharged home to his family for a few months prior to his operation.

Caring for enterocutaneous fistulae

Caring for an enterocutaneous fistula involves the whole of the multidisciplinary team. The most important issues to address are the life-threatening conditions that may result, such as sepsis and electrolyte imbalance. This is covered more fully in

Chapter 12. The nursing care of the appliance required to maintain skin integrity will be discussed, as it is essential to maintain good condition of the skin surrounding the fistula to ensure that the fistula appliance adheres. This can be difficult, as the wound may be large and there are often skin dips and creases, making the skin surface unlevel. Additionally, the fistula output can vary, depending on the site of the fistula. A colonic fistula will have a lower output than a fistula from the ileum, and if the fistula occurs from the jejunum or the duodenum the faecal output will often be very high and corrosive to the skin.

To offer some practical advice, a fistula through a drain site with an output of a few hundred millilitres or less can often be securely contained by an ileostomy appliance, possibly with a seal/washer to help to 'level' uneven skin surfaces and protect the skin near the edge of the fistula from breaking down. In contrast, a large open wound with a fistula may require specialist fistula bags, which are large and costly, but can last for up to seven days (Figure 11.3). The skin can be protected in the same way as skin around the stoma, namely with a skin protector film. Furthermore, unlevel skin, dips and creases may require the use of seals/washers and minimal amounts of paste to 'level' the skin and prevent the appliance leaking. The stoma CNS should be sought for advice on individual patients.

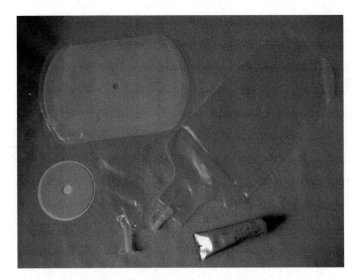

Figure 11.3 Fistula appliances and accessories.

Perianal, ano-rectal or rectovaginal fistula

Inflammatory bowel disease, particularly Crohn's disease, is the second leading cause of these types of fistula. Approximately one-third of all the patients with Crohn's disease will have perianal manifestations at some point in their lives (Person and Norgueras, 2006). Caring for patients with these types of fistula prior to, during and post-treatment involves skin care, management of discharge, care of setons, advice on maximising comfort, pain control and advice about sex. The following is intended to be a guide to assist in the everyday management of perianal, anorectal and rectovaginal fistulae.

Skin care – principles for optimum skin integrity

■ As much as possible keep the area clean and dry, which will help to avoid sore skin in this area (perianal region).
■ Shower/wash the area daily for hygiene.
■ Wash the area with warm water only – avoid using soap/shower gel as this is likely to irritate the area further.
■ Use good-quality toilet tissue or strong non-perfumed/non-lotion disposable wipes or cotton wool to dry.
■ Pat the area dry – do not rub the area vigorously as this will make the skin more irritated.
■ Use a barrier cream as needed to protect the skin around the area, which can become irritated and sore (this will depend on the amount/type of discharge from the fistula). Barrier creams such as Cavilon™ come in different applications (cream and lollipop sticks).
■ Preferably use natural fibre underwear (cotton).

Discharge

It is possible that the fistula may discharge on a regular basis and this can consist of blood, fluid/pus or loose/watery faecal matter.

■ For those who experience discharge from the fistula, it can help to wear a pad/panty liner in their underwear to collect any discharge and maintain hygiene. Scented panty liners can be purchased if there is an issue with odour from the discharge.
■ Frequently changing the pad/panty liner is ideal, as this will again help to maintain skin integrity in this area.
■ A course of oral antibiotics may be advised and can help to reduce the amount of discharge.

- If the fistula opening is very small, occasionally a ball of cotton wool will be sufficient to soak up any discharge.
- Wearing pads will also make it more comfortable to sit down.
- If the faecal matter is more solid then often there is less discharge experienced through the fistula – some patients will alter their diet to encourage more solid stools, but this is not always possible if there is active inflammation.
- The number of pads/panty liners changed in 24 hours can be a helpful measure of any increase or decrease in the amount of discharge from the fistula.

Setons (also see Chapter 9)
- Keep clean by wiping the seton (if loose setons *in situ*) following a bowel motion.
- The surgeon may advise patients further regarding any other techniques necessary to look after setons at the time of having them inserted.

General advice for patients
- Anecdotally it can help for patients to talk to family, including their partner, about their fistula, which helps the individual feel less isolated than when trying to manage this alone.
- Patients should be advised to talk frankly to their doctor (including gastroenterologist and surgeon) about their fistula. It is helpful for medical staff to understand how patients limit their daily activity to manage their own fistulae, as this will be different in each patient.
- Patients can be advised to choose softer seats to sit on.
- Use of cushions/pillows or rings (available from pharmacy) to sit on can help make it more comfortable. For example, donut rings can also help alleviate pressure and make sitting more comfortable.
- Alternatively, lying on one side on the sofa/bed can often be comfortable.
- Looser fitting clothing may be beneficial.
- Observe and report any signs of further skin breakdown, increase pain/ swelling to local nurse/doctor.
- Put together a kit which will allow patients to manage a fistula (when away from home) – such a kit might contain:
  - Disposable wipes/cotton wool
  - A dispenser (filled with water)
  - Pads/panty liners
  - Barrier cream
  - Small plastic bag to dispose of used pads etc.
  - Mirror and scissors if needed

Pain control

Occasionally, perianal fistulae in particular can be painful, making everyday activities such as walking and sitting for extended periods difficult. It is necessary therefore to have adequate pain control, and patients can be advised to contact their gastroenterologist or local specialist nurse for individualised further advice.

Sexual intercourse

How possible it is for patients to engage in sexual intercourse will depend on many factors, but perhaps the most important is the amount of discomfort and discharge experienced from the fistula. Often because of the above factors it is not possible for patients to have sexual intercourse. However, again it is best for patients to discuss this with their partner during these times.

Conclusion

It can be seen that having stoma-forming surgery can lead to many potential problems, but that life for the ostomate can be fulfilling. This is especially true for individuals with support from family, friends, groups and/or healthcare professionals. Furthermore, fistulae can be difficult to care for, but the stoma/IBD CNS is available for help for both patients and members of the multidisciplinary team. It is important to remember that nurses help ostomates, and patients with fistulae, to adjust by giving clear, simple and appropriate information, advice and support to the individual (and those close to them) where and when they need it.

Patient translation summary

For patients with IBD the prospect of having a permanent or temporary stoma may have 'loomed' over their head for a long time, or it might come as a relief of symptoms. Although in many cases a permanent stoma will not be the operation chosen by patients with ulcerative colitis, who may prefer an ileoanal pouch, it is an option and should be discussed to ensure that an informed choice is made. Long-term support for ostomates can be sought from the stoma CNS or the ostomy support groups in relation to their stoma. However, it is important for patients to have realistic expectations of life with a stoma or fistula. The lifestyle of ostomates does often change after their stoma is formed, and in general ostomates cope well with these changes, but periodically may require support from nurses.

Stoma support groups

There are a number of support groups that can be contacted by ostomates. There are national stoma groups for colostomates and ileostomates, and many hospitals also run local groups that may be useful.

Colostomy Association:
Telephone: (+44) (0)800 328 4257
Website: http://www.colostomyassociation.org.uk/

Ileostomy and internal pouch support group:
Telephone: (+44) (0)800 0184 724
Website: http://www.the-ia.org.uk/

References

Black, P. (2009) Cultural and religious beliefs in stoma care nursing. *Br. J. Nursing*, **18**, 790–3.

Borwell, B. (2009) Continuity of care for the stoma patients: psychological considerations. *Br. J. Community Nursing*, **14**, 326–31.

Bradshaw, E. and Collins, B. (2009) Managing a colostomy or ileostomy in community nursing practice. *Br. J. Community Nursing*, **13**, 514–18.

Burch, J. (2008) Stomas: the past, present and future. In: *Stoma Care* (ed. J. Burch). West Sussex: Wiley-Blackwell.

McPhail, J. (2003) Selection and use of stoma care appliances. In: *Stoma Care Nursing* (ed. C. Elcoat). London: Hollister.

Nichols, T. and Riemer, M. (2008) The impact of stabilizing forces on postsurgical recovery in ostomy patients. *J. Wound, Continence and Ostomy Nursing*, **35**, 316–30.

Pearson, M. (2008) Nutrition. In: *Stoma Care* (ed. J. Burch). West Sussex: Wiley-Blackwell.

Person, B. and Norgueras, J. (2006) The management of rectovaginal fistulas in patients with inflammatory bowel disease. *Seminars in Colon and Rectal Surg.*, **17**, 68–75.

Persson, E., Berndtsson, I., Carlsson, E., Hallén, A.-M. and Lindholme, E. (2009) Ostomy related complications and ostomy size – a two year follow-up. *Colorectal Dis.* 'Accepted Article'; doi: 10.111/j.1463-1318.2009.01941.x.

Pittman, J., Rawl, S. M., Schmidt, C. M., Grant, M., Ko, C. Y., Wendel, C. and Krouse, R. S. (2008) Demographic and clinical factors related to ostomy complications and quality of life in veterans with an ostomy. *J. Wound, Ostomy and Continence Nursing*, **35**, 493–503.

Readding, L. A. (2005) Hospital to home: smoothing the journey for the new ostomist. *Br. J. Nursing*, **14**, S16–S20.

Readding, L. (2006) Colostomy irrigation – an option worth considering. *Gastrointest. Nursing*, **4**, 27–33.

Redmond, C., Cowin, C. and Parker, T. (2009) The experience of faecal leakage among ileostomists. *British Journal of Nursing*. **18**(17): S12-S17.

Rudoni, C. and Dennis, H. (2009) Accessories or necessities? Exploring consensus on usage of stoma accessories. *Br. J. Nursing*, **18**, 1106–12.

Rust, J. (2009) Understanding the complexities of the clinical nurse specialist: a focus on stoma siting. *Gastrointest. Nursing*, **7**(4), 18–26.

Slater, R. (2009) Nutritional management of enterocutaneous fistulas. *Gastrointest. Nursing*, **18**(4), 225–30.

Thompson, M. J. (2008) Parastomal hernia: incidence, prevention and treatment strategies. *Br. J. Nursing*, **17**(2), 16–21.

Wade, B. E. (1990) Colostomy patients: psychological adjustment at 10 weeks and 1 year after surgery in districts which employed stoma-care nurses and districts which did not. *J. Adv. Nursing*, **15**, 1297–304.

White, M. and Berg, K. (2005) A new flangeless adhesive coupling system for colostomy and ileostomy. *Br. J. Nursing*, **14**(6), 325–8.

Williams, J. and Da Costa, M. (2006) Cultural aspects of stoma care nursing. *Gastrointest. Nursing*, **4**(1), 12–16.

CHAPTER 12

Intestinal failure

Jeremy Nightingale and Hannah Middleton

Introduction

Intestinal failure (IF) occurs when the gut cannot absorb enough nutrients and/or salt and water to prevent malnutrition and/or dehydration (Nightingale *et al.*, 2006). While this can be due to a failure of any part of the digestive system, including the stomach and pancreas, this chapter will focus on problems due to poor absorption by the intestine itself, with particular reference to inflammatory bowel disease. Most patients with intestinal failure do not require parenteral nutrition.

Crohn's disease certainly constitutes the larger group of patients affected by IF, mainly due to the potential complications associated with the disease. IF can result from intestinal removal, abdominal sepsis (due to a bowel perforation), enteric fistula(e), obstruction (due to current or past inflammation or adhesions) or extensive small intestinal disease. A less common scenario would be the patient with ulcerative colitis being affected by IF. However, surgical complications, including obstruction from adhesions or bowel resections that leave a short remaining length of small intestine can result in IF.

The severity of intestinal failure is based upon the type of nutrition or fluid (in IF fluid refers to sodium and water) support given.

- **Mild**: refers to the need for oral nutrient supplements or dietary modification, with/without a glucose saline solution.
- **Moderate**: when an enteral tube is needed to give a liquid feed and/or a glucose saline solution.
- **Severe**: when parenteral (intravenous) nutrition and/or saline is needed.

Regardless of the severity, the patient with IF will need continuing support from a variety of healthcare professionals, mainly the nutrition support team, including the consultant gastroenterologist, dietitians, nutrition nurse specialists, stoma care nurses and of course, during the acute phase of IF, ward nurses. These relationships will be explored fully later in the chapter.

Intestinal failure is typically classified into three types (Lal *et al.*, 2006):

■ **Type 1** is short-term IF and often occurs immediately after surgery as a paralytic ileus, where the intestine is temporarily paralysed, therefore not allowing any food or fluid to pass. This is common and may be exacerbated by opiate drugs, abdominal sepsis and the excessive administration of 'normal' saline. It is usually managed with parenteral nutrition for up to two weeks and normally resolves spontaneously.

■ **Type 2** or medium-term IF usually follows surgery but can be reversible. IF may be present for much longer than two weeks – often months or years – before it is possible to complete reconstructive surgery. The most common complications post-operatively that result in this type of IF are enterocutaneous fistulae or small bowel obstruction. The potential surgical procedures to reverse the IF could be a resection of a fistula tract or to re-establish bowel continuity.

■ **Type 3** or long-term IF is when the situation is not considered reversible and long-term nutritional support is needed. Type 3 IF is usually due to patients having a short bowel with or without some remaining functioning colon.

Case studies
The following are typical of the cases that present with intestinal failure.

Case 1
Patient with Crohn's disease who has had three previous ileocolonic resections and presents with weight loss and diarrhoea, but no evidence of active Crohn's disease. In this situation, owing to previous surgery, this patient is likely to fall into the category of short bowel with jejunum anatomised to colon.

Case 2
Patient with Crohn's disease who has had a colectomy and the ileostomy refashioned three times. The patient then subsequently presents with dehydration and low magnesium. This patient is likely to behave as having a jejunostomy.

Case 3
Patient post ileal resection has a breakdown of the abdominal wound and small bowel fluid discharges through the wound. This indicates an enterocutaneous fistula.

Understanding the bowel

Understanding the function of the bowel is important when considering the concept of intestinal failure. The gastrointestinal tract has a complex function which relies upon each segment to fulfil its role. It is understandable therefore, that if a proportion is damaged or removed the overall function will be compromised.

Small bowel length

Normal intestinal length, measured at autopsy, at surgery or radiologically, gives a range of small bowel length of 275–850 cm (Figure 12.1). This large range of normal gut length is essential to understanding the variable outcomes after a small bowel resection. For example, a resection of 100–200 cm may have little or no effect on a patient who starts with a small bowel length of 8 metres, but could

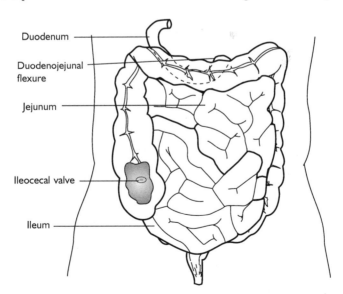

Duodenum
Duodenojejunal flexure
Jejunum
Ileocecal valve
Ileum

Figure 12.1 Duodenum, jejunum and ileum.

225

result in the need for long-term nutritional support if the starting length is less than 3 metres. This demonstrates the importance for surgeons to measure the remaining length of small intestine. This measurement is much more relevant for predicting outcome than the amount removed.

Motility

An example of motility can be demonstrated by considering a meal accompanied by fluid as it passes through the gastrointestinal tract. If an average adult were to have a pancake and orange juice meal, liquids pass quickly out of the stomach (50% within 98 min) and solids more slowly (50% within 150 min). Transit is faster through the jejunum than the ileum and when the food reaches the large bowel, colonic transit is slow and the contents of the caecum take two days before being passed as stool (Figure 12.1).

Secretions

For an average adult, each day about 2 kg of food and drink is consumed. To digest and absorb this, the gut secretes 500 ml saliva, 2000 ml gastric acid and 1500 ml pancreaticobiliary secretions. So each day about 6 litres of chyme (partly digested food) passes the duodenojejunal flexure, and over half of this is absorbed in the first metre of small intestine. Even in the absence of food (nil by mouth) there is secretion into the gut and about 500–1000 ml of secretions will pass the duodenojejunal flexure each day.

Absorptive properties

The distal ileum, extending for approximately 60 cm proximal to the ileocaecal valve, is needed for the absorption of vitamin B_{12}. Therefore, if removed or damaged, B_{12} deficiency is likely and supplementation may be required. The distal ileum (extending 100 cm proximal to the ileocaecal valve absorbs primary and secondary bile acids, and if diseased or removed may result in diarrhoea. Unabsorbed bile acids can have an irritant effect on the colons mucosal cells, inhibiting absorption and causing secretion of salt and water. A SeHCAT scan may be useful to confirm this diagnosis and justify a trial of a bile salt sequestering agent (e.g. cholestyramine).

The intercellular junctions in the jejunum are described as leaky, so allowing salt and water to diffuse into the gut lumen till the gut lumen contents have an osmolality of about 300 mOsm/kg (like plasma) and a sodium concentration of about 100 mmol/l (range 90–140). The jejunal enterocytes have an intracellular pump that moves sodium and glucose (or some amino acids) together from the jejunal lumen into the cell. The intercellular junctions in the ileum are tight, so the luminal contents can be concentrated.

Magnesium is absorbed throughout the large and small bowel. Its absorption is promoted by 1,25 hydroxycholecalciferol (active vitamin D). If a patient is salt- and water-depleted, plasma aldosterone levels will be high. The high aldosterone levels cause sodium absorption within the kidney, but at the expense of magnesium, and also potassium, which are secreted into the urine.

Colonic function

The colon has a large capacity to absorb salt and water (up to 4–6 litres/24 hours), ferment carbohydrate and make some vitamins (e.g. vitamin K). It also slows upper gut transit when exposed to unabsorbed nutrients, and increases upper gut mucosal growth. Thus there are major advantages if a surgeon can preserve all or some of the colon at the time of performing a bowel resection.

Types of short bowel and problems

In clinical practice two types of patient with a short bowel are encountered: those with a jejunostomy (stoma) and those with jejunum anastomosed to part or all of their colon (Figure 12.2). A patient is considered to have a short bowel if less than 200 cm small bowel (measured from the duodenojejunal flexure) remains. Often it is not realised that a patient has a short bowel, but there are clues in the presentation. Both are likely to have had one or more small bowel resections and may already need B_{12} injections. A patient with a jejunostomy often presents to hospital with recurrent 'ileostomy diarrhoea' needing intravenous saline and

Jejunostomy   Jejuno-colic anastomosis

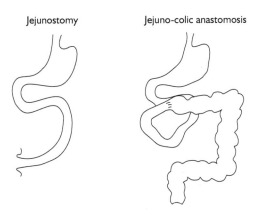

Figure 12.2 Types of patient with a short bowel.

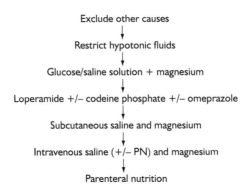

Figure 12.3 Management of patient with jejunostomy and a high-output stoma.

magnesium (Figure 12.3). Malnutrition may be less obvious and is certainly a less immediate problem. This contrasts with a patient with jejunum-colon who may present more insidiously with malnutrition and diarrhoea (steatorrhoea).

Both patient groups have problems of malnutrition and they also have a high risk of developing pigment gallstones (45%), which are often calcified and are more common in men. Jejunum-colon patients have a 25% chance of developing calcium oxalate renal stones and they have a rare risk of D-lactic acidosis if their colonic bacteria manufacture the D (not L) isomer of lactic acid.

It is likely that the patient with a high-output stoma will be suffering a degree of dehydration (in IF this refers to sodium and water depletion). Assessing the state of dehydration can be achieved by asking about thirst, assessing the skin turgor and mucus membranes, performing daily weights at the same time each day (a sudden drop of more than 1 kg in 1–2 days suggests fluid loss), measuring the lying and standing blood pressure (a systolic drop of more than 10 mm Hg with a rise in the heart rate suggests dehydration) and measuring a random urine sodium concentration (less than 10 mmol/l suggests salt depletion). If severely dehydrated creatinine and urea will be raised.

Exclude other causes
High output (more than 2 litres daily) from a stoma can be from causes other than a short bowel and these should be investigated thoroughly. A contrast (BaFT) follow-through radiological examination is most likely to help with both defining other causes and estimating the length of bowel remaining. Based upon the bowel length remaining, the fluid and nutrient requirements can be predicted

Table 12.1 Guide to bowel length and long-term fluid/nutritional support needed by patients with a short bowel (Nightingale *et al.*, 2006).

Jejunal length (cm)	Jejunum-colon	Jejunostomy
0–50	PN	PN + PS
51–100	ON	PN + PS*
101–150	None	ON + OGS
151–200	None	OGS

*: at 85–100 cm may need PS only
PN: Parenteral nutrition
PS: Parenteral saline (± magnesium)
ON: Oral (or enteral) nutrition
OGS: Oral (or enteral) glucose/saline solution

(Table 12.1). The most common reason other than a short bowel is partial or intermittent obstruction (Baker *et al.*, 2009). This is suggested by a history of colicky abdominal pain with or without vomiting during which the stoma may stop working; as the obstruction resolves the stomal output becomes high and it is often then that the patient becomes dehydrated and presents to hospital. When examining such a patient the stoma is inspected and a finger inserted gently into it, as this is the most common site for a stenosis. The treatment is often as simple as advice on a low fibre diet, (Table 12.2) though if persistent, strictures may be treated with endoscopic balloon dilatation, surgery or if at the stoma the regular use of dilators. Some patients with obstruction do additionally have problems of small bowel bacterial overgrowth and they can be helped by a broad spectrum antibiotic (for example co-amoxiclav).

Table 12.2 Low fibre diet.

Avoid	Vegetables/fruit
	Nuts
	Wholemeal products
Eat	Meat/fish/eggs
	Dairy
	White rice/pasta/bread
	Potato without skin
	Jelly

Other causes of a high output stoma include, drug withdrawal (opiates or steroids), certain medications, such as metoclopramide, enteric infection (e.g. clostridium), abdominal sepsis (often associated with a low serum albumin), recurrent disease (including enteroenteric fistulae), duodenal/jejunal diverticulae and other common associated conditions (for example coeliac disease). Treating these will usually resolve the high-output stoma.

Reduce oral intake

This is the most difficult aspect of treatment for a patient to comply with, as they feel thirsty. However, if they drink hypotonic fluids (tea, coffee, orange juice etc.) which contain no sodium they will actually become more thirsty. This is due to the sodium, which will diffuse from plasma into the small bowel lumen to give a luminal concentration of 100 mmol/l. This is then lost from the stoma, so the more that is drunk the more sodium is lost, which results in the patient feeling the continuous need to drink more fluid. At first it is often helpful for the patient to be 'nil by mouth' for 24 hours while rehydrating with saline (to which magnesium has been added). This should allow the patient to be fully rehydrated and no longer thirsty. It also shows the patient that their stomal output is driven by their oral intake. When an oral regimen is restarted normal hypotonic oral fluids are kept to 500–1000 ml daily and an IV fluid regimen sometimes accompanies this. A great deal of support is required when expecting a patient to comply with this regimen, as initially it can be difficult for the patient to understand the physiology. Education is very important: understanding the reasons behind these restrictions help the patient keep to the programme. A strict fluid balance chart should be maintained. It is reasonable to assist the patient to complete this, but it is important that it be an accurate measurement of their progress.

Give glucose–saline solution orally

An electrolyte solution with a sodium concentration of 90–120 mmol/l and glucose (monomer or oligosaccharide) is sipped during the day (Table 12.3), it may be flavoured (e.g. lime) and drunk cold to increase the palatability. When a patient is salt-depleted they often do not notice the saltiness of the solution. However, some find that the removal of tea and coffee is very difficult to cope with. Throughout this process there is a definite transition, and occasionally an element of negotiation is required between medical teams and the patient.

Table 12.3 The modified WHO cholera rehydration solution for patients with a high-output jejunostomy/ileostomy.

Sodium chloride	60 mmol (3.5 gm)
Sodium bicarbonate (or citrate)	30 mmol (2.5 gm) (2.9 gm)
Glucose	110 mmol (20 gm)
Tap water	One litre
Alternative rehydration solution	
Sodium chloride	120 mmol (7 gm)
Glucose	44 mmol (8 gm)
Tap water	one litre

Drug treatment

Loperamide given half an hour before meals (sometimes tipped out of the capsule) slows transit allowing more time for absorption. As loperamide circulates through the entero-hepatic circulation, which is severely disrupted in patients with a short bowel, very high doses may be needed (10 mg or more four times a day, half an hour before food). Codeine phosphate (30–60 mg four times a day, half an hour before food) may give an additional benefit; but it is addictive, sedative and reduces pancreatico-biliary secretion so is not usually given immediately.

When the gut is less than 100 cm, proton pump inhibitors (e.g. omeprazole 40 mg once or twice daily) will reduce gastric acid output and will therefore significantly reduce the stomal output. When given in adequate dose the stomal pH should be more than 5. Octreotide injections (50 μg twice daily) have a similar effect to oral omeprazole in terms of the volume reduction of stomal output, so is rarely given due to the more complicated administration. Other options being developed include clonidine patches and teduglutide (a GLP-2 analogue) injections.

Magnesium

Correction of dehydration and sodium depletion are the most important measures to reduce secondary hyperaldosteronism and thus the urinary magnesium losses. Magnesium oxide is the preferred magnesium salt and may be given as 12 mmol at night. 1-alpha cholecalciferol can be given in gradually increasing doses to promote the gut absorption of magnesium, but care must be taken to avoid hypercalcaemia. If unsuccessful, magnesium may need to be given in saline either subcutaneously or intravenously (Figure 12.3).

231

Oral nutrition

These patients do not have restrictions on the fat, carbohydrate or protein that they eat, as a constant proportion of each is absorbed. A referral to a dietitian should be made for advice on how to maximise the absorption of the remaining bowel. This relationship between dietitian and patient will be significant, as the need to explore different options through diet arises. A hyperosmolar nutrient solution (e.g. elemental diet) should be avoided as it causes water to move by osmosis into the gut lumen. In addition, it contains little salt, so sodium will diffuse into the bowel lumen, which increases water and sodium loss from the stoma. If oral supplements or enteral feeds are required to maintain weight, the ideal solution for these patients would contain 100 mmol/l sodium and have an osmolality of 300 mOsm/kg.

Management of the patient with jejunum-colon anastomosis

Dietary treatment for the patient with jejunum-colon anastomosis

These patients rarely have excess sodium and water losses. They need a high polysaccharide diet to utilise colonic fermentation (Nordgaard *et al.*, 1994) but also one low in oxalate to reduce the risk of making calcium oxalate renal stones (Nightingale *et al.*, 1992). A low oxalate diet generally means avoiding rhubarb, beetroot, spinach and excessive amounts of tea. Fat is a good source of energy and makes food palatable, but unabsorbed fatty acids in the colon cause salt and water secretion and inhibit bacterial fermentation; therefore fat is not encouraged.

Adaptation in patients with a short bowel

Patient's with jejunum-colon show an improvement in absorption with time (up to three years) and will need fewer nutrients. This is probably due to two colonic gut hormones peptide YY and GLP-2 slowing transit and increasing small bowel growth respectively. Analogues of these may be useful in treating these patients in the future. There is no evidence for any improvement in gut function with time in those with a jejunostomy.

Results for small bowel transplantation are improving and carefully selected patients with Crohn's disease may be appropriate for this treatment (Nightingale *et al.*, 2006).

Sepsis and enterocutaneous fistulae

The major cause of mortality in patients with short/medium-term intestinal failure is abdominal sepsis. This is usually from a perforation in the gut due to the Crohn's disease itself, a surgical anastomosis or the surgical repair of a serosal tear. In addition to the obvious signs of sepsis (fever, tachycardia, high white blood count (WBC), low albumin) there may be more subtle indicators, such as the patient's weight/muscle mass not increasing despite adequate oral, enteral or parenteral nutrition, the blood glucose rising (especially on parenteral nutrition) and the patient continuing to look ill with poor or no appetite. Sepsis must be sought with radiological imaging and drained. Other immediate issues relate to hydration (salt and water balance), wound management and pain relief.

The key to managing an enterocutaneous fistula is for the gut contents to drain quickly from the body without them collecting and setting up an inflammatory reaction. If there is a developing collection the patient may present without the clues to sepsis, but being non-specifically unwell. Any patient with ongoing sepsis does not put on weight/muscle with nutritional support, hence sepsis should be drained/treated as a priority. If a patient has taken no food for 5 or more days or is already undernourished (judged by a BMI < 18.5 kg/m² and percentage weight loss > 10%) then nutritional support is needed (National Collaborating Centre for Acute Care group producing NICE guidelines, 2006). This group of patients has a large team involved in their care; this includes specialist gastroenterologists and colorectal surgeons, as well as the nutrition support team. Table 12.4 lists steps taken when managing enterocutaneous fistulae.

Table 12.4 Management of enterocutaneous fistula.

Immediate	Water/electrolytes (Na⁺, Mg⁺⁺)
	Sepsis
	Wound management
	Pain control
Early	Nutrition (refeeding risks) Oral, EN or PN
	Psychosocial
	Mobility
Late	Anatomy (site of fistula, drainage)
	Procedure – Not days 10–100

Oral/enteral or parenteral nutrition for enterocutaneous fistula management

It has been customary to always try to feed into the gut whenever possible. However, this view is being challenged now that parenteral nutrition can be given safely with a low rate of catheter-related sepsis, without giving too much energy (so avoiding liver function abnormalities) and with tight blood glucose control. The evidence that enteral feeding is good because it reduces bacterial translocation and promotes mucosal growth is not definite; however, it does prevent bowel atrophy. An atrophied bowel can be technically difficult to anastomose to the end of normal sized bowel (often a side-to-side anastomosis is needed). If an enteral feed does leak into the abdominal cavity it is an extremely good culture medium that can cause severe sepsis. Thus the old regimen of nil by mouth and parenteral nutrition is often a safe option and at least the amount of energy entering the patient is known (with enteral feeding there is often an unknown amount of absorption, especially when the bowel is oedematous). In considering whether to give oral/enteral nutrition several factors need to be taken into account as described below.

Is the bowel perforation near to the cutaneous exit site?

Most commonly the fistula is from bowel at the abdominal incision site and there is no intra-abdominal leak of intestinal contents, so feeding can be into the gut. If there is a posterior/deep perforation, the bowel contents are likely to collect before finding a way out, either by going round the abdominal wall or through the abdominal cavity. A perforation site is most likely at an anastomotic site or where a mucosal tear has been repaired. A perforation distant from the exit site is likely to be associated with abdominal sepsis and (especially in the first few weeks) radiological or surgical drainage can be performed. In the early stages (first two weeks) a posterior/deep perforation is most safely managed with nil by mouth and parenteral nutrition; oral/enteral nutrition may be introduced later when patient is out of ITU and mobile.

What is the stage of development of the fistula tract?

When the gut first perforates, the bowel contents spread within the abdomen (Figure 12.4). If urgent surgery has not been performed to drain it, fibrous tissue appears and eventually keeps the sepsis fluid more localised. The fluid then finds the easiest way out of the body and this is usually though a suture line (commonly the midline abdominal incision) or a drain site. As a fistula tract matures it is less likely for the bowel contents to leak into the peritoneal cavity and cause sepsis. After several months, small bowel at a fistula site may protrude and look like an ileostomy spout. This is a good sign and means the peritoneal cavity is becoming re-established; it also makes caring for the fistula easier. Stoma care nurses can provide care plans and guidance to assist both the patient/relatives and ward nurses in caring for and managing the fistula.

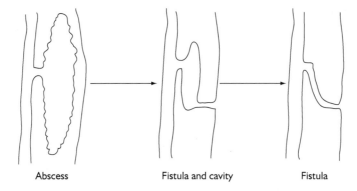

Abscess   Fistula and cavity   Fistula

Figure 12.4 Development of an enterocutaneous fistula.

How far down the gut is the fistula (cm from DJ flexure)
If a fistula tract is within 100 cm of the DJ flexure and if most of the bowel content exits from the tract (no stool or other stomal output), then parenteral support is likely to be needed. This level of nutritional support would be required until the fistula closes spontaneously or is surgically closed. At a greater distance than this oral/enteral nutrition may be used provided the fluid is exiting from the body without collecting.

What is the chance of spontaneous closure?
There are many factors which could hinder spontaneous closure of a fistula. Distal bowel obstruction or active disease at the fistula site will not allow healing. Discontinuity of the bowel ends, an abscess at the site of the fistula or ongoing sepsis will also keep the fistula(e) tract open. Moreover, multiple fistulae or mucocutaneous continuity (the bowel mucosa being visible at the surface of the abdomen) will certainly prevent spontaneous closure.

Once a fistula is draining, there is no associated sepsis, and the patient is nutritionally stable (with oral, enteral or parenteral nutrition) then active inflammatory bowel disease may be treated. This is usually achieved by utilising immunosuppressive drugs, such as azathioprine, mercaptopurine or methotrexate. Recurrent disease may be prevented if these medications are started several months before surgery and then continued for at least six months post-operatively. Occasionally biological treatments are given.

Obstruction

Recurrent episodes of colicky abdominal pain with vomiting suggest bowel obstruction. This can be due to active or inactive Crohn's disease or adhesions. The obstruction can be resulting from one or multiple narrowings.

Management

The activity of Crohn's disease is assessed. Blood tests that suggest activity are high platelets (also WBC), high CRP and low serum albumin. As blood results can be normal if there is only a small area of active disease, imaging is useful and may include a BaFT or MRI. Active Crohn's disease is treated in the usual way depending upon the diseased sites, although care may be needed with biological agents as they may worsen an obstruction. Fibre can cause further blockages as it cannot be easily digested, so a low-fibre diet (Table 12.2) will be recommended. Surgery is performed (resection or stricturoplasty) if the obstructive episodes are frequent or an episode persists despite medical and dietary treatment. Chronic fibrotic strictures may be balloon dilated at endoscopy if short (less than 3 cm), and surprisingly the benefit of a dilatation to 12–20 mm can last for several years, though eventually a surgical resection may be needed.

Active extensive Crohn's disease

If the intestinal failure is due to extensive small bowel Crohn's disease this must be treated in the usual way with immunosuppressive drugs or biological treatments. However, a patient's nutritional status must be maintained with oral, enteral or parenteral nutrition. Liquid diets (elemental, peptide or polymeric) may be effective in inducing and maintaining remission in Crohn's disease, but are not as effective as corticosteroids (Zachos *et al.*, 2007; Akobeng, 2007).

Nursing considerations

As previously mentioned, the patient with intestinal failure holds the attention of many healthcare professionals. Ward nurses are central to the care of the patient in the acute phase of treatment. Some patients at this time will maintain a strong psychological attitude; however, many grieve the loss of function and will need support when adapting to this radical change. Anecdotally, patients who have been chronically unwell tend to adapt to the situation, whereas patients who have suddenly become unwell have difficulty adapting.

The nutrition team will be closely involved, reviewing the patient every day and monitoring blood results. They will also require daily weights, lying and standing BPs and meticulously kept fluid input/output charts to ensure that the patient is receiving the correct fluid balance. Whether the patient is relying upon enteral or parenteral nutrition, the nutrition nurse will be available to assist in teaching, education and ongoing support.

Supporting the patient requiring home parenteral nutrition

During the first few weeks of commencing parenteral nutrition (PN), the regimen may need alteration to reach the ideal requirements for the patient. During this time, if it is known that the patient will need nutritional support on a medium- or long-term basis, teaching should begin and an application for funding requested. This application is made to the patient's primary care trust, as funding for home care needs to be secured prior to discharge. Logistical arrangements can be considered at this point also; for example, the positioning of a fridge at home (specifically for the PN) and storage solutions.

The teaching of the patient and/or relatives is usually instigated by the nutrition nurse specialist. However, ward nurses should assist where possible to ensure that the patient feels confident and well practised at the specific techniques. Local policies need to be adhered to when taking care of central lines and the importance of stringent cleaning should be addressed before any practical competencies are achieved. Catheter-related sepsis can be avoided with a good technique and it is critical that the patient is aware of the potential danger of severe sepsis. Patients with a stoma bag and/or enterocutaneous fistula are required to be especially vigilant due to the possible cross-contamination of the central line.

Once discharged home, great responsibility is placed on the patient and on the family. Having to remember all the procedures and how to deal with serious complications should they arise can be daunting (Lennard-Jones *et al.*, 1992). Each department should therefore provide a comprehensive tool that can be used to troubleshoot. The patient should also be aware of the support available, including the home care company (which employs registered nurses) and the hospital specialist nurses who are available to contact if problems arise.

Psychological implications of intestinal failure and long-term parenteral nutrition

Many patients requiring home parenteral nutrition (HPN) will not take any food orally and their fluid intake may be heavily restricted (Stern *et al.*, 2008). Food and drink are related to many social engagements, but also play an important part in everyday interactions. Many families eat meals together, giving them the opportunity to communicate about their day. Excluding oneself from these experiences can leave the patient feeling incapable of maintaining a social life.

237

The family also has to adapt to the new routine, perhaps finding alternative ways to spend time together. They need to have understanding that the patient will have limited ability to act spontaneously: all activities involve considerable planning (Carlsson *et al.*, 2001). Once well established on parenteral nutrition, quality of life can certainly improve. Patients become independent in dealing with their central line, empowering them to seek a 'normal' way of life. For example, travelling abroad can seem like an extraordinary effort at first, but with help from the nutrition team in secondary care and the home support team who deliver their nutrition, this should prove to be a stress-free and rewarding experience.

Patients with intestinal failure may have concerns about body image. Whether they have a stoma, fistula or central venous catheter (CVC), there may be negative feelings about their body and how others might perceive it. Some people find the concept of forming new relationships a challenge, not knowing how to explain their condition and what the future might hold. Ongoing support from the specialist nurses will assist the patient in dealing with these changes, however, a referral to a psychology service would also be beneficial to most.

Depression associated with long-term conditions is well documented (Department of Health, 2006). Patients reliant on parenteral nutrition are no exception, and therefore psychological support is paramount. Professionals in contact with the patient need to be vigilant with regard to potential self-harm. Recurrent line sepsis might be a sign of intentional cross-contamination. The patient should be reassessed in the tasks related to CVC care and close supervision is required due to the potentially life-threatening complications related to line sepsis. Repeated episodes of line damage should also raise questions. Vigilant staff can be aware of these dangers and try to prevent serious complications through education and psychological input.

Conclusion

Intestinal failure occurs when the body is unable to digest food and absorb the fluids, nutrients and electrolytes essential for life. Crohn's disease is the more common of the inflammatory bowel diseases to cause intestinal failure, due to severely active disease or as the result of surgery or adhesions. The bowel has a complex function which is compromised when a proportion is damaged or removed. If less than 200 cm of small bowel remains, intestinal failure may occur. Patients requiring parenteral nutrition on a medium or long-term basis demand a high level of education and multidisciplinary support.

Patient translation summary

- Intestinal failure occurs when the gut cannot absorb enough nutrients and or salt and water to prevent malnutrition and/or dehydration.
- Crohn's disease is more likely than ulcerative colitis to cause intestinal failure, due to the potential complications and small bowel involvement.
- Understanding how the bowel functions is critical when considering intestinal failure, as each part has a purpose which when removed or damaged compromises the overall function.
- The two types of patient with a short bowel are those with a jejunostomy (stoma) and those with jejunum anastomosed to part or all of their colon.
- With a jejunostomy, fluid restriction will be needed; this is the hardest intervention for the patient to comply with due to excessive thirst.
- Psychological input should not be overlooked.
- Nursing support and training are needed during both the acute phase within the hospital and when the patient is discharged home.

References

Akobeng, A. K. and Thomas, A. G. (2007) Enteral nutrition for maintenance of remission in Crohn's disease. *Cochrane Database Syst. Rev.*, Issue 3: CD005984.

Baker, M. L., Williams, R. N. and Nightingale, J. M. (2009) Causes and management of a high output stoma. *Colorectal Dis.* Nov 3: [Epub ahead of print].

Carlsson, E., Berglund, B. and Nordgren, S. (2001) Living with an ostomy and short bowel syndrome: practical aspects and impact on daily life. *J. Wound, Ostomy and Continence Nursing*, **28**, 96–105.

Department of Health (2006). *Long-term Conditions and Depression: Considerations for Best Practice in Practice Based Commissioning.* http://icn.csip.org.uk/_library/Long-term_conditions_and_depression_PBC.pdf (accessed 29 September 2010).

Lal, S., Teubner, A. and Shaffer, J. L. (2006) Intestinal failure. *Aliment. Pharmocol. Ther.*, **24**, 19–31.

Lennard-Jones, J. E., Allison, S. P. and Brown, P. (1992) *A Positive Approach to Nutrition As a Treatment.* http://www.bapen.org.uk/pdfs/bapen_pubs/pub_kings_fund.pdf (accessed on 29 September 2010).

National Collaborating Centre for Acute Care group producing NICE guidelines (2006) *Nutritional Support in Adults: Oral Supplements, Enteral and Parenteral Feeding.* http://www.nice.org.uk/nicemedia/live/10978/29981/29981.pdf (accessed 29 September 2010).

Nightingale, J. M. D., Lennard-Jones, J. E., Gertner, D. J., Wood, S. R. and Bartram, C. I. (1992) Colonic preservation reduces the need for parenteral therapy, increases the incidence of renal stones but does not change the high prevalence of gallstones in patients with a short bowel. *Gut*, **33**, 1493–7.

Nightingale, J. M. D., Woodward, J. and Small bowel/Nutrition Committee of BSG (2006) Guidelines for the management of patients with a short bowel. *Gut*, **55**(suppl. IV), iv1–iv12.

Nordgaard, I., Hansen, B. S. and Mortensen, P. B. (1994) Colon as a digestive organ in patients with short bowel. *Lancet*, **343**, 373–6.

Stern, J. M., Jacyna, M. and Lloyd, D. A. J. (2008) Psychological aspects of home parenteral nutrition, abnormal illness behavior and risk of self-harm in patients with central venous catheters *Aliment. Pharmacol. Ther.*, **27**, 910–18.

Zachos, M., Tondeur, M. and Griffiths, A. M. (2007) Enteral nutritional therapy for induction of remission in Crohn's disease. *Cochrane Database of Syst. Rev.*, Issue 1. Art. No.: CD000542.

CHAPTER 13

Fertility, pregnancy and IBD

Julie Duncan and Lisa Younge

Introduction

IBD frequently presents in individuals during their reproductive years. It is therefore essential that healthcare professionals caring for people with IBD are familiar with the issues and concerns regarding sexual and reproductive health relating to the diseases and are able to address and discuss these frankly with their patients. Nurses, in particular, will often find themselves in the role of confidante due to their privileged relationship with their patients, requiring both an in-depth knowledge of the issues and the ability to discuss these in an open and non-judgmental way.

Concerns for patients with IBD, both male and female, involve issues relating to fertility, the possibility of passing on their disease to any children they may have, and pregnancy itself, including delivery. It is advisable to initiate these discussions at an early stage of a relationship with a patient, perhaps even soon after diagnosis, to help patients consider the issues before planning pregnancy. A number of well-researched and regularly updated guidelines exist which help the practitioner caring for this patient group and will be referred to within the text.

Case studies

Case I

Katie is a 28-year-old woman who has had a complex course of ileocolonic Crohn's disease (CD) since diagnosis aged 13. Eighteen months ago she had an uncomplicated delivery of her first child followed by a severe and prolonged exacerbation of her Crohn's disease, refractory to medical therapies, with the exception of corticosteroids. She was resistant, psychologically, to surgery due to fears of stoma formation. Due to this, and adherence issues, her disease remained unstable for a prolonged period. During this time she found it difficult to care for her young son and spent significant periods living apart from her partner, with her parents. As a result she felt she had failed her son. When her son was aged 14 months she came to accept that, having failed three immunosuppressants and two biologicals, she required surgery. Following sub-total colectomy and formation of ileostomy, her health was much improved and she wondered why she had been so resistant to surgery, as she felt in control of her life for the first time in a few years. Significantly, she found she had the energy and ability to play with and look after her son, which was a source of great joy. She had managed to leave her parents home and move back in with her partner. Nine weeks following her surgery she contacted the IBD advice line as she had discovered she was four weeks pregnant and had concerns about her medication (azathioprine). An appointment was made in the IBD CNS clinic the following week to discuss her concerns more fully. She attended with her mother. Her main concerns were the potential effects of azathioprine on the foetus; the effect pregnancy might have on her stoma, the possibility of developing a severe flare after delivery and her subsequent ability to look after two young children. Additionally, she was for the first time relishing spending quality time with her son and feared that the progress she had made with her relationship with him would be affected. She wanted to discuss all of these issues and the possibility of opting for a termination of pregnancy.

Case 2
Sam is a 32-year-old man diagnosed with ileal CD aged 24. Five years ago, following ileal resection, he commenced azathioprine. However, an MRI scan showed evidence of disease recurrence and, in an attempt to prevent further surgery, it was planned that he commence infliximab in addition to azathioprine. He raised concerns that infliximab could affect his sperm production having read information on the Internet. As he and his wife were planning pregnancy he was initially not keen to start on a biological medication. However, following discussion with his Consultant Gastroenterologist and IBD CNS he did start infliximab in combination with azathioprine. His disease is currently well controlled, and his wife is 28 weeks pregnant, with the pregnancy progressing well.

Katie's case highlights the complexities of life concerns that people with IBD may face, complicated by individual issues around their health and health beliefs as well as coping strategies and support structures. Focusing on her specific concerns about her unplanned pregnancy, the issues raised are:

- The effects of medications on pregnancy
- The effects of IBD on pregnancy outcomes
- The effects of pregnancy on the course of IBD
- The effects of pregnancy on a stoma

Sam's concerns were chiefly the effect that medications and IBD could potentially have on fertility. This chapter will deal with each of these concerns in addition to inheritance, surgery and the role of the IBD CNS.

Fertility

When discussing fertility with patients it is important to consider the role the disease itself may play on an individual's feelings of self-esteem and sexuality, and the impact this may have on fertility. Although sensitive, intimate and potentially embarrassing for patient and healthcare professional alike, it is important that issues relating to sexuality can be discussed. Nurses involved in the care of IBD patients may find themselves in the position of being the first person with whom the patient feels comfortable to raise such issues. Concerns for individuals might include:

- Reduced or non-existent libido or desire
- Negative feelings about oneself/poor body image
- Pain
- Erectile dysfunction
- Fear of incontinence (faecal or wind)
- Sex following stoma formation
- Fistulating disease
- Hurting their partner (for non-affected individuals)

Although some concerns may be increased and associated with active disease, an IBD diagnosis can impact on an individual's sexuality in mild disease or even when the disease itself is inactive.

The European Colitis and Crohn's organisation (ECCO) report lower levels of childbirth in patients with IBD (Van Assche *et al.*, 2010). It is important, however, to recognise that factors other than sub-fertility may be involved, including the active decision not to have children. IBD can be a debilitating and exhausting condition, and individuals may have concerns about their ability to care for a child when they are struggling to care for themselves. Others may simply choose not to have children for reasons completely independent of their disease.

Evidence suggests issues with fertility in up to 15% of the general population (NICE, 2004), in the absence of any disease, and patients should be made aware of this. Fertility in women with IBD appears unchanged, particularly those with UC (Hudson *et al.*, 1997). Studies have, however, demonstrated possible reduced fertility in patients with active CD, often attributed to mechanisms including inflammation of fallopian tubes and ovaries, previous surgical intervention, reduced libido and reduced levels of general health, including nutritional status (Van Assche *et al.*, 2010; Heetun *et al.*, 2007). On the other hand, fertility in those with quiescent CD is not thought to differ from that of the general population (Woolfson *et al.*, 1990).

There is no evidence that IBD affects male fertility. It is well known, however, that sulphasalazine negatively affects both sperm quantity and quality. This is reversible and therefore male patients wishing to start a family or reporting sub fertility issues taking this as a maintenance medication should consider substitution with an alternative agent (Heetun *et al.*, 2007). The other 5-ASA preparations have not been associated with this finding. Methotrexate is also associated with reversible oligospermia although the United States Food and Drug Administration (FDA) suggest that male patients should discontinue treatment with methotrexate at least three months prior to conception in any case due to concerns about teratogenicity, although there are no controlled studies looking at pregnancy outcomes of female partners to patients on MTX. There is limited evidence that infliximab may decrease sperm motility. How, or even if, this affects male fertility is not known (Mahadevan *et al.*, 2005). There is also a small amount of evidence suggesting that thiopurines might reduce sperm production, and one study showing a higher incidence of birth defects associated with mercaptopurine, although this has not been reproduced in subsequent studies (Francella *et al.*, 2003). Therefore there is no indication for men to stop thiopurine treatment prior to conception. Nonetheless, male patients may wish to discuss the possibility of withdrawing their medications if they are experiencing difficulties with conception, and this should be done, whenever possible, in a controlled way with an agreed approach – if patients feel unsupported they may resort to reducing or stopping therapy without discussion with the team, which can complicate disease management.

Patients who undergo surgery for their IBD may be at increased risk of subsequent impaired fertility. Some men experience problems with erectile dysfunction following surgery for IBD, particularly following colectomy and proctectomy. In women, there is a risk of adhesions and possible tubal damage which may impact on fertility (Van Assche *et al.*, 2010). Cornish *et al.* (2007) demonstrated that the formation of a pouch can result in significantly reduced fertility, a risk which has not been found in women with ileostomies (see Chapter 10); however, rates vary from study to study. These potential outcomes should be discussed with patients who are being considered for surgery, as there can be consideration of timings for the different stages of surgery, such as delaying formation of a pouch until family is complete if the patient prefers. As the fertility issues for women generally relate to potential tubal damage, they are likely to gain benefit from IVF techniques, so in some cases it may be beneficial to refer for fertility discussion pre-operatively.

An IBD nurse is not expected to have all the answers to the above concerns, but it is important to be aware of support organisations which can help and to foster a relationship with patients which encourages them to seek advice if they are experiencing concerns like these. Additionally, if patients discuss their pregnancy plans with their team that should trigger an assessment of their disease control, including nutritional status in preparation for pregnancy, bearing in mind that investigating IBD is less straightforward during pregnancy.

Contraception

For patients who decide not to have children, adequate and appropriate birth control methods are important, and this may also be an area in which the IBD nurse is consulted for advice. Although there has been some association between the use of oral contraception and the development of IBD, a causal relationship has not been found (Faculty of Sexual and Reproductive Healthcare (FSRH), 2009). Cosnes *et al.* (1999) found that oral contraception did not alter the course of CD. In general people with IBD would be wise to consult a family planning specialist, as IBD specific factors (such as malabsorption, medical regimen, pelvic disease, surgical treatment and associated disorders such as osteoporosis) may influence contraceptive choice. It is also important for patients and healthcare staff to recognise that active IBD may interfere with the absorption of the oral contraceptive pill and therefore its efficacy during this time.

The UK Medical Eligibility Criteria for Contraceptive Use have been developed to provide guidance on contraceptive use in specific conditions and, therefore, can be consulted to advise individual patients (Faculty of Sexual and Reproductive Healthcare, 2009).

Inheriting IBD

Both male and female patients with IBD will understandably have concerns about passing on IBD to any children they may conceive. The psychological implications of discovering your child has developed an IBD cannot be underestimated. Children born to individuals with IBD do have a slightly increased risk of developing the condition, a risk of approximately 5% if one parent has IBD, and up to 35% if both parents are affected (see Chapter 1). Generally it is felt that CD is more familial than UC, with up to 14.5% of patients with CD found to have a positive family history for IBD in first-degree relatives (Peeters *et al.*, 1996). An increased genetic risk of developing IBD has been found in Jewish populations, particularly those of Ashkenazi origin compared with those of other Jewish ethnic subgroups (Yang *et al.*, 1993). However, above all it should be emphasised that more than 85% of patients with IBD have no family history of the disease and patients can be reassured.

Impact of IBD on pregnancy

Whenever possible, it is recommended that pregnancy itself is planned for a time when a patient's IBD is quiescent. It is thought that the rate of disease flare during pregnancy is similar to that of non-pregnant IBD patients (Mahadevan, 2007; Morales *et al.*, 2000). Therefore, if a woman becomes pregnant during a stable period of remission she is likely to remain in remission during the pregnancy. In contrast, patients who have active disease at the time of conception are more likely to continue to experience increased activity, and risk further deterioration. Furthermore, it has been shown that active disease at conception is associated with higher rates of spontaneous abortion and preterm birth, and disease activity during pregnancy with low birth weight and preterm birth (Morales *et al.*, 2000; Bush *et al.*, 2004). However, it is felt by some clinicians that the risk of IBD in pregnancy is over-stated and that although babies are, on average, born earlier and smaller than the general population the difference is generally statistically (but not clinically) significant (Smith and Sanderson, 2010). Severe disease flare requiring surgery is associated with very poor pregnancy outcomes, as will be later discussed. Patients need to be aware of these potential risks to their pregnancy and the IBD nurse can engage with the patient to optimise adherence to their medical regimen in order to reduce the likelihood of a flare.

In general, medication used to maintain remission should be continued, the risk of active disease being greater than the risk of complications relating to medicines. Active IBD has been shown to increase the risk of miscarriage, preterm delivery and still births (Van Assche, 2010). Therefore, whether at conception or during pregnancy, disease flares should be treated proactively to reduce this risk. Shared care between the obstetrician and IBD physician is indicated, particularly in those with complex or active disease. Overall, it should be emphasised to the patient that planning is key and the overarching principle is 'healthy mother equals healthy baby'.

Impact of pregnancy on the course of IBD
There is some evidence to show that pregnancy improves disease outcomes in the longer term. For example, it has been shown that women with CD who have multiple pregnancies are less likely to need surgical intervention and that mothers with CD are less likely to relapse in the years following their pregnancy (Van Assche, 2010).

The woman with a stoma may find that as her pregnancy progresses her stoma changes and she needs a different appliance. Therefore pregnant women with a stoma should be advised to visit their stoma nurse (see Chapter 11).

Medication use in pregnancy
Early discussion about intentions of pregnancy give an opportunity to optimise a patient's treatment and to talk about potential concerns that patients may have about their medications prior to conception. Katie was particularly concerned that her medication may cause foetal abnormalities or impact on the outcome of her pregnancy. In general, patients can be reassured that, other than a couple of notable exceptions such as methotrexate and thalidomide, the medications used to treat pregnant women with IBD should be the same as that for non-pregnant patients (see Chapter 6). However, each case should be addressed individually and the risks and benefits for each patient assessed. These discussions can be difficult because there is a genuine paucity of evidence-based literature, with many reports conflicting or small-scale. Much of the evidence is based on case reports, animal studies or clinician experience. Ultimately the patient will make a decision about their medication use depending on a variety of issues, including their own health beliefs, the level of disease activity and the perceived risk. The FDA provides a guide to the use of medications in pregnancy. Table 13.1 lists FDA categories for the drugs commonly used in IBD.

5-Aminosalicylates (5-ASA)
With the exception of olsalazine, which is classified by the as FDA pregnancy category C, all other 5-ASAs, including sulphasalazine, balsalazide and mesalazine, are categorised as B. Initial reports suggested an association between congenital abnormalities and sulphasalazine, but this was refuted in larger studies (Norgard *et al.*, 2001). Sulfasalazine is used less often nowadays in favour of newer 5-ASAs with better side-effect profiles. However, if used there are concerns about potential

Table 13.1 FDA categories for drugs commonly used in IBD.

FDA pregnancy category	FDA definition	Classification of drugs commonly used in IBD management
A	Adequate and well-controlled human studies have failed to demonstrate a risk to the foetus in the first trimester of pregnancy (and there is no evidence of risk in later trimesters)	
B	Animal reproduction studies have failed to demonstrate a risk to the foetus and there are no adequate and well-controlled studies in pregnant women *or* Animal studies have shown an adverse effect, but adequate and well-controlled studies in pregnant women have failed to demonstrate a risk to the foetus in any trimester	5-ASAs **with the exception of Olsalazine** Infliximab Adalimumab Certolizumab Metronidazole
C	Animal reproduction studies have shown an adverse effect on the foetus and there are no adequate and well-controlled studies in humans, but potential benefits may warrant use of the drug in pregnant women despite potential risks	Olsalazine Corticosteroids Natalizumab Ciclosporin A Tacrolimus
D	There is positive evidence of human foetal risk based on adverse reaction data from investigational or marketing experience or studies in humans, but potential benefits may warrant use of the drug in pregnant women despite potential risks	Azathioprine 6-mercaptopurine
X	Studies in animals or humans have demonstrated foetal abnormalities and/or there is positive evidence of human foetal risk based on adverse reaction data from investigational or marketing experience, and the risks involved in use of the drug in pregnant women clearly outweigh potential benefits	Methotrexate Thalidomide

anti-folate effects and women should, therefore, be advised to take folic acid 5 mg daily prior to conception and throughout pregnancy (Smith and Sanderson, 2010). A Danish population-based study suggests no teratogenic risks to the foetus from exposure to mesalazine, although there was an apparent slightly increased risk of premature birth, low birth weight and stillbirth. It is thought, however, that this reflects the effects of disease activity and is not directly attributed to the medication (Norgard *et al.*, 2003). More commonly nowadays, patients are prescribed high-dose 5-ASAs. There is a lack of safety data in pregnancy in these doses and therefore it can be recommended to avoid, if possible, doses higher than 3 g daily due to a reported risk of foetal nephrotoxicity (Smith and Sanderson, 2010).

Thiopurines

Patients are often very concerned about the use of thiopurines at conception and pregnancy as the pharmaceutical leaflet enclosed with their prescription advises against their use in this situation. Azathioprine (AZA) and 6-mercaptopurine (6MP) are, in fact, listed as FDA category D. There is known teratogenicity in animals, but there is a real lack of human data. This makes discussions with patients difficult, as there is no clear-cut answer to their quest for reassurance. Although studies in other disease backgrounds have raised concerns about thiopurine use in pregnancy (in doses higher than used in standard IBD treatment), these concerns have not been substantiated in large IBD cohorts and therefore the generally accepted view is that thiopurines are safe in pregnancy in the IBD context (Heetun *et al.*, 2007). This view is supported by the recent publication of data from the CESAME trial which did not find an increased risk to pregnancy outcomes from exposure to thiopurines (Coelho *et al.*, 2010). AZA is preferred over 6MP as the foetus cannot convert it to 6MP (see Chapter 7) and is thus less exposed to the active metabolite of the drug (Smith and Sanderson, 2010). Any decision to change or stop a thiopurine should be undertaken following frank and open discussion between the patient and IBD physician weighing the risks and benefits for the patient's individual circumstance.

Corticosteroids

Corticosteroids are classed as pregnancy category C. It has been suggested that prednisolone is best avoided in the first trimester of pregnancy if at all possible, as there is a possible small risk of cleft palate (Park-Wylie *et al.*, 2000) but this association has not been confirmed by others (Czeizel and Rockenbauer, 1997). Additionally, this needs to be weighted against the benefits of disease control. There is only one human study on the use of budesonide in pregnancy and this is encouraging (Beaulieu *et al.*, 2009). In the event of an acute episode during pregnancy it is favoured to use prednisolone or hydrocortisone. It is generally considered that rectal preparations may be used until the third trimester (Caprilli *et al.*, 2006); however, again, the balance of risk and benefit must be assessed and rectal preparations used if the condition indicates.

Biologicals

Infliximab and adalimumab (anti-TNFα) are FDA category B. Infliximab does not cross the placenta in early pregnancy but does in the third trimester. It is thought, but not known, that adalimumab will also be able to cross the placenta at this time. Infliximab has been shown to be detectable in cord blood and in infants up to 6 months old when given in the third trimester (Mahadevan, 2007). It is not known what, if any, effects this has on the foetus or infant, although it is advised to avoid administering live vaccines until the infant is 6 months of age if exposed during the third trimester (Smith and Sanderson, 2010). Nonetheless, it is accepted practice to avoid using infliximab in the third trimester, if the mother's health permits. Some have suggested stopping infliximab if the mother is well, and restarting if she flares. However, this in itself carries risk in that she may build antibodies to the drug, increasing the risk of allergy, including anaphylaxis, and loss of response when restarted. There are limited data on the use of these drugs during pregnancy; however, the evidence thus far is that pregnancy outcomes are similar to women with IBD not exposed to anti-TNFα and to the general population (Dubinsky *et al.*, 2008; UKTIS, 2009). Certolizumab is thought to potentially cross the placenta barrier from first trimester and there is limited human data to understand the implications of this. However, it is classed as pregnancy category B. Natalizumab is category C. There is limited experience of this drug during pregnancy in patients with IBD.

Methotrexate

As well as being used in the treatment of cancer and IBD, methotrexate (MTX) is an abortifacient and can be used in the induction of medical abortion. It is strongly associated with congenital abnormalities and foetal mortality and is therefore completely contraindicated in pregnancy (Heetun *et al.*, 2007). Men and women commencing MTX should be advised to use robust contraception and be off MTX for at least 3 months (though many advocate up to 6 months) before planning to conceive.

Thalidomide

Thalidomide is also a pregnancy category X drug due to its well-known teratogenicity. It is contraindicated during pregnancy and in women of childbearing age who are not using two forms of contraceptive during, and one month either side of, treatment.

Ciclosporin A (CyA)

The data relating to CyA use in pregnancy comes from the transplant literature and has demonstrated no increased risk of foetal abnormalities. There was an association with low birth weight and prematurity, but this was not statistically significant, and no different from that of the general population (Bar Oz, 2001). In IBD its use has been in the setting of acute severe colitis unresponsive to corticosteroids. It is considered that CyA may be a better option than surgery with its associated risks in this situation (Dubinsky *et al.*, 2008).

Tacrolimus

Like CyA, tacrolimus is pregnancy category C and, again, most data is from the transplant literature. Van Assche *et al.* (2010) conclude 'apparent safety' with no increase in congenital malformations or other complications, but that prematurity is more common.

Antibiotics

Antibiotics, particularly ciprofloxacin and metronidazole, are often used in the treatment of perianal disease. Metronidazole is classified as Pregnancy category B and population studies have not identified an increased risk of congenital malformations (Heetun *et al.*, 2007). However, recent evidence suggests it may be associated with prematurity and it has been suggested, therefore, that it be used with caution and if there is no alternative (Shennan *et al.*, 2006). Studies of maternal exposure to fluoroquinolones (in which ciprofloxacin is classified) showed no increased risk of spontaneous abortion, prematurity, low birth weight or malformation. The majority of patients were exposed during the first trimester (Loebstein *et al.*, 1996; Schaefer *et al.*, 1996). Overall, it would be considered reasonable to use both these drugs if needed, although some prefer metronidazole to ciprofloxacin as animal studies have linked the latter to arthropathy (Smith and Sanderson, 2010). Amoxicillin also appears safe to use, though Van Assche *et al.* (2010) suggest using the shortest possible antibiotic treatment course to minimise risk. Certainly, in IBD care, antibiotics are often used over a prolonged period and there is limited data in these circumstances, and so caution should be exercised.

Both tetracyclines and sulphonamides should be avoided in pregnancy as they are associated with foetal malformation (Brumfitt and Pursell, 1973).

Although outlining the most common medications used in IBD, this is not an exhaustive list. Many centres have a Medicines Information Service run by the

Pharmacy department. This is an excellent service to access in order to find out the current advice and evidence base to aid patients' decision making.

Investigations during pregnancy

Investigating IBD during pregnancy should essentially be the same as in non-pregnancy. However, it is wise to avoid invasive investigations, if possible, relying rather on clinical signs. Although flexible sigmoidoscopy is thought to be safe during pregnancy, colonoscopy is usually avoided if possible (Heetun *et al.*, 2007). Abdominal X-ray and CT scans should be avoided, with the exception of an acute severe episode during which the risk of incomplete assessment outweighs potential risk. Abdominal ultrasound and MRI are safe. Blood tests can be taken as normal, although it is important to note that erythrocyte sedimentation rate (ESR) is raised in pregnancy and haemoglobin and albumin may be lower (Smith and Sanderson, 2010). C-reactive protein can be used rather than ESR to assess inflammatory markers.

Surgery in IBD

Other than planned elective surgery, the indications for surgery during pregnancy are the same as in non-pregnancy, including intestinal obstruction, perforation, acute severe disease failing to respond to medical therapy, abscesses and fistulae (see Chapter 9). Unfortunately, it has been demonstrated that patients who require surgery for their IBD have an increased risk of spontaneous abortion and preterm delivery, though it is not clear if this relates to the surgery or the disease activity. Indeed, it is considered that the risk to the foetus from continued illness is greater risk than the surgery (Subhani and Hamilton, 1998).

Delivery

A diagnosis of IBD in itself is not considered a reason to modify delivery options for patients. In general, the decision about mode of delivery is made in the usual way, involving discussion between the mother and her obstetric team, and an informed choice made based on their obstetric needs. The exceptions to this include currently active perianal disease, or that which has caused significant perineal scarring (Van Assche, 2010). In these situations it is important to protect the patient's anal sphincters in order to preserve continence. There should be no contraindication in previously active perianal disease and there is no evidence that vaginal delivery reactivates or causes new perianal disease. Previous pouch surgery is a relative contraindication only and there are many reports of vaginal delivery in ileoanal pouch patients in the literature. However, others would advocate caesarean section to minimize risk to anal sphincter function (Lepisto *et al.*, 2007).

Good practice should involve discussion between the patient's obstetrician, gastroenterologist and colorectal surgeon, and in some cases a more formal shared care approach will be adopted, which will encourage confidence for the patient as well as those caring for them. It can be confusing and frightening for patients to find themselves in a situation where they are being given conflicting advice by their specialists. IBD nurses can find themselves in a strong position to facilitate good communication and act as an advocate or spokesperson for the patient. In some centres formal shared care and designated pregnancy clinics have been set up, often delivered and managed by IBD specialist nurses. However, in most cases a more flexible approach is adopted which is tailored to the patient's requirements. It could be argued that this approach is superior as it allows patients to lead their care; however, neither approach has been formally studied.

After the birth

It is important to remember that the care of a patient during pregnancy is just the beginning. Caring for a new baby can be an emotional and stressful time for both female and male patients. A postpartum flare, as well as leaving the patient feeling exhausted and vulnerable, can impact on the ability to care for a baby. In severe cases, mothers may require admission to hospital following childbirth, which can have a substantial impact on the bonding process for mother and child. The IBD team should remain vigilant for problems following the birth of a new baby to an individual with IBD (female or male) and be available in a supportive role as well as a medical one, as required. Links with primary care such as health visitors or the patients GP can help to provide this support. It is good practice to arrange an appointment to see the patient at an agreed point post-delivery to ensure this support and availability is emphasised, in addition to assessing the IBD at this visit.

Breastfeeding

Breastfeeding has been demonstrated to improve immunity and is strongly advocated in maternity care, and indeed is thought to be protective against developing IBD (Mikhailov and Furner, 2009). Unfortunately, some common medications used in the management of IBD are contraindicated in breastfeeding as they are excreted in breast milk, and therefore ingested by the infant, such as metronidazole and ciprofloxacin. Prednisolone is detectable in small amounts and current advice is to have a 4 hour window between dosing and breastfeeding, although it may be difficult on a practical level (Van Assche, 2010). In those instances it may be advisable to discuss between the IBD and obstetric teams whether a combination of breast and bottle feeding is the best solution. It is considered acceptable to breastfeed whilst on infliximab or thiopurines (Van Assche, 2010). The summary of product characteristics for each medication will provide specific information about the drug's use in breastfeeding, and the FDA and hospital's Pharmacy Medicines Information services are also useful resources to ensure the information you provide is current and safe. Discussion about breastfeeding and medication should ideally begin prior to delivery. This, like many issues in fertility and pregnancy, can be an emotive subject, and patients will require information and discussion to help them balance the risks involved and to make an informed decision. They will also require support with the decision they make, and therefore, again, communication with midwives and health visitors is important, to ensure consistency of information.

Conclusion

Overall the message to people with IBD who wish to conceive or who are already pregnant is a positive one. Early discussion with patients about future plans should be encouraged, even if the eventuality may be a long way off. This allows time for the issues around fertility and pregnancy to be discussed and thought about. Thus an actual pregnancy may be planned for a period of optimum health in a woman whilst she is on a treatment not contraindicated in pregnancy. If a patient has a positive relationship with his or her IBD team this is likely to facilitate early and open discussion about matters that can sometimes be embarrassing or difficult. There are a number of well-researched resources to help the clinician give up-to-date and sound advice to enable patients to make informed decisions about their healthcare. However, the decision to stop or continue treatments will ultimately be the patients' choice dependent on their individual beliefs, previous experiences, stability of disease, likelihood of flare and their perception of the risk–benefit ratio for their individual situation. Therefore, fertility and pregnancy, like all aspects of IBD care, should be tailored to that specific patient. In most instances, IBD management is the same in non-pregnant patients, but there are some special considerations around treatments, investigations and modes of delivery depending on the individual situation. Liaison between an obstetrician with a special interest in IBD and the treating team is ideal. Finally, it is important to remember that male patients are affected by issues relating to fertility and pregnancy too.

Patient translation summary

- For most people with IBD, fertility is no different from that of the general population.
- Early discussion with the IBD team should be encouraged in order to plan and optimise health prior to becoming pregnant.
- Most medications used in IBD are safe during pregnancy and do not affect fertility. However, one should always discuss this with the IBD team.
- Pelvic surgery may affect fertility, and discussion about fertility and pregnancy should be initiated prior to surgery.
- In most instances choices around issues such as mode of delivery and breastfeeding are unaffected. However, patients should be encouraged to discuss these factors with their obstetric team early in the pregnancy.
- The IBD CNS is an excellent conduit for information and support.
- Ideally the patient with IBD could be referred to an obstetrician with an interest in IBD and links to the patient's IBD physician.
- Overall, early and frank discussion with the IBD team should be encouraged to ensure the potential issues are considered and addressed.

References

Bar Oz, B., Hackman, R., Einarson, T. and Koren, G. (2001) Pregnancy outcome after cyclosporine therapy during pregnancy: a meta-analysis. *Transplantation*, **71**, 1051–5.

Beaulieu, D. B., Ananthakrishnan, A. N., Issa, M. *et al.* (2009) Budesonide induction and maintenance therapy for Crohn's disease during pregnancy. *Inflammatory Bowel Dis.*, **15**, 25–8.

Brumfitt, W. and Pursell, R. (1973) Trimethropin-sulfamethoxazole in the treatment of bacteriuria in women. *J. Infect. Dis.*, **128**(suppl. 65).

Bush, M. C., Patel, S, Lapinski, R. H. and Stone, J. L. (2004) Perinatal outcomes in inflammatory bowel disease. *J. Maternity, Foetal and Neonatal Med.*, **15**, 237–41.

Caprilli, R., Gassull, M. A., Escher, J. C. *et al.* (2006) European Crohn's and Colitis Organisation. European evidence based consensus on the diagnosis and management of Crohn's disease: special situations. *Gut*, **55**(suppl. 1), i36–i58.

Coelho, J., Beaugerie, L., Colombel, J. F., Hébuterne, X., Lerebours, E., Lémann, M., Baumer, P., Cosnes, J., Bourreille, A., Gendre, J. P., Seksik, P., Blain, A., Metman, E. H., Nisard, A., Cadiot, G., Veyrac, M., Coffin, B., Dray, X., Carrat, F. and Marteau, P. for the CESAME pregnancy study group (France) (2010) Pregnancy outcome in patients with inflammatory bowel disease treated with thiopurines: cohort from the CESAME study. *Gut*. http://gut.bmj.com/, 29 November 2010; accessed 6 December 2010.

Cornish, J. A., Tan, E., Teare, J. *et al.* (2007) The effect of restorative proctocolectomy on sexual function, urinary function, fertility, pregnancy and delivery: a systematic review. *Dis. Colon and Rectum*, **50**, 1128–38.

Cosnes, J., Carbonnel, F., Carrat, F. *et al.* (1999) Oral contraceptive use and the clinical course of Crohn's disease: a prospective cohort study. *Gut*, 45, 218–22.

Czeizel, A. E. and Rockenvauer, M. (1997) Population based case control study of teratogenic potential of corticosteroids. *Teratology*, **56**, 335–40.

Dubinsky, M., Abraham, B. and Mahadevan, U. (2008) Management of the pregnant IBD patient. *Inflammatory Bowel Dis.*, **14**(12), 1736–50.

Faculty of Sexual and Reproductive Healthcare (FSRH) (2009) *FSRH Clinical Guidance: Sexual and Reproductive Health for Individuals with Inflammatory Bowel Disease.* London: Faculty of Sexual and Reproductive Healthcare.

FDA (Food and Drug Administration) (1980) *Regulations*, **44**, 37434–67.

Francella, A., Dyan, A., Bodian, C. *et al.* (2003) The safety of 6-meraptopurine for childbearing patients with inflammatory bowel disease: a retrospective cohort study. *Gastroenterology*, **124**, 9–17.

Heetun, Z. S., Byrnes, C., Neary, P. and O'Morain, C. (2007) Review article: reproduction in the patient with inflammatory bowel disease. *Alimentary Pharmacology and Therapeutics*, **26**, 513–33.

Hudson, M., Flett, G., Sinclair, T. S. *et al.* (1997) Fertility and pregnancy in inflammatory bowel disease. *Int. J. Gynaecol. Obstetr.*, **58**, 229–37.

Lepisto, A., Sarna, S., Tiitinen, A. and Jarvinen, H. J. (2007) Female fertility and childbirth after ileal pouch-anal anastomosis for ulcerative colitis. *Br. J. Surg.*, **94**, 478–82.

Loebstein, R., Addis, A., Ho, E. *et al.* (1998) Pregnancy outcome following gestational exposure to fluoroquinilones: a multicenter porospective controlled study. *Antimicrobial Agents and Chemother.*, **42**, 1336–9.

Mahadevan, U. (2007) Continuing immunomodulators and biologic medications in pregnant IBD patients – Pro. *Inflammatory Bowel Dis.*, **13**, 1439–40.

Mahadevan, U., Terdiman, J. P., Aron, J., Jacobsohn, S. and Turek, P. (2005) Infliximab and semen quality in men with inflammatory bowel disease. *Inflammatory Bowel Dis.*, **11**, 395–9.

Mahadevan, U., Sandborn, W. J., Li, D. K. *et al.* (2007) Pregnancy outcomes in women with inflammatory bowel disease: a population based cohort study. *Gastroenterology*, **133**, 1106–12.

Mikhailov, T. A. and Furner, S. E. (2009) Breastfeeding and genetic factors in the etiology of inflammatory bowel disease in children. *World J. Gastroenterol.*, **15**, 270–9.

Morales, M., Berney, T., Jenny, A. *et al.* (2000) Crohn's disease as a risk factor for the outcome of pregnancy. *Hepato-gastroenterol*, **47**, 1595–8.

National Institute of Clinical Excellence (NICE) (2004) *Assessment and Treatment for People with Fertility Problems. Understanding NICE Guidance – Information for People with Fertility Problems, Their Partners and the Public.* N0465 February 2004. London: NICE.

Norgard, B., Czeizel, A. E., Rockenbauer, M. *et al.* (2001) Population based case control study of the safety of sulfasalazine use during pregnancy. *Alimentary Pharmacol. Therapeutics*, **15**, 483–6.

Norgard, B., Fonager, K., Pedersen, L. *et al.* (2003) Birth outcome in women exposed to 5-aminosalicylic acid during pregnancy: a Danish cohort study. *Gut*, **52**, 243–7.

Park-Wylie, L., Mazotta, P., Patuszak, A. *et al.* (2000) Birth defects after maternal exposure to corticosteroids: a prospective cohort study and meta-analysis of epidemiological studies. *Teratology*, **62**, 385–92.

Peeters, M., Nevens, H., Baert, F., Hiele, M., De Meyer, A.-M., Vlietinck, R. and Rutgeerts, P. (1996) Familial aggregation in Crohn's disease: Increased age-adjusted risk and concordance in clinical characteristics. *Gastroenterology*, **111**, 597–603.

Schaefer, C., Moura-Elefant, E., Vial, T. *et al.* (1996) Pregnancy outcome after prenatal quinolone exposure. Evaluation of a case registry of the European Network of Teratology Information Services (ENTIS). *Eur. J. Obstetr., Gynaecol. Reproductive Biol.*, **69**, 83–9.

Shennan, A., Crawshaw, S., Briley, A. *et al.* (2006) A randomized controlled trial of metronidazole for the prevention of preterm birth in women positive for cervicovaginal fetal fibronectin: the PREMET study. *Br. J. Gynaecol.*, **113**, 65–74.

Smith, M. A. and Sanderson, J. D. (2010) Management of inflammatory bowel disease in pregnancy. *Obstetric Med.*, **3**, 59–64.

Subhani, J. M. and Hamilton, M. I. (1998) Review article: the management of inflammatory bowel disease during pregnancy. *Alimentary Pharmacol. Therapeutics*, **12**, 1039–54.

UK Teratology Information Service (UKTIS) (2009) Use of Infliximab in pregnancy, December 2009. http://www.toxbase.org/ (accessed 13 August 2010).

Van Assche, G., Dignass, A., Reinisch, W., van der Woude, C. J., Sturm, A. *et al.* (2010) The second European evidence-based consensus on the diagnosis and management of Crohn's disease: special situations. *J. Crohn's and Colitis*, **4**, 63–101.

Woolfson, K., Cohen, Z. and McLeod, R. S. (1990) Crohn's disease and pregnancy. *Dis. Colon and Rectum*, **33**, 869–73.

Yang, H., McElree, C., Roth, M.-P. *et al.* (1993) Familial empirical risks for inflammatory bowel disease: differences between Jews and non-Jews. *Gut*, **34**, 517–24.

CHAPTER 14

Care of children and adolescents with IBD

John M. E. Fell

Case study

A 10-year-old boy presented with a four-month history of abdominal pains, loss of energy and more recently loss of appetite. He occasionally passed loose stools. Over the previous four weeks he had been having a significant amount of time off school. He had an older sister aged 12. There was no family history of gastrointestinal disease.

On examination he was prepubertal, his weight was 24 kg (2nd percentile) whilst his height was 138 cm (50th percentile). Abdominal examination revealed fullness in the right iliac fossa. There was a small anal skin tag, but oral examination was normal.

His abnormal investigations were a low haemoglobin 9.2 g/dl and serum albumin 29 g/l, with an elevated sedimentation rate (35 mm/hr) and C-reactive protein (24 mg/l). Upper GI endoscopy was normal, but colonoscopy revealed localised deep ulcers in the caecum and terminal ileum. Mucosal biopsies from this area showed acute and chronic inflammatory changes with granulomas consistent with a diagnosis of Crohn's disease. Magnetic resonance imaging with enteroclysis confirmed the ileocolonic disease, but found no further abnormalities.

He was treated with enteral nutrition (polymeric diet). He managed to take 2 litres prescribed orally for six weeks. At that stage he had gained 4 kg in weight and was asymptomatic. Normal food was introduced over the next three weeks, at which stage he remained well.

Comment

This case, which is typical of a child presenting with Crohn's disease, illustrates some differences (and similarities) in the approach to the

> management of children with early onset IBD. The child may have many years of intestinal inflammation and therapy ahead of him and thus growth needs to be monitored and ionising radiation needs to be avoided, but just as with adult disease, an accurate diagnosis needs to be established and remission needs to be achieved by effective therapy.

Introduction

It is estimated that up to 25% of patients with Crohn's disease and ulcerative colitis present before the age of 18 years (Sawczenko *et al.*, 2001). Although the pathophysiology of these conditions in childhood dose not differ fundamentally from disease presenting in adulthood, managing children with inflammatory bowel disease does differ in some important ways from adult management. A childhood presentation can, for example, result in age-specific complications such as growth failure. Children at different ages also have different emotional and developmental needs which need to be acknowledged when devising their management plans. Against this background this review will cover the overall management of children with inflammatory bowel disease, but focus on areas where the age of presentation has significant implications for outcome, treatment and risk of complications.

Genetics

Following the initial identification of the NOD2/CARD15 polymorphism association with Crohn's disease (see also Chapter 1) (Hugot *et al.*, 2001), advances in technology in the form of genome wide association studies (GWASs) have confirmed and identified a plethora of further associations with Crohn's disease and ulcerative colitis. These span pathways of both adaptive and innate immunity, thus concurring with and expanding our understanding of disease pathogenesis.

The GWAS methodology has also been applies specifically to early onset IBD (Imielinski *et al.*, 2009). In a study of nearly 3,500 affected individuals and 12,000 matched controls from Europe and North America, five new regions associated with early onset IBD were identified, including 16p11 near the cytokine gene interleukin 27. This GWAS also detected 23 of 32 loci previously identified as associated with adult onset and 8 of 17 associated with adult-onset ulcerative colitis. These findings point to the common pathogenesis of early and adult-onset IBD, but also suggest some potential differences.

In a few rare cases of severely affected infants presenting with an indeterminate or Crohn's-like colitis (also termed IBD unclassified or IBD-U), a specific immune defect affecting the inlerleukin-10 receptor has been identified (Glocker *et al.*, 2009). Unlike other cases of inflammatory bowel disease this variant follows a mendelian pattern of inheritance (i.e. single gene cause of a very rare phenotype).

Epidemiology

Up to 25% of cases with inflammatory bowel disease present in childhood or adolescence, with approximately 5% presenting before the age of five (Sawczenko *et al.*, 2001). The reported incidence in children varies between populations studies, with evidence of an increase in children affected over recent decades.

A large prospective survey of children under the age of 16 in Great Britain and Ireland performed in 1998/1999 reported an incidence of 5.2 per 100,000 per year (60% Crohn's, 28% ulcerative colitis, 12% indeterminate colitis), whilst a systematic review of studies in North America estimated an incidence of 3–4 per 100,000 (Heyman *et al.*, 2005). Most paediatric studies report Crohn's disease to be twice as frequent as ulcerative colitis.

An increase in incidence of early onset inflammatory bowel disease over recent decades has been reported in many industrialised countries, such as Scotland and Wales (Barton *et al.*, 1989; Cosgrove *et al.*, 1996; Ahmed *et al.*, 2006), and also from countries in Eastern Europe such as the Czech Republic and Slovenia (Pozler *et al.*, 2006; Orel *et al.*, 2009). These changes in incidence over time and variations in incidence in different geographical areas have led to much speculation as to the changing environmental factors that could explain these phenomena.

Growth

Growth failure has long been recognised as a major potential complication of inflammatory bowel disease in childhood (Walker-Smith, 1996), with the final adult height achieved by these patients being the most obvious manifestation of this problem. Growth is affected by the disease activity and therapy. It is thus an important indicator of well-being of children with chronic disease, and thus a marker of the efficacy of treatment/management approaches being adopted to control disease activity.

Poor growth and reduced final adult height should also be regarded as adverse outcomes in their own right. Final adult height has been shown to influence an individual's success in life. In adolescence short stature and the frequently concomitant delay in puberty often have a significant negative impact on psychological and emotional well-being and quality of life (Otley *et al.*, 2002).

Incidence of growth failure

Studies into growth impairment in IBD fall into two main types: assessment of final adult height in patients who presented in childhood, and assessment of height velocity of children still growing. (Height velocity depends on repeated height measurements over time. It is expressed in cm/year and can be compared to age- and sex-specific standards.) In general growth impairment is more significant in cases with Crohn's disease. Thus up to 46% of children with Crohn's disease have been reported to have reduced height velocity prior to the onset of symptoms, and just 12% having a normal height velocity at diagnosis. In contrast, reduced height velocity is rarer in UC (3–10%). This is reflected in a general reduction in height SDS score at diagnosis in children with CD as opposed to UC in a large national UK cohort of over 700 children (Sawczenko *et al.*, 2001). In general, such single observation studies have their drawbacks since they do not record current growth and can be influenced by parental height, although in this case the large numbers of cases included imply a real effect.

There have been numerous studies into final adult height (Heuschkel *et al.*, 2008). They have focused on Crohn's disease, consistently demonstrating a reduction in final adult height, both in absolute terms and in relation to target height (calculated from parental height). With regard to specific risk factors, steroids during puberty has been shown to be associated with adverse growth outcome (Alemzadeh *et al.*, 2002), as well as delay between symptom onset and diagnosis, and the presence of jejunal inflammation (Sawczenko *et al.*, 2006).

Aetiology of growth failure in inflammatory bowel disease

The aetiology of growth failure in children with IBD is multifactorial and in many aspects not fully understood. Three main related factors – inflammation, under-nutrition and corticosteroid therapy – have, however, been identified. Since growth failure is more marked in CD, much of the subsequent discussion refers to this disease, although the adverse effects of corticosteroids therapy in particular are as pertinent to ulcerative colitis as Crohn's.

Under-nutrition has in the past been felt to be the major cause of growth failure. It is caused by a combination of reduced intake, excess energy expenditure and malabsorption. Of these, reduced energy intake appears to be the dominant factor. Dietary intake of children with active CD is relatively insufficient when compared with healthy children of the same age (Thomas *et al.*, 1993), and indeed nutritional supplementation has been shown to improve their linear growth (Aiges *et al.*, 1989). This reduction in intake may in part be 'voluntary' to reduce symptom such as pain, but may also be as a result of inflammation-induced anorexia, mediated by cytokines such as tumour necrosis factor α (TNFα). The role of changes in energy expenditure in growth failure is less clear. Resting energy expenditure does not differ markedly from controls, but malnourished adolescents with CD fail to reduce resting energy expenditure when compared to adolescents with anorexia nervosa (Azcue *et al.*, 1997).

The linkage between inflammation and growth has become clearer in recent years. Not only are there indirect effects on energy expenditure and appetite, but several of the cytokines implicated in CD inflammation also have several direct affects on growth. Pro-inflammatory cytokines disrupt the growth hormone, insulin-like growth factor 1 axis (Walters and Griffiths, 2009). TNFα and interleukin-1 have been shown to increase chondrocyte death (Martensson *et al.*, 2004) which will impair the formation of new bone, whilst interleukin-6 has an adverse effect on growth by several mechanisms including a reduction in IGF-1 production (De Benedetti *et al.*, 1997).

Corticosteroid therapy adversely affects growth by a variety of mechanisms and results in a state of functional growth hormone deficiency (Ballinger *et al.*, 2003). The dose, preparation, duration and scheduling of treatment can all influence the degree of growth suppression. A dose of prednisolone as low as 3–5 mg/m^2 (Allen, 1998) can impair growth in pre-pubertal children. The effect can, however, be partially mitigated by an alternated day dosage regimen.

Pubertal delay can be a consequence of previous poor growth and under-nutrition. There is, however, evidence that pro-inflammatory cytokine TNFα can directly influence puberty down regulate androgen secretion (Mizokami *et al.*, 2000)

Clinical assessments of growth

Clinical assessment of growth (Heuschkel *et al.*, 2008) requires regular, accurate measurement of height and weight, performed by staff trained in these measurements. Recording parental height, to enable a mid-parental height centile to be calculated, and obtaining records of pre-morbid weight and height are helpful in defining growth potential.

In order to follow growth over time height and weight needs to be plotted sequentially (4–6 monthly) on a centile chart. Data can also be presented as a standard deviation score (SDS or Z score). For a Z score the height (or weight) is calculated as a number of standard deviations from the mean height (weight) for that age and sex compared to a reference population, as opposed to the percentage of children with height (weight) less than the subject at that age, which is the centile score. Further calculation should be made of height velocity and body mass index (BMI). Children need to be followed until early adulthood, by which time final adult height has been achieved. In view of the influence of puberty on growth and growth potential, regular accurate pubertal assessment by Tanner staging (which grades individuals 0–5, depending on the development of secondary sexual characteristics) and assessment of testicular volume is essential. Bone age should be obtained at diagnosis, and annually in cases with suspected growth delay.

Bone health

Children with inflammatory bowel disease, particularly Crohn's disease are predisposed to developing osteopaenia. There is a wide range of reported prevalence of between 11% and 50% in children with Crohn's disease (Beattie *et al.*, 2006; Burnham *et al.*, 2004; Boot *et al.*, 1998; Herzog *et al.*, 1998; Semeoa *et al.*, 1999). This variability probably reflects variable disease severity, treatment regimens, age and pubertal status, as well as highlighting the difficulty in interpreting bone mineral density scans (DEXA), since reference values that take account of weight, height and pubertal status are limited.

There are several factors which affect bone mineral density. Broadly speaking, as with growth impairment, these factors relate to therapy (such as corticosteroids), disease activity (such as interleukin 6) and nutrition (vitamin D and calcium). Although studies of children have failed to quantify the relative contribution of each factor, corticosteroid use in general has been shown to be linked with the main complication of reduced bone mineralisation, namely fracture risk in both children and adults (Boot *et al.*, 1998; Dinca *et al.*, 1999).

Bone mass accumulates to a significant degree during the pubertal growth spurt; thus preventative strategies in childhood are important. Although there is little objective data in the paediatric age group (Wilson *et al.*, 2010), apart from trying to minimise corticosteroid use some centres will recommend routine supplementation with calcium and vitamin D (Sandhu *et al.*, 2010).

Clinical features of inflammatory bowel disease in children

The clinical features of IBD presenting in childhood are in general the same as those of adult cases, although in younger children in particular the ascertainment of symptoms will typically by via a parent/carer. The impact of IBD on growth and development does, however, result in some features specific to paediatric cases.

In children with UC, blood loss, diarrhoea and abdominal pain are the main symptoms, occurring in the majority of cases. The most commonly reported extra-intestinal manifestation is arthropathy, whilst skin involvement is rare. Inflammatory bowel disease unclassified (IBD-U) also presents with predominantly colitis symptoms. The child with Crohn's disease, on the other hand, can present in different ways, depending on the site of disease involvement. The classical Crohn's presentation is with abdominal pain, diarrhoea and weight loss. This occurred in 80% of cases reported from The Hospital for Sick Children, Toronto from 1980–1989 (Griffiths, 2004). More recently, in a large UK survey of children with IBD in the Great Britain and Ireland only 25% of cases presented this way. Abdominal pain was still the main symptom, but only 56% of children had diarrhoea. In addition to weight loss, Crohn's disease is associated with more non-specific symptoms such as lethargy, anorexia, nausea and growth failure. Extra-intestinal manifestations such as erythema nodosum, arthropathy and fever, as well as more Crohn's-specific physical signs such as mouth ulcers and perianal disease (skin tags, fissures, fistulae and abscesses) are all features of Crohn's disease, but occur in only a minority of cases (Sawczenko and Sandhu, 2003).

Distinct paediatric disease pattern and evolution

The Montreal classification of inflammatory bowel disease (Silverberg *et al.*, 2005) was devised to further subdivide Crohn's disease and ulcerative colitis according to characteristics such as age at onset, disease location, behaviour and severity. By definition, IBD presenting in childhood is 'early onset'. (Early onset according to the Montreal classification is 16 years or younger, but applies only to Crohn's.)

Cosnes *et al.* (2002) described the evolution of the Crohn's disease phenotype (in adults) over time in a large cohort in Northern France followed for 20 years. At diagnosis 80% of cases had an inflammatory phenotype. Over time, however, the proportion with stricturing and penetrating disease increased so that at 20 years only 12% still had an inflammatory phenotype. Initial indications for early onset disease, from cohorts being monitored in Europe and New Zealand, indicate that disease behaviour at diagnosis is similar, and evolves over time in the same fashion (Van Limbergen *et al.*, 2008; Vernier-Masouille *et al.*, 2008; Tarrant *et al.*, 2008).

Inflammatory bowel disease in childhood does, however, appear to have more extensive intestinal involvement. For Crohn's disease, pan-enteric distribution (ileocolonic plus upper gastrointestinal: Montreal L3 + L4) has been reported in 43% of cases at presentation as opposed to 3% in adults (Van Limbergen *et al.*, 2008), although this higher incidence of upper intestinal disease may reflect more extensive initial investigation in these cases with upper gastrointestinal endoscopy (as per Porto criteria: see below) (IBD Working Group, 2005). In the case of ulcerative colitis, however, it is well recognised that extensive or pan-colonic (Montreal E3) disease is considerably more common at presentation in childhood

(80–90%) (Van Limbergen *et al.*, 2008; Sawczenko and Sandhu, 2003; Heyman *et al.*, 2005), when compared to adult cases (24% pancolitis, 33% extensive colitis) (Witte *et al.*, 2000; Henriksen *et al.*, 2006). Furthermore children with distal and left-sided disease progress to more extensive disease over time (Van Limbergen *et al.*, 2008).

Diagnosis and investigation

History and examination

A full history in children with suspected IBD needs to include details of stool frequency, consistency, urgency and the presence or absence of blood or mucus. In younger children this will be by parental observation, which may affect the accuracy of the reports, whilst adolescents may not be forthcoming in reporting changes in bowel habit. Other symptoms to be explored include abdominal pain, a common symptom in school-age children, weight loss, nausea, malaise and anorexia. The history should also include a family history, and a history of foreign travel, diet, and features that could relate to extra-intestinal manifestations (joints, eyes, skin).

The physical examination needs to include an assessment of general well-being and vital signs as well an assessment of the abdomen. The oral cavity should be inspected in particular for changes that occur in Crohn's disease, such as deep mouth ulcers, lip swelling and buccal cobble stone appearance. The perianal area should be examined for evidence of skin tags, fissures and fistulae. Measurement of weight and height, and assessment of pubertal status are important, since not only is growth failure a feature of IBD (particularly Crohn's disease), but it also defines the growth potential and thus helps make an overall framework within which future treatments can be selected and monitored; see Table 14.1.

Investigation

Investigation of children with suspected IBD is, as with adults, aimed at establishing a diagnosis, which includes distinguishing between ulcerative colitis and Crohn's disease, and defining the extent and severity of the disease. The 'Porto criteria' (IBD Working Group, 2005) devised by the European Society of Paediatric Gastroenterology, Hepatology and Nutrition (ESPGHAN) define the recommended investigations that need to be undertaken in children (Figure 14.1). The criteria in particular emphasise the importance of upper gastrointestinal endoscopy, and colonoscopy with terminal ileal intubation for both diagnosis and discrimination between ulcerative colitis and Crohn's.

Table 14.1 Presenting clinical features of Crohn's disease and ulcerative colitis in childhood. This list is not exhaustive but demonstrates the relative frequency of the clinical features of ulcerative colitis (predominantly colitic) and Crohn's disease (can be colitic, but often include other general/constitutional features and growth failure).

		Crohn's disease	Ulcerative colitis
Common symptoms	Abdominal pain	+ + +	+ + +
	Diarrhoea	+ +	+ + +
	Blood loss per rectum	+	+ + +
	Anorexia	+ +	+
	Weight loss	+ +	+
	Malaise/lethargy	+ +	+
Other symptoms	Arthropathy	+	+
	Nausea/vomiting	+	
Physical signs	Growth failure/ pubertal delay	+	
	Perianal disease, e.g. abscess, fistula	+	
	Erythema nodosum	(+)	(+)
	Liver disease	(+)	(+)

Investigations should thus include standard laboratory tests such as a full blood count, erythrocyte sedimentation rate, C-reactive protein and liver function tests (including albumin). Stool needs to be tested for potential infectious causes of symptoms, including the presence of *Clostridium difficile* toxin. This will also need to be repeated if symptoms relapse at a later date. Tuberculosis needs to be excluded, particularly for children from areas where this infection is prevalent (Sandhu *et al.*, 2010).

Serological markers such as perinuclear antineutrophil cytoplasmic antibody (pANCA) and anti-*Sacchromyces cerevisiae* antibody (ASCA) can be used to aid discrimination between ulcerative colitis and Crohn's, although a positive pANCA does not preclude Crohn's; neither does a positive ACSA preclude ulcerative colitis (Ruemmele *et al.*, 1998; Hoffenberg *et al.*, 1999). In clinical practice, however, these markers are not universally tested or available due to the limitations of their

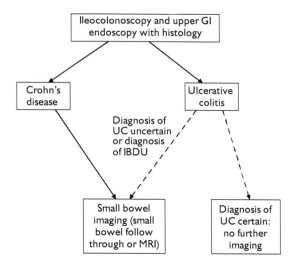

Figure 14.1 Porto criteria for the diagnosis of IBD in children (modified to include assessment of small bowel by MRI).

predictive value and because disease differentiation can usually be achieved by other means (histology etc).

The Porto criteria recommend upper GI endoscopy and colonoscopy with intubation of the terminal ileum for assessment of children with suspected IBD. This requires an appropriately skilled endoscopist, particularly for younger children, and a safe sedation or general anaesthetic environment, which will usually require a practitioner with anaesthetic skills to manage the sedation/ anaesthetic. The macroscopic appearances of IBD in childhood are the same as for adults with the disease, and the histological criteria adopted are the same (Jenkins *et al.*, 1997).

Assessment of the small intestine, which according to the Porto criteria is mandatory in cases where Crohn's disease is suspected, has traditionally been by means of contrast radiology: barium follow through or small bowel enema. Recent advances in imaging techniques and the advent of capsule endoscopy mean that the small bowel can be assessed by alternative methods.

Ultrasonography, in skilled hands, is a valuable technique for the assessment of bowel wall thickness in particular, as well as identifying abscesses or free fluid (Bremner *et al.*, 2004). Computed tomography and magnetic resonance imaging (MRI) are also useful in evaluating disease activity and complications, for example perianal fistulae. Distension of the intestine during MRI (MRI enterography) has further improved the sensitivity of this imaging technique, particularly in relation to small bowel disease (Laghi *et al.*, 2003). The risks associated with lifetime exposure to ionising radiation from contrast radiology and CT scanning become more significant with repeated investigation for disease re-evaluation, and thus MRI and ultrasound are becoming more widely used, particularly for evaluating disease progression.

Capsule endoscopy is becoming more widely available, particularly for small bowel assessment (Seidman *et al.*, 2004). In a condition which is prone to stricture formation, there is inevitably a small risk of capsule retention, a complication which one would suspect to be greater in smaller patients (many reported studies have a minimal age requirement of 6 or 8 years). Swallowing the capsule may not be possible for younger children, a problem that needs to be pre-empted to avoid waste of the capsule, but can be avoided by endoscopic placement into the duodenum. For further details see Chapter 4.

Treatment

Treatment approaches for inflammatory bowel disease in children (Beattie *et al.*, 2006; Sandhu *et al.*, 2010), including those published as consensus guidelines such as the European Crohn's and Colitis Organisation (ECCO) (Caprilli *et al.*, 2006; Biancone *et al.*, 2008), are (not surprisingly) similar to those devised for adults with the disease, given that the aim in general is to control the inflammatory process, which will essentially be the same in the different age groups. Furthermore, a systematic review of paediatric therapeutic trials conducted up until December 2006 identified only a limited number of such studies, of which very few were of 'good quality' (Wilson *et al.*, 2010). There are, however, certain aspects of inflammatory bowel disease (such as its impact on growth; Newby *et al.*, 2005) and of treatments (such as their impact on growth or their associated risk of malignancy) that may influence treatment choices in the younger patient.

Nutritional therapy

Nutritional therapy with liquid diet as the sole source of nutrition has been shown to be effective in inducing remission in children with Crohn's disease. Treatment courses of four to eight weeks have recommended, followed by a period of food reintroduction. The treatment has been shown to induce mucosal healing (Fell *et al.*, 2000) and reduce inflammation which will impair growth (Bannerjee *et al.*, 2004), both of which are major objectives of therapy in inflammatory bowel disease.

When compared with corticosteroids in a systematic review of trials with adult patients, enteral nutrition was not as effective as corticosteroids in achieving remission (Zachos *et al.*, 2004) although in children efficacy is similar (Heuschkel *et al.*, 2000). Furthermore in trials which included growth as an outcome, corticosteroids have a significantly greater adverse impact than enteral nutrition (Sanderson *et al.*, 1987; Thomas *et al.*, 1993).

Despite these potential advantages the therapy is not universally used as first line therapy. In Europe it is often used as first-line therapy, but in North America much less frequently. In practice adherence is variable, even with more palatable polymeric feeds, and requires a significant investment in emotional/psychological support, assisted by a well-motivated nursing and dietetic team. Treatment will often have to be started as an in-patient to provide this support, which has significant impact on overall treatment cost.

In the longer term, general objectives of therapy are growth maintenance and prevention of relapse. Relapse rates of between 50% and 80% have been reported following remission with enteral nutrition (Yamamoto *et al.*, 2010). Cyclical nutritional therapy has been used to promote growth (Belli *et al.*, 1988). Maintenance nutritional therapy with significant, but not exclusive enteral nutrition resulted in a reduced relapse rate, with a greater beneficial effect reported with larger volumes of feed (Yamamoto *et al.*, 2010). For further details on nutritional therapy see Chapter 8.

Corticosteroids

Corticosteroids are effective therapy for induction of remission in both ulcerative colitis and Crohn's disease (Wilson *et al.*, 2010). Numerous adverse effects have however been reported in children with inflammatory bowel disease as well as other chronic inflammatory conditions (Leonard *et al.*, 2004; Boot *et al.*, 1998; Gokhale *et al.*, 1998). The effect on growth and bone health is a recognised concern, particular with chronic usage. Attempts have been made to mitigate these effects by the selection of a corticosteroid with fewer side-effects, such as budesonide for ileocaecal disease (Escher, 2004), or topical use for distal colitis. Alternatively, treatment strategies have been developed to reduce or avoid corticosteroid use, such as enteral nutrition to induce remission in Crohn's, or azathioprine for maintenance therapy. Even with this understanding of complications with corticosteroid therapy, steroid dependency rates one year after diagnosis of 31% and 45% have been reported from large North American series of children with Crohn's disease and ulcerative colitis, respectively.

5-Aminosalicylates

5-Aminosalicylates (5-ASA) are widely used in paediatric ulcerative colitis. In active Crohn's disease, although used, the evidence for efficacy is less clear (Caprilli *et al.*, 2006) . Despite the lack of paediatric trial data they appear to be as useful in management as they are in adult practice (Wilson *et al.*, 2010). They can be administered orally or topically (enema or suppository) for left-sided disease, although adolescents may be reluctant to consider topical therapy. Since the disease presentation is often more severe (and extensive) in children, 5-ASAs are often initially administered in combination with other therapy. Higher doses are now typically used (e.g. for children over 12 years, mesalazine 50–75 mg/kg/day, maximum 4 g/day), in line with adult practice (Biancone *et al.*, 2008). Maintenance therapy is recommended in ulcerative colitis. In children, taking large 5-ASA tablets can often be a difficult. This problem can be overcome by using sulphasalazine, which is available in liquid form, or a 5-ASA granule preparation.

Immunomodulator therapy

Azathioprine and 6-mercaptopurine are widely used to maintain remission in children with inflammatory bowel disease (Markowitz *et al.*, 2002). In a randomised trial of 55 children with newly diagnosed mild-to moderate Crohn's disease who were randomised to receive an initial course of prednisolone and either 6-mercaptopurine or placebo, there was no difference in remission rate, but a striking difference in relapse rates over the 18 months of follow-up (9% with 6-MP versus 47% with placebo) (Markowitz *et al.*, 2000). Methotrexate also has a role as maintenance therapy. Its use has largely been confined to azathioprine non-responsive or intolerant cases (Uhlen *et al.*, 2006). More recently concerns regarding the lymphoma risk of combination therapy, with anti-TNF monoclonal therapy plus azathioprine, may influence the choice of the maintenance immunomodulatory drug used in some cases (Rosh *et al.*, 2007).

Biological therapy

There is a wealth of data from adult studies on the efficacy of anti-TNF monoclonal therapy as a treatment for Crohn's disease (and also ulcerative colitis); severe and/or refractory to other therapies (Hanauer *et al.*, 2002, 2006; Lawson *et al.*, 2006; Colombel *et al.*, 2007). Recent NICE guidelines (2010) in the UK state that in children (6–17 years) infliximab, within its licensed indication, is recommended for the treatment of severe active Crohn's disease which has not responded to conventional therapy, or for patients who are intolerant of or have contraindications to conventional therapy. The need for treatment should be reviewed every 12 months.

The randomised, multicentre, open-label, REACH study (Hyams *et al.*, 2007) of 112 children aged 6–17 years, which set out to compare two infliximab dosing regimens, is the major source of confirmatory data as to the efficacy of infliximab for induction and maintenance of remission of Crohn's disease in the younger age group. In this trial 88.4% achieved a response to the standard induction regimen (5 mg/kg at weeks 0, 2 and 6) and 58.9% were in remission at 10 weeks. Following maintenance therapy (5 mg/kg 8 weekly) for 54 weeks, 63.5% did not require a dose adjustment, and 55.8% were in clinical remission. This response was associated with a significant improvement in quality of life and a marked reduction in corticosteroid usage. Furthermore, children receiving infliximab showed a significant increase in height Z-score compared to pre-treatment baseline.

The beneficial effect of infliximab on perianal Crohn's disease observed in adults has also been demonstrated in children. In the REACH study, 22 children had concurrent perianal disease; 9/22 (41%) responded at 2 weeks, and 16/22 (73%) responded at 52 weeks (15 complete) (Crandall *et al.*, 2009). For ulcerative colitis the paediatric data is more limited, although it has been used in a similar fashion to adult practice for severe and refractory cases.

Despite these encouraging responses, there are limitations to the use of anti-TNF therapies in Crohn's disease which relate in part to potential adverse effects. This therapy has been associated with an increased risk of infection (particularly tuberculosis) and infusion-related hypersensitivity reactions (Lichtenstein *et al.*, 2007). In younger patients, however, it is the potential for the development of malignancy that has been a particular cause for concern. This has to some extent been mitigated by observations from the large TREAT registry of adult subjects, where similar rates of malignancy (and lymphoma) were observed in infliximab and non-infliximab treated patients. In younger patients, however, a rare but aggressive lymphoma (hepato-splenic T cell lymphoma: HSTCL) has caused significant concern. A review in 2009 of 14 cases of HSTCL, usually with a fatal outcome, in patients who had received anti-TNF therapy (Cucchiara *et al.*, 2009), showed this condition to occur in younger patients (12 to 31 years), nearly all of whom were male (13/14). In this series nearly all had Crohn's disease, and all had received concomitant azathioiprine or 6-MP therapy. This observation, and the occasional occurrence of HSTCL in individuals with IBD (ulcerative colitis and Crohn's disease) who had not received anti-TNF therapy (but had received azathioprine/6-MP) has led to discussion as to the true causal association. The potential association of anti-TNF therapy and HSTCL has in practice resulted in a somewhat more cautious approach to the use of biological therapy in children.

Surgery

The indications for surgery in IBD are generally the same as those for adult patients. Thus in ulcerative colitis, colectomy with a view to ileoanal pouch formation is undertaken where medical management has failed. In Crohn's disease surgical resection may similarly be undertaken due to failure of medical management or mounting side-effects of treatment, such as excessive corticosteroid dosage. Local resection or strictoplasty may also be necessary for local complications such as stricture formation. Growth and pubertal status in particular need to be considered when deciding the timing of resection, since in cases where growth potential remains, catch-up growth can occur following surgery (Evans *et al.*, 1991; Heuschkel *et al.*, 2008).

Psychosocial impact and age appropriate management

The young person with IBD is faced with several potential personal and emotional issues that are specific to their age group. During puberty in particular, they have to face the physical demands of their disease and therapies, with their potential lifetime implications, at a time when their personal life is undergoing significant transition. Some consequences of IBD are of specific concern to some children. Short stature and pubertal delay can be a cause of anxiety and affect relationships between adolescents and their peers. Weight gain and cosmetic changes as a result of corticosteroid therapy are a particular concern for some, and influence the choice of therapy that are accepted or will be taken. Compliance with therapy is a difficulty in the management of the chronic features of IBD, and there is some data to indicate that it is a particular problem for some adolescents (Hommel *et al.*, 2009).

Hospital/medical services

Paediatric gastrointestinal services for the management of children with IBD are optimally provided in a multidisciplinary fashion. Endoscopy and other in-patient procedures/admissions need to take place in an age-appropriate setting. Thus, wherever possible, investigation and treatment should be in a 'paediatric or adolescent-friendly' environment, which will usually be led by a paediatric gastroenterologist. Key members of the multidisciplinary team are paediatric nurses, nurse specialists, dietitians and psychologists, with support from pharmacists, play specialists and teachers. Appropriate linkages to local services are also important to maximise the amount of care that can be delivered close to home.

Children and families will deal with the problem of living with IBD in a wide range of ways and in some cases the psychologist can be of great assistance. The variety of problems encountered by young patients range from the specific, such

273

as needle phobia and fear of procedures, to the more general, often underpinned by anxieties relating to the condition. These will need to be viewed in the wider family context, the aim typically being to assist the coping strategies of the child and family.

Transition to adult services represents a further challenge to young persons with IBD (see Chapter 15). The challenge is to maintain continuity of support, but also to evolve the managing team from 'paediatric' to 'adult'. A model of joint clinics has been suggested as optimal, but this may not be possible if paediatric services are congruent with adult services. One of the aspirations of joint clinics is that they can facilitate the evolution from parental management of the child's condition to the young person taking fuller responsibility for their health and treatment. The age at which transition occurs or indeed should occur depends on several factors. The 'paediatric' age range varies in different healthcare systems (typically up to 16 or 18 years), and similarly the expectation of transition age varies. Furthermore, individuals vary in their maturity. Physically, puberty and growth may be delayed and thus represent a significant reason for remaining within paediatric services. Emotionally, individuals vary widely in their aspiration for independence, which attendance at an adult clinic may represent.

Schooling and other support

Outside of hospital a degree of support may be accessible for children and carers. For example, in the UK financial support for carers is available via the Disability Living Allowance system. The process for accessing financial support in some circumstances may, however, be lengthy and complex. This can be facilitated if a named social worker is attached to the gastroenterology team.

Frequent hospital visits for clinic appointments and diagnostic tests, as well as periods of ill health, can significantly affect school attendance. This can to some extent be mitigated by timely contact with the school. Home tuition can be organised where necessary. Similarly, the embarrassment of diarrhoeal symptoms can be mitigated by sensitively addressing access to toilets.

Conclusion

Although the pathophysiology of IBD in childhood does not differ fundamentally from that in adults, the paediatric age group presents some specific challenges in management. Growth and pubertal delay represent major factors in management since they can be influenced by the disease and need to be accounted for in the therapeutic choices adopted. In common with other chronic disease in childhood it is important to take account of the fact that symptom reporting and treatment administration will depend to a greater or lesser extent, depending on the child's age and maturity, on a parent or carer. Thus the basis of the relationship between the child and health professionals is an evolving, and sometimes challenging, interaction.

Patient translation summary

- 25% of patients with Crohn's disease and ulcerative colitis present before the age of 18 years.
- Early onset ulcerative colitis and Crohn's disease tend to be more severe than later onset disease.
- Ulcerative colitis is usually more extensive at diagnosis, and surgery (when required) tends to occur sooner after diagnosis.
- Crohn's disease tends to be more extensive at diagnosis, but progress to stricturing/fistulating complications is the same as for adult onset disease.
- Growth failure is a major potential complication of IBD (particularly Crohn's disease) and also some of the standard treatments (corticosteroids).
- Treatment of IBD thus needs to be aimed at achieving remission, but also needs to minimise potential adverse effects on growth.
- Children need to be managed in an age-appropriate fashion. This means providing appropriate in-patient and out-patient environments. Furthermore, it is important to meet their (and their family's) more general psychosocial needs, as well as facilitating their specific educational requirements.

References

Ahmed, M., Davis, I. H., Hood, K. *et al.* (2006) Incidence of paediatric inflammatory bowel disease in South Wales. *Arch. Dis. Child.*, **91**, 344–5.

Aiges, H., Markowitz, J., Rosa, J. and Daum, F. (1989) Home nocturnal supplemental nasogastric feedings in growth-retarded adolescents with Crohn's disease. *Gastroenterology*, **97**, 905–10.

Allen, D. B. (1998) Influence of inhaled corticosteroids on growth: a pediatric endocrinologist's perspective. *Acta Paediatr.*, **87**, 123–9.

Alemzadeh, N., Rekers-Mombarg, L. T., Mearin, M. L. *et al.* (2002) Adult height in patients with early onset of Crohn's disease, *Gut*, **51**, 26–9.

Azcue, M., Rashid, M., Griffiths, A. and Pencharaz, P. B. (1997) Energy expenditure and body composition with Crohn's disease: effect of enteral nutrition and treatment with prednisolone. *Gut*, **41**, 203–8.

Ballinger, A. B., Savage, M. O. and Sanderson, I. R. (2003) Delayed puberty associated with inflammatory bowel disease. *Pediatr. Res.*, **53**, 205–10.

Bannerjee, K., Camacho-Hubner, C., Babinska, K. *et al.* (2004) Anti-inflammatory and growth-stimulating effects precede nutritional restitution during enteral feeding in Crohn's disease. *J. Pediatr. Gastroenterol. Nutr.*, **38**, 270–5.

Barton, J. R., Gillon, S. and Ferguson, A. (1989) Incidence of inflammatory bowel disease in Scottish children between 1968 and 1983: marginal fall in ulcerative colitis, threefold increase in Crohn's disease. *Gut*, **30**, 18–22.

Beattie, R. M., Croft, N. M., Fell, J. M. *et al.* (2006) Inflammatory bowel disease. *Arch. Dis. Child.*, **91**, 426–32.

Belli, D., Seidman, E. G., Bouthillier, L. *et al.* (1998) Chronic intermittent elemental diet improves growth failure in children with Crohn's disease. *Gastroenterology*, **94**, 603–10.

Boot, A. M., Bouquet, J., Krenning, E. P. *et al.* (1998) Bone mineral density and nutritional status in children with chronic inflammatory bowel disease. *Gut*, **42**, 188–94.

Biancone, L., Michetti, P., Travis, S. *et al.* (2008) European evidence-based consensus on the management of ulcerative colitis: special situations. *J. Crohn's Colitis*, **2**, 63–92.

Bremner, A. R., Pridgeon, J., Fairhurst, J. *et al.* (2004) Ultrasound scanning may reduce the need for barium radiology in the assessment of small bowel Crohn's disease. *Acta Paediatr.*, **93**, 479–81.

Burnham, J. M., Shults, J., Semeao, E. *et al.* (2004) Whole body BMC in paediatric Crohn's disease: independent effects of altered growth, maturation, and body composition. *J. Bone Miner. Res.*, **19**, 1961–8.

Caprilli, R., Gassull, M. A., Escher, J. *et al.* (2006) European evidence based consensus on the diagnosis and management of Crohn's disease: special situations. *Gut*, **55**(suppl.), i36–i58.

Cosgrove, M., Al-Atia, R. F. and Jenkins, H. R. (1996) The epidemiology of paediatric inflammatory bowel disease. *Arch. Dis. Child.*, **74**, 460–1.

Cosnes, J., Cattan, S., Blain, A. *et al.* (2002) Long term evolution of disease behaviour of Crohn's disease. *Inflamm. Bowel Dis.*, **8**, 244–50.

Colombel, J. F., Sandborn, W. J., Rutgeerts, P. *et al.* (2007) Adalimumab for maintenance of clinical response and remission in patients with Crohn's disease: the CHARM trial. *Gastroenterology*, **132**, 52–65.

Crandall, W., Hyams, J., Kugathasan, S. *et al.* (2009) Infliximab therapy in children with concurrent perianal Crohn's disease: observations from REACH. *J. Pediatr. Gastroenterol. Nutr.*, **49**, 183–90.

Cucchiara, S., Escher, J. C., Hildebrand, H. *et al.* (2009) Pediatric inflammatory bowel disease and the risk of lymphoma: should we revise our treatment strategies? *J. Pediatr .Gastroenterol. Nutr.*, **48**, 257–67.

De Benetti, F. *et al.* (1997) Interleukin 6 causes growth impairment in transgenic mice through a decrease in insulin-like growth factor-1. A model for stunted growth in children with chronic inflammation. *J. Clin. Invest.*, **99**, 643–50.

Dinca, M., Fries, W., Luisetto, G. *et al.* (1999) Evolution of osteopenia in inflammatory bowel disease. *Am. J. Gastroenterol.*, **94**, 1292–7.

Evans, C. M., Kirk, J. M., Savage, M. O. *et al.* (1991) Growth after gut resection for Crohn's disease. *Arch. Dis. Child.*, **66**, 370.

Escher, J. C. (2004) Budesonide versus prednisolone for the treatment of active Crohn's disease in children: a randomized, double blind, controlled, multicentre trial. *Eur. J. Gastroenterol. Hepatol.*, **16**, 47–54.

Fell, J. M., Paintin, M., Arnaud-Battandier, F. *et al.* (2000) Mucosal healing and a fall in mucosal pro-inflammatory cytokine mRNA induced by a specific oral polymeric diet in paediatric Crohn's disease. *Aliment. Pharmacol. Ther.*, **14**, 281–9.

Glocker, E. O., Kotlarz, D., Boztug, E. M. *et al.* (2009) Inflammatory bowel disease and mutations affecting the interleukin-10 receptor. *N. Engl. J. Med.*, **362**, 2091–3.

Gokhale, R., Favus, M. J., Karrison, T. *et al* (1998) Bone mineral density assessment in children with inflammatory bowel disease. *Gastroenterology*, **114**, 902–11.

Griffiths, A. M. (2004) Specificities of inflammatory bowel disease in childhood. *Best Pract. Res. Clin. Gastroenterol.*, **18**, 509–23.

Hanauer, S. B., Feagan, B. G., Lichtenstein, G. R. *et al.* (2002) Maintenance infliximab for Crohn's disease: the ACCENT 1 randomised trial. *Lancet*, **359**, 1541–9.

Hanauer, S. B., Sandborne, W. J., Rutgeerts, P. *et al.* (2006) Human anti-tumor necrosis factor monoclonal antibody (adalimumab) in Crohn's disease: the CLASSIC-I trial. *Gastroenterology*, **130**, 323–33.

Henriksen, M., Jahansen, J., Lygren, I. *et al.* (2006) Ulcerative colitis and clinical course: results of a 5-year population based follow-up study (the IBSEN study). *Inflamm. Bowel Dis.*, **12**, 543–50.

Herzog, D., Bishop, N., Glorieux, F. *et al.* (1998) Interpretation of bone mineral density values in pediatric Crohn's disease. *Inflamm. Bowel Dis.*, **4**, 261–7.

Heuschkel, R. B., Menache, C. C., Megerian, J. M. and Baird, A. E. (2000) Enteral nutrition and corticosteroids in the treatment of acute Crohn's disease in children. *J. Pediatr. Gastroenterol. Nutr.*, **31**, 8–15.

Heuschkel, R., Salvestrini, C., Beattie, R. M., Hildebrand, H., Walters, T. and Griffiths, A. (2008) Guidelines for the management of growth failure in childhood inflammatory bowel disease. *Inflamm. Bowel Dis.*, **14**, 839–49.

Heyman, M. B., Kirschner, B. S., Gold, B. D. *et al.* (2005) Children with early onset inflammatory bowel disease (IBD): analysis of a pediatric IBD consortium. *J. Pediatr.*, **146**, 35–40.

Hoffenberg, E. J., Findanza, S. and Sauaia, A. (1999) Serological testing for inflammatory bowel disease. *J. Pediatr.*, **134**, 447–52.

Hommel, K. A., Davis, C. M. and Baldassano, R. N. (2009) Objective versus subjective assessment of oral medication adherence in pediatric inflammatory bowel disease. *Inflamm. Bowel Dis.*, **15**, 589–93.

Hugot, J. P., Chamaillard, M., Zouali, H. *et al.* (2001) Association of NOD2 leucine-rich repeat variants with susceptibility to Crohn's disease. *Nature*, **411**, 599–603.

Hyams, J., Markowitz, J., Lerer, T. *et al.* (2006) The natural history of corticosteroid therapy for ulcerative colitis in children. *Clin. Gastroenterol. Hepatol.*, **4**, 1118–23.

Hyams, J., Crandall, W., Kugathasan, S. *et al.* (2007) Induction and maintenance infliximab therapy for the treatment of moderate-to-severe Crohn's disease in children. *Gastroenterology*, **132**, 863–73.

IBD working group of the European Society of Paediatric Gastroenterology Hepatology and Nutrition (ESPGHAN) (2005) Inflammatory bowel disease in children and adolescents: Recommendations for diagnosis – the Porto criteria. *J. Pediatr. Gastroenterol. Nutr.*, **41**, 1–7.

Imielinski, M., Baldassano, R. N., Griffiths, A. *et al.* (2009) Common variants at five new loci associated with early-onset inflammatory bowel disease. *Nature Genetics*, **41**(12), 1335–40.

Jenkins, D., Balsitis, M., Gallivan, S. *et al.* (1997) Guidelines for the initial biopsy of suspected chronic idiopathic inflammatory bowel disease. The British Society of Gastroenterology Initiative. *J. Clin. Path.*, **50**, 93–105.

Laghi, A., Borrelli, O., Paolontonio, P. *et al.* (2003) Contrast enhanced magnetic resonance imaging of the terminal ileum in children with Crohn's disease. *Gut*, **52**, 393–7.

Lawson, M. M., Thomas, A. G. and Akobeng, A. K. (2006) Tumour necrosis factor alpha blocking agents for induction of remission in ulcerative colitis. *Cochrane Database Syst. Rev.*, 3:CD005112.

Leonard, M. B., Feldman, H. I., Schults, J. *et al.* (2004) Long-term, high-dose glucocorticoids and bone mineral content in childhood glucocorticoid-sensitive nephritic syndrome. *N. Engl. J. Med.*, **351**, 868–75.

Lichtenstein, G. R., Cohen, R. D., Feagan, B. G. *et al.* (2007) Safety of infliximab and other Crohn's disease therapies – TREAT Registry data with nearly 20,000 patient-years follow up. *DDW*, S1124.

Martensson, K., Chrysis, D. and Savendahl, L. (2004) Interleukin-1β and TNF-α act in synergy to inhibit longitudinal growth in fetal rat metatarsal bones. *J. Bone Miner. Res.*,

19, 1805–12.

Markowitz, J., Grancher, K., Kohn, N. *et al.* (2000) A multicenter trial of 6-mercaptopurine and prednisone in children with newly diagnosed Crohn's disease. *Gastroenterology*, **119**, 895–902.

Markowitz, J., Grancher, K., Kohn, N. and Daum, F. (2002) Immunomodulatory therapy for pediatric inflammatory bowel disease: changing patterns of use, 1990–2000. *Am. J. Gastroenterol.*, **97**, 928–32.

Markowitz, J., Hyams, J., Mack, D. *et al.* (2006) Corticosteroid therapy in the age of infliximab: acute and 1-year outcomes in newly diagnosed children with Crohn's disease. *Clin. Gastroenterol. Hepatol.*, **4**, 1124–9.

Mizokami, A., Gotoh, A., Yamada, H. *et al.* (2000) Tumor necrosis factor-α represses androgen sensitivity in the LNCaP prostate cancer cell line. *J. Urol.*, **164**, 800–5.

Newby, E. A., Sawczenko, A., Thomas, A. G. *et al.* (2005) Interventions for growth failure in childhood Crohn's disease. *Cochrane Database Syst. Rev.*, 3:CD003873.

Orel, R., Kamhi, T., Vidmar, G. *et al.* (2009) Epidemiology of pediatric chronic inflammatory bowel disease in central and western Slovenia, 1994–2005. *J. Pediatr. Gastroenterol. Nutr.*, **48**, 579–86.

Otley, A., Smith, C., Nicholas, D. *et al.* (2002) The IMPACT questionnaire: a valid measure of health-related quality of life in pediatric inflammatory bowel disease. *J. Pediatr. Gastroenterol. Nutr.*, **35**, 557–63.

Pozler, O., Maly, J., Bonova, O. *et al.* (2006) Incidence of Crohn's disease in the Czech republic in the years 1990 to 2001 and assessment of pediatric population with inflammatory bowel disease. *J. Pediatr. Gastroenterol. Nutr.*, **42**, 186–9.

Rosh, J. R., Gross, T., Mamula, P. *et al.* (2007) Hepatosplenic T-cell lymphoma in adolescents and young adults with Crohn's disease: a cautionary tale? *Inflamm. Bowel Dis.*, **13**, 1024–30.

Ruemmele, F. M., Targan, S. R., Levy, G. *et al.* (1998) Diagnostic accuracy of serological assays in pediatric inflammatory bowel disease. *Gastroenterology*, **115**, 822–9.

Sanderson, I. R., Udeen, S., Davies, P. S. *et al.* (1987) Remission induced by an elemental diet in small bowel Crohn's disease. *Arch. Dis. Child.*, **62**, 123–7.

Sandhu, B. K., Fell, J. M. E., Beattie, R. M. *et al.* (2010) Guidelines for the management of inflammatory bowel disease (IBD) in children in the United Kingdom. *J. Pediatr. Gastroenterol. Nutr.*, **50**, S1–S13.

Sawczenko, A., Sandhu, B. K., Logan, R. F. *et al.* (2001) Prospective survey of childhood inflammatory bowel disease in the British Isles. *Lancet*, **357**, 1093–4.

Sawczenko, A. and Sandhu, B. (2003) Presenting features of inflammatory bowel disease in Great Britain and Ireland. *Arch. Dis. Child.*, **88**, 995–1000.

Sawczenko, A., Ballinger, A. B., Savage, M. O. *et al.* (2006) Clinical features affecting final adult height in patients with pediatric – onset Crohn's disease. *Pediatrics*, **118**, 124–9.

Seidman, E. G., Sant'Anna, A. M. and Dirks, M. H. (2004) Potential applications of wireless capsule endoscopy in the pediatric age group. *Gastrointest. Endosc. Clin. N. Am.*, **14**, 207–17.

Semeao, E. J., Jawad, A. F., Stouffer, N. O. *et al.* (1999) Risk factors for low bone mineral density in children and young adults with Crohn's disease. *J. Pediatr.* **135**, 593–600.

Silverberg, M. S., Satsangi, J., Ahmad, T. *et al.* (2005) Towards an integrated clinical, molecular and serological classification of inflammatory bowel disease: report of a working party of the 2005 Montreal world congress of gastroenterology. *Can. J. Gatrroenterol.*, **19**(suppl.), 5A–36A.

Tarrant, K. M., Barclay, M. L., Frampton, C. M. A. *et al.* (2008) Perianal disease predicts changes in Crohn's disease phenotype- results of a population-based study of inflammatory bowel disease phenotype. *Am. J. Gastroenterol.*, **103**, 3082–93.

Thomas, A. G., Taylor, F. and Miller, V. (1993) Dietary intake and nutritional treatment in childhood Crohn's disease. *J. Paediatr. Gastroenterol. Nutr.*, **17**, 75–81.

Uhlen, S., Belbouab, R., Narebski, K. *et al.* (2006) Efficacy of methotrexate in pediatric Crohn's disease: a French multicenter study. *Inflamm. Bowel Dis.*, **12**, 1053–7.

Van Limbergen, J., Russell, R. K., Drummond, H. E. *et al.* (2008) Definition of phenotypic characteristics of childhood-onset inflammatory bowel disease. *Gastroenterology*, **135**, 1114–22.

Vernier-Masouille, G., Balde, M., Salleron, J. *et al.* (2008) Natural history of pediatric Crohn's disease. *Gastroenterology*, **135**, 1106–13.

Walker-Smith, J. A. (1996) Management of growth failure in Crohn's disease. *Arch. Dis. Child.*, **75**, 351–4.

Walters, T. D. and Griffiths, A. M. (2009) Mechanisms of growth impairment in pediatric Crohn's disease. *Nat. Rev. Gastroenterol. Hepatol.*, **6**, 513–23.

Wilson, D. C., Thomas, A. G., Croft, N. M. *et al.* (2010) Systematic review of the evidence base for the medical treatment of paediatric inflammatory bowel disease. *J. Pediatr. Gastroenterol. Nutr.*, **50**, S14–S34.

Witte, J., Shivananda, S., Leonard-Jones, J. E. *et al.* (2000) Disease outcome in inflammatory bowel disease: mortality, morbidity and therapeutic management of a 796-person inception cohort in the European collaborative study on inflammatory bowel disease (EC-IBD). *Scand. J. Gastroenterol.*, **35**, 1272–7.

Yamamoto, T., Nakahigashi, M., Umegae, S. and Matsumoto, K. (2010) Enteral nutrition for the maintenance of remission in Crohn's disease: a systematic review. *Eur. J. Gastroenterol. Hepatol.*, **22**, 1–8.

Zachos, M., Tondeur, M. and Griffiths, A. M. (2001) Enteral nutritional therapy for induction of remission in Crohn's disease. *Cochrane Database Syst. Rev.*, **3**, CD000542.

CHAPTER 15

Managing the transition from paediatric to adult care

Kay Greveson and Vikki Garrick

Introduction

Around 10–15% of inflammatory bowel disease presents in childhood (Biancone *et al.*, 2008) and, as with all chronic disease, this requires a multidisciplinary, multi-faceted approach in order to deliver care effectively. Children and adolescents with chronic disease such as inflammatory bowel disease (IBD) are surviving longer as a result of advances in paediatric care (Carson, 2001). The point where the adolescent becomes an adult represents a milestone not only in healthcare delivery, but also in the wider context, such as education, employment, sexual and psychosocial development. The transition from paediatric to adult care is integral to this development, but is often poorly done. Effective transition is recognised as a core standard in the National Service Framework for Children, Young People and Maternity Services (Department of Health, 2004). A generally accepted definition of transition is:

> A purposeful, planned process that addresses the medical, psychosocial and educational/ vocational needs of adolescents and young adults with chronic physical and medical conditions as they move from child-centred to adult orientated health care systems (Blum *et al.*, 1993, p. 570)

Many confuse transition with transfer; but this is just a single component, occurring at one point along the transition pathway, and should not be the main focus (Hait *et al.*, 2006). The aim should be to provide effective coordinated care which promotes independence, communication and decision making skills in preparation for adult life. The cyclical nature of IBD and treatment means that patients should be transferred with as much continuity as possible. Well-organised transition is vital and has been shown to have measurable benefits in terms of improved follow-up, increased disease control, adherence and quality of life (Department of Health, 2006; Biancone *et al.*, 2008).

There are marked differences between child-centred and adult-orientated healthcare which can impact on transition. Paediatric healthcare is very family focused, and when the child is still young the care tends to be parent-led, with consultations and clinical decisions predominantly made by the parent. There are marked differences in treatment: for example, the use of enteral feeding instead of corticosteroids. Much more emphasis is put on physical growth and pubertal development, including the use of growth charts. As the child progresses through puberty and into adolescence, consultations are directed much more towards the young person; however, the parent is always present. Conversely, adult-orientated healthcare is directed towards patients who have fully developed in terms of autonomy, independence and ability to make treatment decisions (Hait *et al.*, 2009; Robertson *et al.*, 2006). Adult gastroenterologists also encounter long-term issues such as fertility, colorectal cancer risk and surveillance more frequently than their paediatric counterparts, and therefore have familiarity in addressing these issues. The transition period should be used to educate young people in these differences and equip them with the knowledge and skills needed to interact effectively in the new heath care system (Robertson *et al.*, 2006). Here we focus on various issues surrounding the management of young adults through the transition from child-centred to adult-orientated healthcare and give practical insight into how to manage services in order to facilitate this process.

Case study

Jane was diagnosed with Crohn's disease at 9 years old. Growth and puberty had been delayed as a result of aggressive disease and she had struggled to cope with this emotionally. Both she and her family required significant support as she progressed through adolescence, and there were problems with medication adherence and acceptance of her condition.

By the time Jane was ready for transition to adult services, she had experienced several hospital admissions and was maintained on biologic therapy after failing to respond to standard second line therapies. The transition process started when she was 15 and entering the last year of school. Both she and her parents felt she was ready to take more control in managing her own disease. Initially she was sent a letter by the IBD nurses identifying how best to achieve this. In essence this involved:

- coming into the clinic room alone at appointments
- arranging her own blood monitoring at the GP
- arranging repeat prescriptions at the GP

In addition, the letter was addressed to Jane herself (this does not usually happen in the paediatric setting: the letters are addressed to the parent or guardian). Following attendance at the clinic, Jane had further input from the IBD nurses addressing issues such as sexual health and other social pressures often experienced by teenagers – mainly advice on smoking and alcohol intake.

The next clinic took place in the paediatric setting with the adult gastroenterologist, adult IBD nurse, paediatric gastroenterologist and paediatric IBD nurse, with the consultation led by the paediatric team. Summary documentation was prepared and sent to the adult centre before the first joint consultation so that all parties were aware of the patient and her journey to date. In addition, a pre-clinic meeting was held to further discuss the case and highlight any current issues which had arisen between appointments. In this way both teams were appropriately prepared before the patient arrived in the clinic room.

Jane was introduced to those taking over her care in an environment familiar to her and in the presence of staff she was familiar with. During this appointment, practical issues, such as differences in medical management, in particular endoscopy, were discussed. Many paediatric centres use general anaesthetics for endoscopy, while most adult centres use sedation. This is a particular source of anxiety at transition both for young people and their parents and Jane was no exception to this.

Finally, the handover process was completed with a further appointment in the adult setting. This was attended by the paediatric gastroenterologist and IBD nurse, but was led by the adult team. Jane therefore had the experience of attending the adult hospital for the first time in a supported manner. She attended the appointment herself, with her parents being invited in at the end of the session to allow them the forum to raise any concerns they may have had between appointments. The whole process took around one year and both Jane and her family were positive about this experience.

Role of the healthcare worker

Transition requires multidisciplinary and multi-agency input (including but not exclusive to adult and paediatric doctors and nurses, social services, educational agencies and dietitians), with all involved understanding the roles of different professionals within the team and how to access services (Department of Health, 2008). Paediatric and adult healthcare providers are pivotal in guiding young people though the transition to adulthood. For transfer to be successful there has to be effective collaboration between both teams at the transition interface (McDonagh, 2005), and the development of an appropriate and effective model of care.

Developing models

Several models have been proposed for transfer and are highlighted in Box 15.1. They vary significantly and can include an intermediary step model where adolescents are seen at sequential visits by both paediatric and adult teams, or where they are seen at one visit by both teams and then immediately transferred over to adult care. The model adopted depends on local resources, such as the availability of a specialist nurse or presence of on-site paediatric gastroenterology department. Joint paediatric and adult transition clinics, where the adolescent is seen by both teams for as long as appropriate are considered optimal (Biancone *et al.*, 2008, Sandhu *et al.*, 2008) as this enables developmental transition and serves to reassure the young person and their family that the teams are working together. This also provides a conducive environment for experiential learning for both teams (McDonagh 2005).

Whichever model of transitional care is adopted, continuous audit is imperative to ensure outcomes are improved and maintained (Royal College of Nursing, 2004). Services must be evaluated against measures of development; extent of adolescent/ parent involvement in planning and delivering services; and the quality of experiences and outcomes. This ensures a tailored, age-appropriate service that meets the needs of adolescents and their families. Assessment measures, such a developmental frameworks, checklists or educational tools must be evaluated to ensure they are appropriate and useful in the context of transition.

Box 15.1 Transition models

- **Handover clinic**: One-off direct transfer – single step from paediatric to adult clinic with little face-to-face communication.
- **Parallel clinic**: Paediatric and adult clinics run at the same time but independently, allowing for communication between teams.
- **Transition clinic**: Adolescent patients seen by both teams so that all involved develop familiarity and transfer of expertise.

The key worker

The introduction of a named key worker to oversee and coordinate the process is pivotal in ensuring a positive outcome (Royal College of Nursing, 2004). The role is often taken by the IBD clinical nurse specialist or paediatrician who is familiar with the adolescent and the family, and is therefore in a position to assess the need for additional input such as social worker or emotional/ psychological support along the pathway. IBD nurses trained in dealing with adolescents have a pivotal role in coordinating care between the service, the patient and their family during the transition period (Biancone *et al.*, 2008). Paediatric IBD nurses are ideal key workers as they are already familiar with the adolescents and their families. Further training for those not formally trained in paediatrics may come from in-house programmes or standalone modules, which may be available from educational institutions. Alternatively experience can be gained from working alongside paediatric colleagues. Key workers can develop a transition plan to coordinate care and facilitate the decision for formal handover in conjunction with the patient (NACC and CICRA, 2008). They may also help adolescents and their families overcome the perceived barriers to transition, such as meeting new teams and having appropriate clinical expectations; by being a constant familiar face and point of contact; and by helping to educate and empower them to be more independent.

Healthcare professionals from adult teams working with adolescents often perceive barriers in having adequate knowledge and confidence to deal sensitively with the needs of the young person – for example, pubertal and educational development (Hait *et al.*, 2009). Close communication between both adult and paediatric teams is essential and an excellent way of ensuring two-way learning in dealing with these issues.

Setting up the service

The reality of setting up an effective transition service depends on many factors, not least of which is the availability of key personnel to be involved. These personnel would be:

- Adult gastroenterologist
- Adult IBD nurse
- Adult GI dietitian (where available)
- Adult psychologist (where available)

The pathway proposed by the Royal College of Nursing (2004) is a helpful document for outlining the process for the patient. A pathway which outlines clear

285

lines of responsibility within the local healthcare team is also helpful when setting up the service. In addition, condition specific transition documentation ensures effective communication of all relevant stages in the patient's paediatric medical history to the adult setting.

Patient advocacy

Forging relationships

The move from paediatric to adult care is a time of great upheaval for both the adolescent and their family. All parties involved in the process will have concerns which must be addressed. Strong links have often been forged between the young person, their family and the paediatric team, particularly during periods of ill health. The adolescent and parents will initially have a lack of familiarity with the adult team. They may also be concerned that the team will not have adequate knowledge about the medical history, or not be as sensitive to developmental or social issues, and that the issues arising may be too complex for the adult team to deal with (Tuchman *et al.*, 2008; Baldessano *et al.*, 2002). These issues need to be dealt with over the course of the transition process by encouraging open and frank discussions and forging relationships with open effective lines of communication with the adult team. Research has shown that adolescents prefer to be prepared for eventual transfer early so that they can become accustomed to the idea and have time to meet the new team (Tuchman *et al.*, 2008). The literature also suggests that transition should be introduced long before it becomes an issue, and should be done in an open, consistent manner that is flexible and allows for any setbacks, for example, as a result of ill health (Department of Heath, 2006). The Royal College of Nursing advocates this and suggests a pathway whereby the concept of transition to adult healthcare is introduced from the age of 12 (See Figure 15.1). Issues may be complicated when there is geographical distance between the paediatric and adult clinics. In these cases it is important to forge excellent communication links between teams in each department and ensure the concept of transition is introduced one year before the formal transfer to allow at least two visits to the adult clinic (Department of Heath 2006).

Promoting autonomy

Adolescents report a desire for autonomy (Tuchman *et al.*, 2008; Baldessano *et al.*, 2002). Despite being a family-focused event, the transition framework should encourage adolescents to attend at least part of the clinic independently of their parents, as this encourages them to develop essential communication skills,

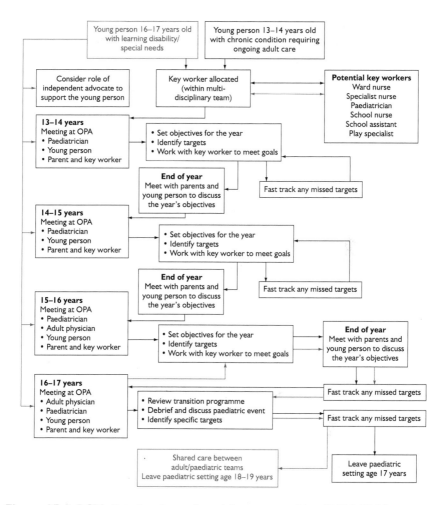

Figure 15.1 RCN clinical pathway for adolescent transition (RCN, 2004; reproduced with kind permission from the RCN).

exercise autonomy and feel respected and involved in their own care (Department of Health, 2004; Shaw *et al.*, 2004). It also enables then to discuss topics such as alcohol, drug use, smoking and safe sex, which they may be reluctant to with parents present. This is an important concept, but requires a careful balance to ensure that the parents feel included while at the same time giving the adolescent more control and independence. This approach is clearly not ideal for all adolescents, as there is a tremendous variation in maturity and education which must be taken into consideration throughout. A clear understanding of the adolescent developmental framework is critical to providing appropriate care and forming an effective partnership with patients and their family (Hait *et al.*, 2009).

Adolescents with chronic disease such as IBD have the same issues about their health and body as their healthy counterparts, but often this can be overshadowed by disease and illness (Soanes and Timmons, 2004). Baldessano *et al.* (2002) suggest that adolescents with IBD may have more age-related concerns, for example alcohol consumption, sexual activity, medication side-effects or restrictions such as those imposed by corticosteroids or methotrexate. The predominant focus of transition is for the young person to develop autonomy and be educated in disease awareness, self-management and decision-making within the healthcare setting (Department of Health, 2006), as is the case with adults diagnosed with IBD. This includes principles such as having an understanding of medications they are taking and potential side-effects, how to contact the hospital, how to recognise symptoms of a flare and what to do in this situation. It is also important to acknowledge life beyond the young person's disease; they should be assisted in managing social, educational and employment issues in the wider context of their growth and development. This is not a simple task and takes considerable time and effort through education, discussions with the adolescent and their family and structured transition planning by those directly involved in the transition process. The Royal College of Nursing has developed useful guidance for transitional care which can be adapted to local needs and include checklists for key areas of development and stages of the transition process (RCN, 2004). This covers early, middle and late stage transition and incorporates various aspects, including sexual health, psychological support and self-advocacy at each stage. The guidance provides structure and goals for the adolescent to achieve at each stage, further empowering and preparing them for the transfer to adult care. This should always be implemented gradually, discussed and documented throughout to enable the adolescent to have a structure and future goals towards final transfer. Hand-held patient records have been suggested as being a useful tool to aid in this framework and promote involvement (Hait *et al.*, 2009). McDonagh (2005) suggests a useful acronym, 'HEADS', which can be used in clinical practice to help address generic health issues (see Box 15.2). This starts with easy topics and moves to more sensitive issues and can provide a strong foundation for addressing adolescent issues.

Steps can be taken during transition to facilitate the process and encourage autonomy. Parents have equally valid concerns about the process. During childhood they are the predominant decision makers for their child. Transition sees a gradual shift in this relationship, where the adolescent gains more control

---

Box 15.2 HEADS acronym (McDonagh, 2005)
H   Home: relationships, social support, household chores
E   Education: school, exams, work experience, career
E   Exercise: general
A   Activities: peers
A   Affect
A   Ambitions
D   Dental care
D   Diet: calcium, vitamin D, weight, caffeine
D   Driving
D   Drugs, cigarettes, alcohol
S   Sex: concerns, periods, contraception
S   Sleep
(Reproduced with kind permission from John Wiley & Sons Ltd)

---

and autonomy. Parents may have feelings of being shut out or ignored and may be reluctant to 'let go'. For this reason it is essential for transition to be a family-focused event, with a triad of communication between the young person, parent and healthcare professional (Department of Health, 2006).

Education

Education is at the forefront of promoting autonomy, with the clinical nurse specialist ideally situated to deliver developmentally appropriate information to arm adolescents with the necessary skills to function in the adult service. Early and repetitive teaching of important concepts, including disease, medication and issues such as smoking, fertility and pregnancy, are integral to self-management and have been shown to improve not only coping mechanisms for chronic disease but also quality of life and adherence (McDonagh, 2005; Shaw *et al.*, 2004). Assessment of understanding is equally important in order to identify individual barriers or setbacks with learning and implement a strategy for intervention (Hait *et al.*, 2009). The transition framework should mirror this.

Timing of transition

Adolescents should be encouraged to have an active role in planning and delivering services, particularly with regard to determining the timing of transfer (Department of Health, 2006). Optimal timing should not be based on chronological age and should instead be flexible, focusing on developmental readiness with regard to

289

self-management behaviours, communication skills and disease awareness, in addition to health status and readiness for transition (Department of Health, 2006; McDonagh, 2005; Callahan *et al.*, 2001). These can all be assessed using a framework such as one proposed by the RCN (2004), which mirrors developmental stages and assesses progress toward transition. Transfer should ideally take place when the disease is in remission and also when there are no coinciding social or educational transitions (such as starting university), as this may be too much change at once and have a negative impact (Tuchman *et al.*, 2008). Adolescents and parents should feel ready and prepared for the transfer to adult care and should not feel under pressure from such deadlines. This aspect can be challenging, as often there are institutional barriers, such as a cut-off age for admission or service provision, which can negatively affect this preferred flexibility.

Guidance produced from the National Association for Colitis and Crohn's Disease (NACC) and CICRA (2008) also suggest adopting a mentoring or buddy scheme, where the young person is put in contact with someone who has been though the transition process, as a way of facilitating the move and reducing anxiety about the situation. This again depends on the individual and stage of development and confidence. It is also important to note that the issues surrounding transition, including the steps that can be taken to resolve surrounding issues, can be tailored to the majority of settings, including those overseas. This will obviously depend on local delivery, role boundaries and national guidance.

Support groups

The collaboration of IBD support groups such as the NACC (now known as Crohn's and Colitis UK) and CICRA, with working groups involving societies such as the British Society of Gastroenterology (BSG), British Society of Paediatric Gastroenterology Hepatology and Nutrition (BSPGHAN), and the Royal College of Nursing have produced excellent transition guidance based on current evidence. This guidance is available for healthcare professionals, parents and young people, advising on current best practice and informing adolescents what they should be expecting from their transition service. For further information on the role of support groups, refer to Chapter 13.

Connexions Direct is a local authority run service in England available to all young people between the ages of 13 and 19 which provides diverse information and guidance on a range of issues including health, relationships, employment, and social issues including alcohol and drug use. Services can be accessed online, including web chat, message boards and confidential advice, or through local connexions centres. This encourages adolescents and their parents to be proactive in dealing with everyday issues that include and impact on their health.

Box 15.3 summarises some support groups and organisations available for young people.

Conclusion

The purpose of this chapter is to give nurses either already working with adolescents or considering setting up a transitional service an insight into the considerations that need to be made and provisions set up in order to deliver effective coordinated care. This type of service promotes independence, communication and decision-making skills needed by the adolescent for eventual transfer to adult services. Well-organised transition has the ability to provide measurable benefits in terms of improved follow-up, increased disease control, adherence and quality of life, and should be done in a careful, planned and consistent manner. Multidisciplinary and multi-agency working is an essential component of an effective transition clinic. Nurses should be encouraged to forge links with units with established transition clinics in order to learn from their experience, develop supportive networks and share protocols in order to develop an effective model of care that reflects their patients and local service needs.

Box 15.3 Useful contacts

National Association for Crohn's and Colitis Disease
http://www.nacc.org.uk/

Crohn's in Childhood Research Association
http://www.cicra.org/

Connexions direct
http://www.connexions-direct.com/

Transition in IBD: guidelines for healthcare workers, adolescents and parents
http://www.ibdtransition.org.uk/

Patient translation summary

Inflammatory bowel disease (IBD) is being diagnosed more frequently in children and young people. This group of people have very different needs from the adult population and healthcare providers have a responsibility to ensure these needs are being met. Transition is the process where the responsibility for the young person's care is moved from the children's hospital to the adult hospital. It is important to realise that transition is a process, not an event, and this has to be planned in conjunction with the young person and their family. This can be a time of significant anxiety for the young person and their parents, and healthcare staff must make sure that they are adequately prepared for this change in their care. Within the team, the IBD nurse is best placed to act as the coordinator for transition. She or he is frequently the interface between the families and the healthcare providers and is therefore more able to assess when the young person is ready for transition from both of these perspectives. Timing for transition has to be flexible and patient driven where possible. Ideally, transition would be a staged process and the final point of handover to the adult services would be at a time where the young person's IBD is well controlled and they are adequately prepared to take on the responsibility for their condition. This can be challenging in the healthcare setting. Effective communication between the child and adult teams is vital if the process is to be effective, and there are several models of transition available for the healthcare providers to use as a guide. In addition, support groups such as Crohn's and Colitis UK and CICRA are a great resource for the families.

References

Baldassano, R., Ferry, G., Griffiths, A. *et al.* (2002) Transition of the patient with inflammatory bowel disease from pediatric to adult care: recommendations of the North American Society for Pediatric Gastroenterology, Hepatology and Nutrition. *J. Pediatr. Gastroenterol. Nutr.*, **34**, 245–8.

Biancone, L., Michetti, P. and Travis, T. (2008) European evidence-based Consensus on the management of ulcerative colitis: special situations. *J. Crohn's and Colitis*, **2**, 63–92.

Blum, R. W., Garell, D., Hodgman, C. H. *et al.* (1993) Transition from child centred to adult health care systems for adolescents with chronic conditions. A position paper of the Society for Adolescent Medicine. *J. Adolesc. Health*, **14**, 570–6.

Callahan, S. T., Winitzer, R. F. and Keenan, P. (2001) Transition from pediatric to adult-orientated health care: a challenge for patients with chronic disease. *Curr. Opinion Gastroenterol.*, **13**, 310–16.

Carson, A. R. (2001) Adult paediatric patients. *Am. J. Nursing*, **101**(3), 46–54.

Department of Health (2004) *National Service Framework for Children, Young People and Maternity Services*. http://www.dh.gov.uk/en/Publicationsandstatistics/Publications/PublicationsPolicyAndGuidance/DH_4089101 (accessed 6 September 2010).

Department of Health (2006) *Transition: Getting it Right for Young People*. http://www.dh.gov.uk/en/Publicationsandstatistics/Publications/PublicationsPolicyAndGuidance/DH_4132145 (accessed 6 September 2010).

Department of Health (2008) *Transition: Moving on Well*. http://www.dh.gov.uk/en/Publicationsandstatistics/Publications/PublicationsPolicyAndGuidance/DH_083592 (accessed 6 September 2010).

Hait, E., Arnold, J. and Fishman, L. (2006). Educate, communicate, anticipate – practical recommendations for transitioning adolescents with IBD to adult care. *Inflamm. Bowel Dis.*, **12**, 70–3.

Hait, E., Barendse, M., Janis, H. *et al.* (2009) Transition of adolescents with inflammatory bowel disease from pediatric to adult care: a survey of adult gastroenterologists. *J. Pediatr. Gastroenterol. Nutr.*, **48**, 61–5.

McDonagh, J. E. (2005) Growing up and moving on: transition from pediatric to adult care. *Pediatr. Transplant.*, **9**, 364–72.

National Association of Crohn's and Colitis and CICRA (2008) *Inflammatory Bowel Disease Transition to Adult Health Care. Guidance for Health Care Professionals*. http://www.ibdtransition.org.uk/ (accessed 6 September 2010).

Royal College of Nursing (2004) *Adolescent Transition Care: Guidance for Nursing Staff*. http://www.rcn.org.uk/__data/assets/pdf_file/0011/78617/002313.pdf (accessed 6 September 2010).

Robertson, L. P., McDonagh, J. E. and Southwood, T. R. (2006) Growing up and moving on. A multicentre UK audit of the transfer of adolescents with juvenile idiopathic arthritis from paediatric to adult centred care. *Ann. Rheum. Dis.*, **65**, 74–80.

Sandhu, B. K., Fell, J. M. E., Beattie, R. M. and Mitton, S. G. (2008) *Guidelines for the Management of Inflammatory Bowel Disease (IBD) in Children in the United Kingdom*. http://bspghan.org.uk/working_groups/documents/IBDGuidelines_000.pdf (accessed 27 August 2010).

Shaw, K. L., Southwood, T. R. and McDonough, J. E. (2004) Transitional care for adolescents with juvenile idiopathic arthritis: a Delphi study. *Rheumatology*, **43**, 1000–6.

Soanes, C. and Timmons, S. (2004) Improving transition: a qualitative study examining the attitudes of young people with chronic illness transferring to adult care. *J. Child Health Care*, **8**, 102–12.

Tuchman, L. K., Slap, G. B. and Britto, M. T. (2008) Transition to adult care: experiences and expectations of adolescents with a chronic illness. *Child: Care, Health and Development*, **34**, 557–63.

CHAPTER 16

Psychosocial aspects of inflammatory bowel disease

Sonya Chelvanayagam and Anton Emmanuel

The active mind is difficult to tame, flighty and wandering wherever it wills; taming it is essential, leading to the joy of well-being.

The Buddha (Dh 35)

Introduction

Inflammatory bowel diseases (IBD) are regarded as chronic disorders which typically present in early adulthood. These diseases are not curable, although symptoms may be ameliorated by surgical or medication intervention (see Chapters 6–9). The person with IBD will experience periods of remission and relapses with their condition (Younge and Norton, 2007). There is an unpredictability regarding the course of the disease, so a person cannot identify when an exacerbation of their symptoms will occur (Schneider and Fletcher, 2008). The symptoms are painful, socially disabling and involve bowel function, which remains a taboo area (Pihl-Lesnovska *et al.*, 2010). Corrective surgery can lead to the formation of a stoma which will alter body image and will require a period of readjustment (Williams, 2005). Therefore all of these factors will undoubtedly have a profound effect on psychosocial functioning. This chapter will discuss the impact of IBD on a person's psychological, physical and social functioning and discuss interventions to help improve their quality of life.

Effects of chronic illness on health

The Expert Patient Programme, developed in 2001 by the UK's Department of Health, stated that 17.5 million people in the UK live with a chronic disease (Department of Health, 2001). Sixty per cent of people in England report living

295

with a chronic health problem, with 9% of the population reported living with a 'digestive health problem', which includes stomach, liver and kidneys (Department of Health, 2004). Living with chronic illness has an effect on physical and psychological functioning, causes social and economic difficulties and can make individuals feel socially excluded, especially when suffering from a stigmatising condition. These effects also have ramifications for the person's family.

Prolonged physical illness has a direct effect on mental health (NHS Information Centre, 2009). Unfortunately, symptoms related to mental health problems may not be recognised. For example if a person is suffering from an exacerbation of their ulcerative colitis they may report feeling tired and lethargic, with loss of energy and motivation. They may also report not eating properly, sleeping difficulties, loss of libido or interest in usually enjoyable activities. These are also symptoms of depression. The clinician will be able to objectively measure the person' disease index, but depression is measured much more subjectively, although the use of rating scales can help to formulate a diagnosis. Also, people with mental illness state that, when reporting physical symptoms to staff within primary or secondary services, their symptoms are disregarded or are attributed to their mental health problems and related medication (Seymour, 2003). Head *et al.* (2008) discovered, when examining predictions of mortality in relation to diagnosis of certified sickness, that sickness absences due to mental health problems, particularly depression, had increased mortality related to cancer and cardiovascular disease. They felt that this may be due to depression causing a delay in health seeking, and cancer survival is closely related to early detection of symptoms. They postulated that possibly the early symptoms of cancer such as tiredness could be presumed to be a mental health diagnosis rather than physical illness.

Health-related quality of life in IBD

Health-related quality of life (HRQOL) examines the effect of a symptom or disorder on physical, psychological and social functioning from the person's perspective (Irvine, 2008). Health-related quality of life measures are most frequently used to evaluate the outcome of medical or surgical interventions, but also examine the impact of living with a specific disorder. They can influence decision making and directly inform practice and are usually in the form of self-report questionnaires rather than clinician-directed interviews (Higginson and Carr, 2001).

HRQOL measures are global, generic or disease-specific. Global measures examine overall quality of life (not necessarily health related) rather than specific areas. Generic measures, such as Medical Outcomes Scale Short Form 36 (MOS – SF36) (Stewart *et al.*, 1989) can compare changes across a range of disorders and have been used to examine HRQOL in gastrointestinal conditions including IBD (Guthrie *et al.*, 2002).

Disease-specific instruments examine the effect of a particular condition on the related patient population. The disease-specific measures used to assess quality of life with IBD which have been well validated are:

- Inflammatory Bowel Disease Questionnaire (IBDQ) (Guyatt *et al.*, 1989)
- Rating Form for Inflammatory Bowel Disease Patients' Concerns (RFIPC) (Drossman *et al.*, 1989)
- Gastrointestinal Quality of Life Index (GQLI) (Eypasch *et al.*, 1995)

The IBDQ is the most widely used and felt to be most suitable for assessing treatment outcome. It has 32 items, covering four domains – bowel symptoms, systemic effects and effects on social and emotional functioning. Each question is answered by a seven point Likert scale. It can be self-administered or completed by the clinician. However, Canavan *et al.* (2006) recommend that a clinician completes it rather than the patient.

The Rating Form for Inflammatory Bowel Disease Patients' Concerns consists of 25 questions which examine four domains – impact of IBD, sexual relationships, complications of the disease and body stigma. For each answer there is a 10 cm visual analogue scale on which the person marks their response 0 cm (not at all) – 10 cm (a great deal). This measure is more focused on psychological aspects associated with living with IBD and is self-administered.

The Gastrointestinal Quality of Life Index is not specific to IBD but can be used to assess HRQOL across a population with gastrointestinal disorders (Eypasch *et al.*, 1995). It contains 36 questions which are scored on a five-point Likert scale.

HRQOL has been examined extensively in both ulcerative colitis and Crohn's disease across age and gender groups and socioeconomic status, from diagnosis to longstanding disease. Although there are some variations, generally:

- People with IBD have a poorer quality of life than the general population at all stages of the disease (i.e. newly diagnosed or ongoing disease) (Lix *et al.*, 2008; Canavan *et al.*, 2006; Sainsbury and Heatley, 2005; Bernklev *et al.*, 2004).
- Women with IBD report poorer quality of life than men particularly in Crohn's disease (Sainsbury and Heatley, 2005; Rubin *et al.*, 2004; Bernklev *et al.*, 2004).

- Crohn's disease has a greater negative impact on HRQOL than ulcerative colitis and is equally poor in those newly diagnosed and with longstanding disease (Canavan *et al.*, 2006; Berklev *et al.*, 2004).
- HRQOL worsens with disease severity/relapse (Pihl-Lesnovska *et al.*, 2010; Vidal *et al.*, 2008).
- Individuals with IBD who have a lower socioeconomic status report worse HRQOL. Also those living in more deprived districts reported significantly lower HRQOL which was not related to extent of disease (Rubin *et al.*, 2004).
- Co-morbidity of psychiatric illness/psychological disorder will adversely affect HRQOL (Irvine, 2008; Vidal *et al.*, 2008; Guthrie *et al.*, 2002).

Social function and IBD

Effect of symptoms

The symptoms of IBD, due to their stigmatising nature, and especially during a relapse, will certainly affect social functioning. The frequency of defecation, with a fear of faecal incontinence, will mean that the person affected will need to remain within close proximity to a toilet and plan their journeys to ensure that they are always near a toilet to avoid episodes of faecal incontinence (Wolfe and Sirios, 2008). Even if a person has never experienced an episode of incontinence, there remains a fear of this occurring (see also Chapter 19) and there is a curtailment or reduction of certain social activities. In addition, the other symptoms of IBD, such as abdominal pain, fatigue and side-effects of medication, may inhibit activity and therefore adversely affect social functioning (Clearfield, 2008).

Employment

Not surprisingly work and employment can be affected by IBD. Anecdotal accounts from IBD nurses have shown that most individuals with IBD try to maintain employment and report many positive benefits of doing so, such as financial stability and improved quality of life (O'Connor 2010). Work can cause stress, however, which will impact on physical and mental health. Individuals may also find that certain employment positions are difficult to maintain due to lack of adequate toilet facilities or the nature of the job, such as working in a catering/hospitality role, where it may be difficult to make frequent visits to the toilet and maintain the level of energy required to fulfil the requirements of the post. People with IBD could be perceived as disabled due to the chronic nature of their condition and its effects on everyday functioning. Directgov (2010a) states:

The Disability Discrimination Act (DDA) defines a disabled person as someone who has a physical or mental impairment that has a substantial and long-term adverse effect on his or her ability to carry out normal day-to-day activities

The Disability Discrimination Act (1995) stated that a person cannot be discriminated against due to their disability unless this can be justified. In addition, the employer has to make 'reasonable adjustments' to ensure that the person is not disadvantaged by the employment arrangements or the workplace environment (Directgov, 2010b). This may entail transferring the person to another position or place of work, making adjustments to the building and being flexible about the hours worked, including time at hospital appointments.

This act is being replaced by the Equality Act 2010, which aims to provide a simpler and stronger legislative process to address discrimination and ensure a 'fair and more equal society' (Government Equalities Office, 2010).

However, due to the nature of IBD symptoms, employees may have some difficulty discussing their condition with their employer or decide that they are unable to continue with their job. 'I used to cook... but you can't just leave the cooking while you're messing about in the loo' (Chelvanayagam and Norton, 2000). Further information for patients about employment issues can be found on the Crohn's and Colitis UK website: http://www.nacc.org.uk/downloads/factsheets/employment.pdf.

Personal and family relationships

Support from family and friends can be seen as a significant factor in coping with the stressors of IBD, and positive social support can positively impact on psychological and physical health improving health outcomes (Rogala *et al.*, 2008). How their family and friends respond to their symptoms is crucial, and the impact of their symptoms on their friends and family can also cause feelings of guilt in the person with IBD (Fletcher *et al.*, 2008).

The fear of faecal incontinence can lead to an avoidance of sexual activity for many people with IBD. Women diagnosed with IBD may report dyspareunia (Clearfield, 2008; Sainsbury and Heatley, 2005). Although men and women with IBD report issues regarding body image and sexuality as important, women express greater concerns surrounding these issues. (Sainsbury and Heatley, 2005).

Stress and development of IBD/brain–gut axis

The exact causes of the inflammatory bowel diseases, what precipitates relapse, and what determines the response to treatment remain unknown. However, it is now widely accepted that a complex interaction between genetics and the environment is central to aetiopathogenesis. Psychological stress has for many years been cited by patients and doctors as worsening disease activity in IBD. Several reports have suggested that unpleasant life events, chronic stress and acute daily stress can increase the frequency of relapse in patients with IBD (Maunder and Levenstein, 2008; Maunder, 2005). To understand this better it is important to understand the relationship between personality factors and these environmental stressors, as it is clear that not all individuals with IBD are vulnerable to stress-induced exacerbations.

Stress

It is important first to define what is meant, biologically, by the term stress. To maintain homeostasis, a living organism constantly adapts at behavioural, physiological, cellular and molecular levels to environmental alterations. Stress is defined as a state of threatened or perceived threatened homeostasis. The function of the stress response is to maintain homeostasis; it involves integration of the hypothalamus, amygdala and periaqueductal grey matter in the brain. This network receives inputs from both the visceral and somatic nervous systems, and also receives input from higher cortical structures. In other words, this brain network is what integrates personality factors with environmental stressors. In turn, this nerve network governs the neuroendocrine stress response via the autonomic nervous system (ANS) and the hypo-pituitary axis (HPA). Stress stimulates the sympathetic nervous system leading to the immediate release of noradrenaline and adrenaline from the adrenal medulla, the so-called 'fight or flight response'. In addition the hypothalamus secretes corticotrophin releasing factor (CRF), which stimulates the pituitary to release ACTH and subsequently cortisol from the adrenal cortex.

The brain–gut axis and inflammation

The enteric nervous system (ENS) contains 100 million neurones and regulates the motility, exocrine and endocrine functions and the microcirculation of the GI tract. It communicates via efferent and afferent neurones of the sympathetic and parasympathetic ANS (the 'brain–gut' axis); unlike the other nervous systems in the body it can work without central input from the brain (the 'brain-in-the-gut'). It is increasingly recognised that the HPA, ANS and ENS can interact directly with the immune system systemically and in the gut wall. Nerve fibres of the ANS form close associations with immunoregulatory cells in lymph glands, bone marrow, thymus, spleen and mucosa-associated lymphoid tissue. These immunoregulatory cells are known to carry receptors for several neurotransmitters of the ANS and HPA systems.

Stress as a pathogenetic factor in UC

There is increasing epidemiological data demonstrating that both acute and chronic stresses have a role in relapse in IBD (Irvine, 2008). Surveys show that 50–75% of patients with IBD believe that stress plays a role in causing relapse of their disease (Taft *et al*., 2009) Supportive data comes from the therapeutic trials of CD and UC, where there is a high placebo response of about 35% (Sands, 2009). These rates not only relate to subjective self-reported symptomatology but also to objectives measures such as endoscopic findings.

Few studies have examined experimental stress in man. The reason for the paucity of data is that accurate studies examining the effects of psychological stress in IBD are challenging to design and perform. The data available suggests that psychological stress in active UC may lead to worsening inflammation. In addition, patients with quiescent UC who perceive higher levels of external stress had a greater rate of subsequent relapse than those with lower perceived stress scores.

Psychological problems seen in patients with IBD

Case study I

Giles is a commercial lawyer who was diagnosed with ulcerative colitis age 28. He had a relatively quiescent course until a major flare-up aged 30, which almost required colectomy. As a last ditch therapy he was commenced on a novel biological agent medication as part of a drug trial and improved dramatically. Subsequently he was discharged taking azathioprine and a 5-ASA drug only. Over the following six months he re-presented 11 times as an emergency, with a history of diarrhoea, abdominal pain and feeling ill. Blood tests remained normal despite weight fluctuations, and the colonic mucosa always looked absolutely normal. He was keen to have further doses of the trial medication (which had long-since ended), and on one occasion he persuaded the team to give him prednisolone, which made him 'dramatically' better, although his symptoms rapidly returned on weaning. He was eventually persuaded that his recurrent symptoms reflected loss of confidence in his health rather than actual inflammation. He began a course of cognitive behavioural therapy (CBT), recognising that his anxiety about bowel urgency when with clients was a significant factor. He fared well and remains well following the end of CBT.

Case study 2

Tamara presented with her first signs of Crohn's disease of perianal pain and bloody diarrhoea at the age of 17. She was found to have perianal and colonic Crohn's disease and commenced on steroids after an examination under anaesthesia. The appearances rapidly improved but she remained upset and often anxious at out-patient review. Following gentle discussion on several occasions it became clear that the onset of symptoms was after her first consensual sexual contact whilst on holiday. She felt the disease was caused by this contact, and it evoked unhappy buried memories of unwanted sexual touching as a child by her step-brother. Despite attempts at engagement she declined follow-up and presented again at age 21 with severe perianal disease, which she had tried to ignore for two years. She underwent emergency surgery and has ended up with an ileostomy which she has remained unwilling to take responsibility for.

These two case histories reflect the spectrum of psychological burden that accompany IBD. In some circumstances the distress arises from the disease, and in some cases the distress evokes past unhappy experiences. The vignettes also illustrate the role of medication in the psychology of patients with IBD. Treatments that are rapidly and powerfully effective are very much favoured by some patients for future treatments (typically corticosteroids or biological agents), even when the advice is that they may not be useful. Furthermore, treatment with corticosteroids can induce mood disorders and other psychiatric symptoms. The latter include feelings of paranoia and overt psychosis: most specialists who have looked after patients with IBD will have in their memory at least one patient who has had a major psychiatric adverse effect following intravenous or oral corticosteroids. In fact, such symptoms occur in only 5% of patients who receive steroids, and they almost always cease on withdrawing the steroid.

Anxiety and depression

Anxiety and depression are more common in patients with IBD than control subjects (but less frequent than in patients with functional gastrointestinal disorders) (Guthrie *et al.*, 2002). In hospital-based studies between 10% and 60% of IBD patients have depression (Fuller-Thomson and Sulman, 2006) – the wide range reflecting the method of case ascertainment (questionnaire or formal interview) as much as the population (secondary or tertiary care). Equally, anxiety is reported in up to 80% of IBD patients at some point in their illness (Walker *et al.*, 2008).

Altered mood

Unsurprisingly, such mood and anxiety symptoms are more severe during periods of active disease. It does not seem as though anxiety and depression are risk factors for IBD, but it is clear that the course of the disease is worse in depressed patients (Szigethy *et al.*, 2004; Fuller-Thomson and Sulman, 2006). Since depression represents a risk for IBD relapse, it is important to account for mood when considering optimal maintenance management of IBD patients. It is also evident from prospective cohort studies that patients with chronic active disease have greater impairment of mood and quality of life than those with relapsing-remitting illness (Graff *et al.*, 2009). When this knowledge is coupled with the observation that disease activity is only weakly associated with psychological functioning, it suggests that chronic IBD adversely affects patients' quality of life even when the disease is in remission. Interestingly, these prospective studies suggest that patients become less anxious with time, possibly as they get more used to their disease and their coping strategies improve. The exception to this trend seems to be in relation to aversive reactions to pain, which increase with time. Possibly pain processing tends to catastrophisation in IBD patients because of the difficulty in treating abdominal pain (compared to the relative efficacy of drugs in improving diarrhoea and blood loss).

Eating disorders

In paediatric IBD practice, and to a lesser extent in adults, there is anecdotal evidence of an association with eating disorders. One particular reason for this has been speculated as being related to use of corticosteroids, with their body shape modifying as well as brain effects. Conversely the problem could be over-diagnosed by specialists, confronted by a patient with weight loss who declines to eat more since it exacerbates her or his symptoms. In either case the situation needs to be addressed both from the point of view of managing the risks of osteoporosis (associated with both IBD and eating disorders) as well as optimally managing the patient's psyche. Specialist assessment by an expert in the field, at an early stage, is essential to identify typical or atypical eating disorders.

Obsessional behaviour/obsessive compulsive disorder

Another anecdotal association, and certainly one which presents management challenges, is co-morbidity of IBD with obsessionality (as a personality trait or a formal obsessive-compulsive disorder). Such feelings about bowel function in patients with a diarrhoeal condition, especially if a stoma is present, can result in perseveration of thinking and ritualisation of behaviour which can paralyse the patient, grossly limiting their ability to look after their chronic inflammatory disease. Once again, early specialist psychiatric input is essential to diagnose the issue, along with subsequent psychological input if that is deemed appropriate.

Assessment and management of psychological distress

The gold standard for assessment of gut symptoms will always be a focused comprehensive clinical history. Research tools, however, require quantitative assessment methods, both for confirmation of the inclusion or entry criteria, and as a monitor of outcome with intervention. Increasingly, the role of these instruments is extending into the clinical setting. Such assessments may encompass both symptom questionnaires and quality of life assessment, the latter being either generic or IBD-specific. The Inflammatory Bowel Disease Questionnaire (IBDQ) is the most widely studied quality of life questionnaire in patients with IBD. It evaluates general activities of daily living and intestinal, social and emotional status. This 32 item questionnaire has been translated into several languages and validated in a variety of cultures. It has been shown to be both reflective of disease activity and, more importantly, responsive to treatment.

Other self-assessment instruments are widely used in gastrointestinal practice, usually to assess specific symptoms such as incontinence, abdominal discomfort and eating behaviour. Whilst none of these is validated in patients with IBD, they may represent an objective way of quantifying change in specific symptomatology in IBD patients. What this highlights, however, is the vital importance of empathic clinical interaction with the IBD patient, to assess not only the physical symptoms but also the potential psychological co-morbidity:

- Eating behaviour
- Perceptions about body appearance/size
- Concerns about sexual life
- Cognitions regarding chronic pain
- Lifestyle adjustments/avoidances undertaken to tackle IBD symptoms

One other area of emerging importance with regard to identifying psychological co-morbidity is in relation to compliance with maintenance treatment. It is known that one-third of IBD patients are poorly adherent (Jackson *et al.*, 2010); a worryingly high rate given the increasing recognition of the role of maintenance medication in reducing cancer and relapse risk. The presence of past psychiatric diagnoses has been revealed to be an important factor in non-adherence, and stresses the role of detailed psychiatric history taking as part of the IBD assessment.

With regard to treatment, antidepressants are frequently prescribed to IBD patients for either pain, sleep disturbance, depression or anxiety. Indeed, patients feel they are useful in improving psychosocial well-being and quality of life. No evidence is available for the role of selective serotonin reuptake inhibitors as opposed to tricyclic antidepressants. Recent observations that the tricyclics can alter the gut's response to stress (Thoua *et al.*, 2009) highlight one mechanism through which these drugs may help improve symptoms in IBD patients. Amelioration of the stress response, and secondary alterations of the neuro-immune system described above, may represent a viable target for tackling some of the troublesome symptoms that existing anti-inflammatory drug therapies do not target.

Complementary therapies are being used increasingly by patients with chronic illnesses. These therapies include acupuncture, aromatherapy, naturopathy, Chinese medicine, herbal therapies, homeopathy, osteopathy, Reiki and hypnotherapy. For patients with gastrointestinal symptoms the use of complementary and alternative therapies ranges from 9–50% (Langmead and Rampton, 2006). Younger, single patients with IBD particularly will tend to try complementary therapies, as well as those who report poorer quality of life in relation to psychosocial functioning (Langmead *et al.*, 2002).

Hypnotherapy, even as a single session, has been shown to reduce the systemic and mucosal inflammatory response in active ulcerative colitis toward levels found in inactive disease. Controlled trials of hypnotherapy in UC are under way to assess the potential therapeutic effect in a formal way.

Other interventions

The Expert Patient highlighted that empowering patients to self manage their condition could help improve symptoms, disease outcomes and quality of life (Hall *et al.*, 2007). Within IBD care, self-management programmes have been developed and recommended as one of service standards for IBD services (IBD Standards Group, 2009). Self-management programmes consist of education regarding IBD, diagnosis and treatment, management of exacerbations of the disease and health promotion. Each patient is provided with a guidebook providing them with information on IBD and their own individualised plan of care for management of their IBD. Patients are also able to access a rapid access clinic and there is a telephone helpline usually operated by a nurse. Stansfield and Robinson (2008)

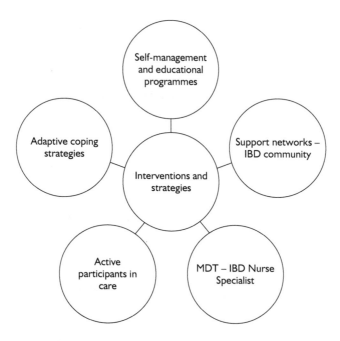

Figure 16.1 Strategies and interventions to support people with IBD.

found that 90% of their patients involved in this programme reported it as good/ excellent. However, although patients report it as beneficial, Kennedy *et al.* (2003) found that it did not improve anxiety or depression and had no effect on quality of life. Also, those who participate in these programmes are more likely to have active coping styles. People with active or adaptive coping styles are able to adjust appropriately to changing situations, learning from the experience and solving problems well (Gross and Kinnison, 2007). Therefore they are more likely to access such programmes and to find them beneficial. Barlow *et al.* (2010) reviewed self-management and educational interventions. They discovered that education alone is insufficient to change behaviour and impact on health. A combination approach using interventions to help the person adapt to learning to live with IBD and adapt their lifestyle accordingly have lead to improved physical and psychological state (Barlow *et al.*, 2010). Therefore interventions include a range of psychological therapies, such as problem-solving techniques, cognitive behavioural techniques to manage anxiety, and stress management programmes, which include relaxation techniques, yoga and meditation. The development of adaptive coping strategies in order to manage their symptoms and the effect on their lifestyle is also a key intervention. These strategies and the nursing role in supporting and educating patients are also discussed in Chapter 19.

Support networks such as Crohn's and Colitis UK provide information about IBD as well as local support groups and a confidential telephone service. Many of the people involved in this organisation have experience of living with IBD. Crohn's and Colitis UK produce a range of publications and are a well known and respected organisation (Terry, 2006). Such organisations and self-help groups demonstrate that individuals living with the disorder are able to function well and provide support for others. Therefore they act as role models for those who are currently adjusting to their diagnosis and the impact of this on their lifestyle.

Role of the nurse

As this chapter highlights, IBD can detrimentally affect all aspects of a person's life – socially, psychologically and physically. This is not only due to the physical effects of the disorder, but because it concerns what remains a taboo and stigmatising subject – bowel function (Clearfield, 2008). However, there are a range of interventions and strategies which can enable a person to maintain a good quality of life and may even help to reduce reoccurring episodes of their symptoms. In line with evidence-based principles, not all interventions will suit all people. Therefore to provide appropriate individualised care holistic assessment is required.

In order to achieve an effective assessment it is imperative to develop a therapeutic relationship. The aim of a therapeutic relationship is to initiate supportive interpersonal communication in order to understand the perceptions and needs of another person to empower and enable them to manage their symptoms and altered lifestyle (Barker, 2003).

A therapeutic interaction (Cutcliffe and McKenna, 2005, p. 310):

...is a conversation with a purpose that aims to explore, understand, interpret, and appreciate what for the individual patient is causing distress, in order to facilitate assessment of need and negotiation of approach and to plan for interventions to promote development and recovery

Holistic assessment involves asking questions from the patient's perspective about their physical symptoms, psychological effects of their illness or previous mental health problems, and social effects, which include employment and education (Bach and Grant, 2009). This addresses all aspects of a person's life, which enables the nurse to assess the ramifications of IBD.

As well as asking relevant questions to address each area, the nurse may wish to include the use of an HRQOL measure as discussed earlier. If possible it is useful to send this to the patient with their appointment letter as it can form the focus of the assessment. People often find it difficult to introduce sensitive topics, but using the questionnaire can facilitate the discussion. It also ensures that all aspects of a patient's quality of life are discussed and can avoid directly asking them questions that may seem very intrusive. The nurse is able to gauge a person's response to a certain question – for example about sexual function – and decide whether they are ready to discuss this currently or at another time. Not all information can be gleaned from one assessment discussion, but developing a therapeutic relationship with the person will enable the patient to feel comfortable to raise or discuss these topics at a later date.

Another tool which is frequently used in research studies to assess mood and anxiety in patients with physical illnesses is the Hospital and Depression Scale (Zigmond and Snaith, 1983). This is a very simple tool to use: it consists of 14 questions which ask specific questions related to anxiety and mood and is completed by the patient. However, this tool needs to be introduced sensitively with a clear rationale for its use, otherwise patients may perceive that their symptoms are being judged as 'psychological' and may be fearful that their responses may affect the care provided. Therefore it is important, when providing education about IBD, that nurses can discuss how stress, anxiety and depression can impact on their disease, both in reoccurrence of symptoms and coping on a daily basis.

Therefore the role of the nurse is:

- To develop a therapeutic relationship with the patient and their families
- Provide a holistic assessment from the patient's perspective of the impact of IBD on their life
- Provide ongoing support and link with the MDT and psychological services if required
- Be aware of the range of resources available to offer ongoing support and advice

Conclusion

This chapter has demonstrated that to optimise health and quality of life for the person living with IBD a balance needs to be maintained between physical and mental health. A person with mental health problems and IBD may have increased difficulty adhering to treatment programmes, which will impact on their physical health status. In addition, the role of increased stress and maladaptive coping strategies can affect the pathophysiology of the disease and may precipitate re-emergence of IBD symptoms. Additionally, living with IBD and its stigmatising symptoms will affect a person's functioning, particularly their quality of life.

Therefore the role of the nurse and MDT is to provide a therapeutic relationship which is supportive and educational. The care they provide has to be patient-centred and must focus on providing a range of evidence-based interventions in order to enhance and optimise health and quality of life.

Patient translation summary

Nurses may feel reluctant to address psychological and social aspects. This is frequently related to a fear of not possessing adequate skills or knowledge about relevant services. Failing to address these issues can have an impact on both physical and mental health, lead to maladaptive coping styles and result in poorer health outcomes. Addressing these issues by demonstrating understanding and empathy facilitates the development of a therapeutic relationship. This enables the person with IBD to ventilate their concerns and work collaboratively with the nurse and the MDT to ensure they lead more fulfilling lives.

References

Barker, P. (2003) *Psychiatric and Mental Health Nursing: The Craft of Caring.* London: Hodder Arnold.

Barlow, C., Cooke, D., Mulliagan, K., Beck, E. and Newman, S. (2010) A critical review of self-management and educational interventions in inflammatory bowel disease. *Gastroenterol. Nurs.*, **33**(1), 11–18.

Bach, S. and Grant, A. (2009) *Communication and Interpersonal Skills for Nurses.* Exeter: Learning Matters Ltd.

Bernklev, T., Jahnsen, J., Aadland, E., Sauar, J., Schulz, T., Lygren, I., Henriksen, M., Stray, N., Kjellevold, Ø., Vatn, M., Moum, B. and the IBSEN Group (2004) Health-related quality of life in inflammatory bowel disease five years after the initial diagnosis. *Scand. J. Gastroenterol.*, **4**, 365–73.

Canavan, C., Abrams, K. R., Hawthorne, B., Drossman, D. and Mayberry, J. F. (2006) Long-term prognosis in Crohn's disease: factors that affect quality of life. *Aliment. Pharmacol. Therapeutics*, **23**, 377–85.

Chelvanayagam, S. and Norton, C. (2000) Quality of life with faecal continence problems. *Nursing Times*, **96**(31)(suppl.), 15–17.

Clearfield, H. R. (2008) How does IBD affect quality of life? *Inflamm. Bowel Dis.*, **14**(suppl. 2), S45–S46.

Cutcliffe, J. R. and McKenna, H. P. (2005) *The Essential Concepts of Nursing*. London: Elsevier.

Department of Health (2001) *The Expert Patient: A New Approach to Chronic Disease Management for the 21st Century*. London: Department of Health.

Department of Health (2004) *Chronic Disease Management: A Compendium of Information*. London: Department of Health.

Directgov (2010a) *Definition of 'Disability' Under the Disability Discrimination Act (DDA)*. http://www.direct.gov.uk/en/DisabledPeople/RightsAndObligations/DisabilityRights/DG_4001069 (accessed 5 September 2010).

Directgov (2010b) *Employment Rights and the Disability Discrimination Act*. http://www.direct.gov.uk/en/DisabledPeople/Employmentsupport/YourEmploymentRights/DG_4001071 (accessed 5 September 2010).

Drossman, D. A., Patrick, D. L., Mitchell, C. M., Zagami, E. and Applebaum, M. I. (1989) Health-related quality of life in inflammatory bowel disease. *Digestive Dis. Sci.*, **34**, 1379–86.

Eypasch, E., Williams, J. I., Wood-Daupinee, S., Ure, B. M., Schmulling, C., Neugebauer, E. and Troidl, H. (1995) Gastrointestinal Quality of Life Index: development, validation and application of a new instrument. *Br. J. Surg.*, **82**, 216–22.

Fletcher, P. C., Schneider, M. A., Van Ravenswaay, V. and Leon, Z. (2008) I am doing the best I can! Living with inflammatory bowel disease and/or irritable bowel syndrome. *Clin. Nurse Specialist*, **22**, 278–85.

Fuller-Thomson, E. and Sulman, J. (2006) Depression and inflammatory bowel disease: findings from two nationally representative Canadian surveys. *Inflamm. Bowel Dis.*, **12**, 697–707.

Government Equalities Office (2010) *Equality Act 2010*. http://www.equalities.gov.uk/equality_act_2010.aspx (accessed 5 September 2010).

Graff, L. A., Walker, J. R. and Bernstein, C. N. (2009) Depression and anxiety in inflammatory bowel disease: a review of comorbidity and management. *Inflamm. Bowel Dis.*, **15**, 1105–18.

Gross, R. and Kinnison, N. (2007) *Psychology for Nurses and Allied Health Professionals*. London: Hodder-Arnold.

Guthrie, E., Jackson, J., Shaffer, J., Thompson, D., Tomenson, B. and Creed, F. (2002) Psychological disorder and inflammatory bowel disease health-related quality of life in ulcerative colitis and Crohn's disease. *Am. J. Gastroenterol.*, **97**, 1994–9.

Guyatt, G., Mitchell, A., Irvine, E.J., Singer, J., Williams, N., Goodacre R. and Tomkins, C. (1989) A new measure of health status for clinical trails in imflammatory bowel disease. *Gastroenterology*, **96**, 804–10.

Hall, A., Porrett, T. and Cox, C. (2007) Self management in the care of patients with inflammatory bowel disease. *Gastrointest. Nurs.*, **5**(5), 34–8.

Head, J., Ferrie, J. E., Alexanderson, K., Westerlund, H., Vahtera, J. and Kivimäki, M. (2008) Diagnosis-specific sickness absence as a predictor of mortality: the Whitehall II prospective cohort study. *Br. Med. J.*, **337**, 1469.

Higginson, H. J. and Carr, A. J. (2001) Using quality of life measures in the clinical setting. *Br. Med. J.*, **322**, 1297–300.

IBD Standards Group (2009) *Quality Care: Service Standards for the Healthcare of People who have Inflammatory Bowel Disease (IBD)*. Oyster Healthcare Communications Ltd.

Jackson, C. A., Clatworthy, J., Robinson, A. and Horne, R. (2010) Factors associated with non-adherence to oral medication for inflammatory bowel disease: a systematic review. *Am. J. Gastroenterol.*, **105**, 525–39.

Kennedy, A., Nelson, E., Reeves, D., Richardson, G., Roberts, C., Robinson, A., Rogers, A., Sculpher, M. and Thompson, D. (2003) A randomised controlled trial to assess the impact of a package comprising of a patient-orientated evidence-based self-help guide-book and patient-centred consultations on disease management and satisfaction in inflammatory bowel disease. *Health Technol. Assess.*, **7**(28).

Irvine, E. J. (2008) Quality of life of patients with ulcerative colitis: past, present and future. *Inflamm. Bowel Dis.*, **14**, 554–65.

Langmead, L. and Rampton, D. S. (2006) Review article; complementary and alternative therapies for inflammatory bowel disease. *Aliment. Pharmacol. Therapeut.*, **23**, 341–9.

Langmead, L., Chitnis, M. and Rampton, D. S. (2002) Use of complementary therapies by patients with IBD may indicate psychosocial distress. *Inflamm. Bowel Dis.*, **8**, 174–9.

Lix, L. M., Graff, L. A., Walker, J. R., Clara, I., Rawsthorne, P., Rogala, L., Miller, N., Ediger, J., Pretorius, T. and Bernstein, C. N. (2008) Longitudinal study of quality of life and psychological functioning for active, fluctuating and inactive disease patterns in inflammatory bowel disease. *Inflamm. Bowel Dis.*, **14**, 1575–84.

Maunder, R. G. (2005) Evidence that stress contributes to inflammatory bowel disease: evaluation, synthesis, and future directions. *Inflamm. Bowel Dis.*, **11**, 600–8.

Maunder, R. G. and Levenstein, S. (2008) The role of stress in the development and clinical course of inflammatory bowel disease: epidemiological evidence. *Curr. Molec. Med.* **8**, 247–52.

NHS Information Centre (2009) *Adult Psychiatric Morbidity in England 2007. Results of a Household Survey.* http://www.ic.nhs.uk/webfiles/publications/mental%20health/other%20mental%20health%20publications/Adult%20psychiatric%20morbidity%2007/APMS%2007%20%28FINAL%29%20Standard.pdf (accessed 19 February 2009).

O'Connor, M. (2010) Unpublished observations.

Pihl-Lesnovska, K., Hjortswang, H., Ek, A.-C. and Frisman, G. H. (2010) Patients' perspective of factors influencing quality of life while living with Crohn's disease. *Gastroen-*

terol. Nurs., **33**(1), 37–44.

Rogala, L., Miller, N., Graff, L. A., Rawsthorne, P., Clara, I., Walker, J. R., Lix, L., Ediger, J. P., McPhail, C. and Bernstein, C. N. (2008) Population-based controlled study of social support, self-perceived stress, activity and work issues and access to healthcare in inflammatory bowel disease. *Inflamm. Bowel Dis.*, **14**, 526–35.

Rubin, G. P., Hungin, A. P. S., Chinn, D. J. and Dwarakanath, D. (2004) Quality of life in patients with established inflammatory bowel disease: a UK general practice survey. *Aliment. Pharmacol. Therapeut.*, **19**, 529–35.

Sainsbury, A. and Heatley, R. V. (2005) Review article: psychosocial factors in the quality of life of patients with inflammatory bowel disease. *Aliment. Pharmacol. Therapeut.*, **21**, 499–508.

Sands, B. E. (2009) The placebo response rate in irritable bowel syndrome and inflammatory bowel disease. *Digestive Dis.*, **27**(suppl. 1), 68–75.

Schneider, M. A. and Fletcher, P. C. (2008) 'I feel as if my IBS is keeping me hostage!' Exploring the negative impact of irritable bowel syndrome (IBS) and inflammatory bowel disease (IBD) upon university-aged women. *Int. J. Nurs. Pract.*, **14**, 135–48.

Szigethy, E., Levy-Warren, A., Whitton, S., Bousvaros, A., Gauvreau, K., Leichtner, A. M. and Beardslee, W. R.(2004) Depressive symptoms and inflammatory bowel disease in children and adolescents: a cross-sectional study. *J. Pediatr. Gastroenterol. Nutrition*, **39**, 395–440.

Seymour, L. (2003) *Not All in the Mind: The Physical Health of Mental Health Service Users*. Radical Mentalities: Briefing Paper 2. London: Sainsbury Centre of Mental Health.

Stansfield, C. and Robinson, A. (2008) Implementation of an IBD nurse-led self-management programme. *Gastrointest. Nurs.*, **6**(3), 12–18.

Stewart, A. L., Greenfield, S., Hays, R. D., Wells, K., Rogers, W. H., Berry, S. D., McGlynn, E. A. and Ware, J. E. (1989) Functional status and well being of patients with chronic conditions: results from the Medical Outcomes Study. *J. Am. Med. Assoc.*, **262**, 907–13.

Taft, T. H., Keefer, L., Leonhard, C. and Nealon-Woods, M. (2009) Impact of perceived stigma on inflammatory bowel disease patient outcomes. *Inflamm. Bowel Dis.*, **15**, 1224–32.

Terry, H. (2006) Improving the life for people affected by colitis and Crohn's disease. *Gastrointest. Nurs.*, **4**(7), 14–15.

Thoua, N. M., Murray, C. D., Winchester, W. J., Roy, A. J., Pitcher, M. C., Kamm, M. A. and Emmanuel, A. V. (2009) Amitriptyline modifies the visceral hypersensitivity response to acute stress in the irritable bowel syndrome. *Aliment. Pharmacol. Therapeut.*, **29**, 552–60.

Vidal, A., Gomés-Gil, E., Sans, M., Portella, M. J., Salamero, M., Piqué, J. M. and Panés, J. (2008) Health-related quality of life in inflammatory bowel disease patients: the role of psychopathology and personality. *Inflamm. Bowel Dis.*, **14**, 977–83.

Walker, J. R., Ediger, J. P., Graff, L. A., Greenfeld, J. M., Clara, I., Lix, L., Rawsthorne, P., Miller, N., Rogala, L., McPhail, C. M. and Bernstein, C. N. (2008) The Manitoba IBD cohort study: a population-based study of the prevalence of lifetime and 12-month anxiety and mood disorders. *Am. J. Gastroenterol.*, **103**, 1989–97.

Williams, J. (2005) Psychological considerations in gastrointestinal nursing *Br. J. Nurs.*, **14**(17), 931–5.

Wolfe, B. J. and Sirois, F. M. (2008) Beyond standard quality of life measures: the subjective experiences of living with inflammatory bowel disease. *Qual. Life Res.*, **17**, 877–86.

Younge, L. and Norton, C. (2007) Contribution of specialist nurses in managing patients with IBD. *Br. J. Nurs.*, **16**(4), 208–12.

Zigmond, A. S. and Snaith, R. P. (1983) The Hospital Anxiety and Depression Scale. *Acta Psychiatrica Scandinavica*, **67**, 361–70.

CHAPTER 17

Living with inflammatory bowel disease – a patient's experience

Sneha Wadhwani and Marian O'Connor

Introduction

As healthcare professionals working in the field of inflammatory bowel disease, most of us can only imagine what it is like to live with IBD, and the immense impact this has on the person. Therefore it is imperative that we try to understand what it might be like to live with IBD and empathise with the person.

Adjusting

As a lifelong condition, it means that patients have to come to terms with the diagnosis of IBD, gain an understanding of the disease and the treatments used, and then find a way to manage their disease in conjunction with their daily life. This is a steep learning curve, and one which requires the person to be supported adequately during this time.

Accepting a diagnosis of this magnitude could be likened to Kubler-Ross's work on the experience of death and dying (Kubler-Ross, 1969), in which she outlined a process by which people deal with grief and loss. This work explored the way in which some individuals coped with dying, and Kubler-Ross proposed stages of grief and loss that people experience on the way towards acceptance of their situation. These five stages, in the context of chronic disease, might also be related to IBD and how people adjust to living with their condition (see Table 17.1). For example, an individual with IBD may feel a sense of grief in relation to the loss of their usual lifestyle, a change in bowel function, an altered body image, loss of sexual function, or a change in their social functioning. It can be useful for healthcare professionals to identify what stage patients are experiencing, and also to recognise that some patients can move back and forth between these stages, sometimes taking years to get to acceptance. Until patients reach the acceptance stage, this may impact, largely negatively, on the management of

315

Table 17.1 The five stages of grief in relation to IBD (adapted from information in Kubler-Ross, 1970).

1. Denial	'I feel fine' 'No, not me, it's not true'	Denial is usually only a temporary defence for the individual.
2. Anger	'Why me?' 'It's not fair' 'How can this happen to me?'	The individual recognises that denial cannot continue. This stage of anger can be very difficult to deal with from the point of view of the family and healthcare staff as the individual can displace and project the anger in various directions (can be towards family members and healthcare staff).
3. Bargaining	'I'll do anything for more years' 'For good behaviour'	If individuals have been unable to accept the facts in Stage 1, and have been angry at people in the second stage, in this stage individuals may try to enter into some agreement in order to delay the inevitable. The bargaining is an attempt to postpone.
4. Depression	'I'm so sad, why bother with anything?' 'I'm going to die... What's the point?'	The individual begins to understand the certainty of their illness. When the individual is forced to undergo further medical/surgical therapies and hospitalisations, and continues to have symptoms, it can be difficult to smile it off, and be 'cheered up'. This is, however, an important time for feelings to be acknowledged and to be processed. Added to that the financial burden associated with illness meaning that luxuries and later even necessities may not be afforded. Whilst important to observe, psychological assessment is also paramount, and where indicated, further support and/or treatment is offered. This is discussed in detail in Chapter 16.
5. Acceptance	'It's going to be okay' 'You can't give into it – I can keep fighting it' (unidentified patient with Crohn's disease) 'I am learning to live with this'	If the individual has enough time, and is given support to work through the above stages, then this stage of acceptance may be reached, in which the individual is accepting of their situation and has adjusted to living with the condition, using support offered and seeking help when it is required.

their disease; such as patients who find it difficult to adhere with treatment regimes or follow-up appointments.

Therefore it is of vital importance that all people with IBD are supported adequately, in terms of social (family and friends), healthcare (the wider team) and the other agencies such as the patient support groups (e.g. Crohn's and Colitis UK).

The patient's experience

Although we all see patients every day with IBD, for the purpose of this chapter a patient has kindly provided us with her experience of living with IBD. This provides a look at this patient's experience through her eyes, highlighting what has been important to her in living with IBD.

My experience – Sneha Wadhwani

I was a fit and well 14-year-old at the time my symptoms started in 1994, and really these came on quite suddenly. There was no gradual change in bowel habit, loss of weight or lethargy that is often noted with the onset of IBD. Rather, I suddenly started noticing blood in the toilet pan whenever I went to pass stool, which alarmed me. As such I duly reported it to my mum, and after a few days of observation that it wasn't resolving my mother took me to the doctor, where it all started.

After a rigid sigmoidoscopy (most traumatic for a teenage girl) and a trial of various rectally delivered treatments for suspected proctitis, I underwent a full colonoscopy, which confirmed ulcerative colitis.

On reflection I'm not really sure I understood the diagnosis too well. Since both my parents are doctors, the biology of it all was actually quite straightforward, and though the consultant kindly and delicately told me that I would likely require medication for the rest of my life, I don't think I fully appreciated what the impact of having this problem was really to be. However, he did his best to educate me and gave me a video to watch (narrated by John Cleese) which talked about colostomy bags and having sex with IBD. It all seemed a world very distant from the one in which I was living.

I commenced a course of IV hydrocortisone and oral prednisolone and then sulphasalazine – and for the first couple of years things seemed to be fine. I made regular visits to clinic and saw the consultant, who monitored me closely. The possibility of the disease burning out in later life was raised, and on reflection perhaps I held on to this somewhat. I was able to do all the things that an average teen would, but eating meals was fraught with avoidance of certain foods, and I was often reminded when I had eaten the wrong thing.

Strangely, a year after my diagnosis, it came to light that IBD ran in my family. My paternal aunt in India was quite unwell with ulcerative colitis, and shortly after becoming aware of this, my father was diagnosed with ulcerative colitis too. I realised I wasn't alone, but having my dad go through the same thing was upsetting. I didn't want him to have to cope with this, especially since he had had a heart attack just a few months previously.

Facing GCSEs and A-levels was demanding, and just before sitting my A-levels I began to feel extreme tiredness – so much so that I would find it difficult to put on my seat belt in the car. My hair had started to fall out in quite considerable quantities, and I was losing weight, although I was unaware of this until much later. My tongue had become so swollen and sore that I was salivating so much that I couldn't speak properly. My mother took me to a colleague of hers in the hospital, where blood tests showed significant anaemia, with a haemoglobin of 7. I started taking iron tablets and returned to the gastroenterologist, who altered my medication to azathioprine – an immunosuppressant. Initially again all seemed well, and I went off to university some distance away to study medicine, while keeping my gastroenterology follow-up at home. In those days I wasn't 'allocated' a specialist nurse to call if things went wrong or I wanted advice, and this made accessing care from a distance difficult. However, my consultant was always kind and considerate, returned my calls, and accommodated seeing me in university holidays, or even at short notice. This made things much more manageable.

In my first year things were pretty stable and I kept up with regular blood tests, sending the results to my consultant at home and maintaining telephone contact with him. After a severe episode of sinusitis rendered me bed-bound for a few days, I received a call from the consultant instructing me to stop the azathioprine as I was neutropenic. I did so and carried on with sulphasalazine as normal until I could return home to see him. My bowels were OK; I would go to the loo 3–4 times a day but felt relatively well systemically. He changed my medication after a repeat colonoscopy found a mesalazine tablet in my colon which clearly hadn't been absorbed!

The following four years of university passed with frequent flares. There were long spells of diarrhoea and having to visit the loo immediately after eating. I started to feel rough, with nausea, abdominal pains and lethargy, and at times I struggled to cope with medical school and my health. As such I had frequent visits to the gastroenterologist when home for the holidays. On many of these occasions colonoscopies were done and I was told they were normal. I began to feel like perhaps I wasn't being taken seriously. I felt as if I was being viewed as an over-sensitive or emotional teen who just couldn't cope very well. However, things continued in this manner and eventually it all came to a head with spectacular timing in my final year.

After a particularly bad flare, I returned home and was admitted for observation, IV hydrocortisone therapy and colonoscopy. During that colonoscopy the gastroenterologist made particular efforts to scope the whole colon, and as such found something new – skip lesions – and a repeat biopsy confirmed indeterminate colitis – likely Crohn's colitis.

I was tearful when the consultant gave me the news. It was a mixture of relief (that my symptoms had been justified) and fear. Until then I had lived with the idea that ulcerative colitis could be cured with a colectomy – and though I didn't want that, it had always been a possibility if things got really bad. Crohn's, I knew, was a different entity, and all of a sudden it felt more like a life sentence. With the IV hydrocortisone and high dose oral prednisolone, after returning home from the admission I began to feel really low. I couldn't sleep at night and was tearful all the time, but couldn't understand why. I realise now that these were probably side-effects of the steroid therapy, but they hadn't been made clear to me. My mum and dad were great. They looked after me at home and reassured me that the feelings would pass once I was off the steroids, and indeed they did.

My gastroenterologist started me on IM methotrexate and recommended transferring my care to a gastroenterologist near university. I was apprehensive about this. I had developed a rapport with my consultant – I could trust him and I felt he understood me. I was worried about the prospect of a new consultant and how I would be looked after somewhere new, but I reluctantly agreed, understanding that on this new medication I would need closer monitoring. In transferring my care I met an enthusiastic bubbly consultant who had a specialist nurse. I felt vulnerable for the first time, taking responsibility for my own care, rather than being led by my parents, and the specialist nurse was fantastic in supporting me through this period of change. Until this time I had never even thought about support groups. I knew about NACC (Crohn's and Colitis UK) but didn't ever feel as if I needed support. While at school and college things had been fine, but now things were different.

By the time I transferred my care away from home I felt as if I had been unwell for so long, and with finals looming I accessed the British Medical Association (BMA), who provide a sick doctors' matching scheme. They find you a doctor of a similar level who's suffering with a similar condition, so that you can support and empathise with each other. However, the person who I was matched with sent email after email detailing traumatic flares and described 'haemorrhaging on the floor' whilst on a ward round. After a while I realised it really wasn't my thing. I just wanted to get on with my life rather than wallowing in the inconveniences of it.

But it seemed the rocky road has still not come to an end, and things didn't go so well on the methotrexate. My bleeding continued, and I was readmitted, three months before my final exams, with an episode of shortness of breath. After a variety of investigations, including VQ scans etc., it was put down to the effect of the methotrexate, which was subsequently stopped.

Now I was in trouble. It was 2001 and there wasn't much else available other than surgery. Ciclosporin was a possibility, but the team weren't optimistic it would work. Thalidomide was another option, but as a woman of childbearing age the potential teratogenicity soon excluded it. Then my consultant raised the possibility of a new drug called infliximab, which could control my symptoms. It would be given via eight weekly IV infusions in hospital.

I grabbed the opportunity, as surgery was always my last resort, and the thought of living with a colostomy seemed so inhibiting on my life. What clothes would I wear? Would I be able to go on holidays and sit on the beach in a bikini? How would I ever meet someone with a colostomy bag – who would want me? How would I work as a junior doctor and deal with a colostomy bag? I wasn't ready to deal with all of this, so infliximab was an obvious choice regardless of the unknown future consequences. I was living for now and wanted to do so with the very best quality of life that I could, even if it meant sacrificing poorer health later on.

In those days the process of getting the infliximab infusions was somewhat long-winded, and on reflection rather strange. Due to the high cost of the drug, the therapy had to be authorised by two gastroenterology consultants on a case-by-case basis. So my own Consultant was the first to sign, and I was packed off to see another consultant with my notes and colonoscopy photos in my hand. I always struggled and felt I had to fight hard for the drug. My inflammatory markers had almost always been normal since diagnosis, despite severe flares of the disease. This made my case a difficult one to prove, and with no one to go with me, each time was as traumatic as the one before. However, being a medic sometimes worked in my favour, and every eight weeks, after battling with varying consultants, I had my infusions.

I remember my first infusion... and it changed my life. Within three days of sitting there hooked up to the drip, it seemed as if my bowels just switched off! I could eat normally and went to the loo three times a day instead of seven or eight. I had appetite again and was pain-free – I felt great.

During my house jobs (called FY1 these days I believe!) I began to suffer some odd symptoms. I had episodes of arthralgia with redness and swelling, and a very strange episode of numbness in my L3/4 dermatomal area, which nobody could explain. However, these soon settled and toward the end of my houseman year I was stable and very happy – I had my life back.

With this I moved to London to train to be a GP, and thus transferred my care. I thought being a houseman was tough, but being an SHO was even tougher. The responsibility was greater and the night shifts busier: I needed to be well.

When I transferred my care, the first consultant who looked after me felt that Infliximab wasn't appropriate for indeterminate or Crohn's colitis and so decided to stop it after a rectal biopsy done under rigid sigmoidoscopy showed ulcerative colitis changes. He started me back on the sulphasalazine, which was wildly ineffective and I felt my flares were becoming out of control again. I struggled to work and eat. Long on-call periods and night shifts as a junior doctor with active Crohn's disease were so difficult. I felt awful, and in my first job I was signed off as unfit for work for a few weeks by Occupational Health. After a gradual recovery following steroid treatment I returned to work, but Occupational Health were unhappy with me doing nights for a further few weeks. This wasn't received well by my colleagues in the hospital who had to cover my shifts, and thus things were difficult. I went back to the gastroenterologist and was changed to azathioprine, and this time the nausea was overwhelming. I had now moved to working in A+E and couldn't keep anything down. The A+E nurses kept giving me IM cyclizine just so that I could cope – I couldn't go on like this.

So I returned to clinic one day and saw the registrar who, unfortunately and probably unfairly, bore the brunt of my frustration. I couldn't understand why such a successful treatment had been taken from me. After a long discussion about the impact the disease was having on my life, my inability to work or eat, and needing to go to the toilet so often, she discussed it with the consultant. He agreed to put me back on infliximab, and sure enough within 2–3 days after the infusion, I felt normal again.

A year or so later I transferred my care to a fantastic new gastroenterologist, within the same hospital, supported by a strengthened and expanded specialist nursing team. They were pivotal in my recovery.

That was five years and more than 20 infusions ago.

And I'm here. Fit and well. In 2006 I got married after completing my training in General Practice. A year later I became a Partner in General Practice, and moved out of London to the countryside.

Aged 30 I faced the dilemma of whether I would be able to have children. For many years I had been subtly warned that it might not be straightforward, but given little more information than that. Adhesions in the abdomen from the inflammation may cause problems with the fallopian tubes and such. And there was also the issue of the medication. At the time I started therapy with infliximab, little in the way of long-term studies had been done. The effect on pregnancy and the unborn baby was relatively unknown at that time.

I knew I wanted to try for a baby so spoke to my specialist nurse and the consultant. They presented up-to-date research to me and suddenly the prospect didn't seem so bleak. The evidence had shown successful pregnancies on infliximab with no evidence of teratogenicity. Together we planned how we would handle the infliximab infusions during pregnancy. With all that on board I went away to try...

... and now, at the time of writing, I'm 28 weeks into pregnancy facing the last infusion before we take a break. It's advised to stop the infusions three months before the due date so that the antibodies don't cross to the foetus. At the moment I feel well, my IBD has been well controlled on the infusions and despite the pregnancy. Time will tell how I'll be off treatment, and I will be unable to use the infliximab if I want to breast feed, so we'll have to wait and see how things go.

My journey with IBD has been a long and, at times, turbulent one filled with uncertainty. I'm now at an age where it has contributed to more than half of my life, but on infliximab and with the care and support of my consultant and specialist nurse I foresee many more years of a normal life.

While I have been fortunate to avoid surgery, and have been able to complete my education and further studies without any big gaps, I've often pushed myself harder than I should have. My medical school years left me resenting the disease and feeling unwell, such that to do what was required of me was such a struggle. I recall living on a diet of boiled egg for three weeks, as it was all I could tolerate. I look back now on those years when food was a necessity and not an enjoyment and can't imagine how I existed like that. On infliximab I can eat whatever I like, and have done! I can go out to restaurants and enjoy experimenting with cooking. I never realised that food was such a passion of mine until infliximab allowed me to be introduced to this world.

My father however, wasn't so fortunate. Like me, after repeated failed trials of various oral medications his ulcerative colitis continued to flare. He tried infliximab, but that too didn't work. So, two years ago, he elected to have a total colectomy. It was tough surgery to go through, especially given his history of ischaemic heart disease. And he was really quite sick afterward, requiring treatment on a High Dependency Unit and medication to support his cardiac and circulatory function. However, he got through it, and as a family we helped him to come to terms with his colostomy bag. We named it 'Burt' and slowly, Burt became part of the family. My dad too has a new life now. One he enjoys free of IBD, and he still works full time as a hospital consultant.

Life with IBD has been difficult. We take for granted things like eating and toileting when we are well, but when these things become disturbed it can have a significant impact on life, and it did on mine.

My family supported me throughout – and still do. The gastroenterology teams under whose care I have been have always delivered high quality care and an empathic approach. However, my most recent consultant and specialist nurse have provided me with outstanding, flexible, high quality care which has allowed me to work through difficult patches in both life and disease circumstances. They have ensured that I've had the best treatment available, such that I've been able to achieve whatever I have wanted to. Life has been possible because of the care they and my family have given me – oh, and a fair bit of bloody mindedness and determination on my part too!

As a medic, having IBD has given me more than it's taken away. Though life has been really really hard at times, physically and emotionally, in living with the disease I've been given precious insight into the life of the patient, and that's made me a better doctor. In addition, living with the disease has taught me to appreciate the simple things in life, often the things we take for granted, and embrace them.

For those who have been just diagnosed with IBD, my message to them would be, don't tolerate the symptoms, but rather be honest with your team so that they can help you. When you have IBD you tend to plod on, comparing each flare with the really bad one you had in the past and consoling yourself that really it's not so bad. You tend to think you have to cope, and actively push yourself beyond your limits despite the disease. For me it was only when my disease became well controlled by infliximab, and I was able to have a normal life, that I could appreciate how sick I had been and indeed how much better life could be.

I don't know what the future holds for me in terms of my IBD. Will I be able to carry on with infliximab for ever? Will I stop it and have the disease miraculously disappear? Will my child inherit this condition? There are still so many uncertainties. But I play it day by day and with the support of my consultant and specialist nurse, I'm sure I'll be just fine. With my fantastic team behind me – anything is possible!

Reference

Kubler-Ross, E. (1970) *On Death & Dying*. London: Routledge.

CHAPTER 18

Living with IBD – the role of patient support organisations

Helen Terry

Introduction

> Treatment involves more than routine medical diagnosis, hospitalised care
> or even the prescription of drugs. When confronted by illness, patients
> seek professional help and advice from their doctors, and also rely on
> support from family members, peers and fellow patients.
> (World Health Organization, 2010)

Much of the formal supportive care available to patients is healthcare based, with
exceptions such as patient support organisations or support groups. Such groups
are an excellent resource for patients to gain access to further information on all
aspects of their disease, but can also provide a safe forum for patients to meet,
share information on living with the disease and generally support each other.
Patient support organisations can play an important role in providing support and
disseminating information to patients and those who care for them, and also by
raising public and political awareness of specific conditions, acting as advocates
for those affected, campaigning for improved health and social care services, and
raising funds for vital research.

The aim of this chapter is to outline the nature of patient support organisations,
providing insight into the type of activities undertaken and their effects. The
activities of Crohn's and Colitis UK will be used in particular to illustrate the work
of a UK patient organisation for the purposes of this chapter. A list of national and
international organisations can be found at the end of the book.

Crohn's and Colitis UK (National Association for Colitis and Crohn's Disease – NACC)

The National Association for Colitis and Crohn's Disease (NACC) is the major UK charity offering information and support to people affected by IBD. The working name for this association is now Crohn's and Colitis UK, hence this title will be used throughout the chapter to depict the present day organisation. The NACC title will be used when discussing past activities, research or local groups.

Aim – improving life for people affected by colitis and Crohn's disease

Established in 1979 as a partnership between patient, their families, friends and the health professionals who care for them, the organisation known as NACC was created as a voluntary association of members working at national level and through local groups to provide mutual support and to help all those affected by colitis and Crohn's disease. Anyone affected by IBD is invited to join the organisation.

Volunteering and supporting Crohn's and Colitis UK provides opportunities for people living with IBD to develop their skills and personal confidence, helping them to overcome the barriers or disadvantages imposed on them by their illness and to fulfil or enhance potential achievements in their education, employment or daily activities. The information and support services are open to anyone affected by colitis or Crohn's disease. The questions people ask and the experiences shared inform and shape all areas of Crohn's and Colitis UK's work.

The Crohn's and Colitis UK Plan 2010–2012

Meeting needs for information and support

Good quality information and emotional support, both early in their illness and at critical stages in their lifelong experience of IBD, help patients to understand and manage their illness with more confidence and support them in achieving

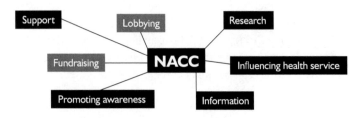

Figure 18.1 NACC plan spider diagram.

their individual potential so far as possible within the constraints imposed by their illness.

Access to Crohn's and Colitis UK's national helpline services and the opportunity to take part in local group activities helps patients and their families feel less alone and enables them to benefit from sharing experiences.

1. Information Service – 0845 130 2233

> ...great knowledge of my condition... I feel like no one around me understands how I am feeling and what I am going through. It was such a relief... I will definitely call again. (Lancaster, 2007)

Crohn's and Colitis UK's Information Officers respond to telephone or email queries on all aspects of IBD and related services. The Information Line is open every weekday morning, and an answerphone service is provided outside of opening times.

2. Publications

The organisation is committed to the production of accurate, reliable and timely information to help people understand their illness and make informed choices about their care and treatment. In 2009, NACC became one of the first organisations to be accredited against the Information Standard, a nationally recognised way of reassuring people that the health and social care information they receive comes from a credible source.

3. National support services

Crohn's and Colitis UK's support services are offered by volunteers who are carefully selected and trained for each role. As patients or relatives of patients, they offer a very personal quality of understanding.

3.1 Crohn's and Colitis Support – 0845 130 3344

> I cannot fault the [Contact] for her calming influence and attitude. (Lancaster, 2007)

Managed and delivered by volunteer 'Contacts', This national support line is a confidential supportive listening service for patients and their families. The support line is open on weekday afternoons from 1 p.m.–3:30 p.m. and evenings from 6:30 p.m.–9 p.m.

3.2 Disability Benefit Support Service

> You have been very kind and helpful and understanding at a very frustrating time in my family's life. Thank you for making things seem a lot clearer. (Lancaster, 2007).

Disability benefits can make a big difference to people's lives. They can give people back some of their feelings of independence and control. But making a claim can be a long drawn-out and emotionally draining process with no guarantee of success at the end. (Donnison and Whitehead, 2007). Appointments can be made through the information line for telephone support and general guidance on claiming disability benefits (Disability Living Allowance or Attendance Allowance).

3.3 Parent to Parent
This service is available by appointment and offers confidential telephone support and information to parents of children with IBD. Further information about support and patient groups for adolescents and children can be found in Chapter 15.

3.4 Personal grants
Grants are awarded to help people with the cost of items needed as a result of their illness. A Young Person's Assistance Fund supports young people with vocational or educational needs.

4. NACC Groups – the local face of NACC
Many people become isolated after being diagnosed with IBD and often choose only to tell close family and friends about their illness. Consequently, they can find it quite difficult to identify other patients with similar interests and share experiences. Crohn's and Colitis UK supports a network of 70 local volunteer-run groups, bringing people together by holding meetings and events and keeping members informed by producing a local newsletter and maintaining a local group website. Some groups raise funds to support local projects, provide additional facilities or equipment for patients in IBD clinics, or provide training for specialist nurses.

5. iNACC
The Internet offers information and opportunities for people to come together and be involved in the organisation through sharing experiences and giving mutual support in flexible ways.

5.1 Website
Information on IBD and all aspects of NACC activities can be found on the website at http://www.crohnsandcolitis.org.uk/.

5.2 IBD and Me
Web-based communities enable sharing of information, experiences and mutual support through online communities or virtual networks. IBD and Me

is an online discussion forum where young people between the ages of 16 and 29 come together to share their stories, feelings and practical ideas on living with IBD.

Promoting awareness

An Ipsos Mori (2009) survey of public awareness (Figure 18.2), commissioned by NACC, confirmed a much lower awareness and understanding of IBD than other equally or less prevalent conditions such as Parkinson's disease or multiple sclerosis. Awareness of ulcerative colitis was significantly lower than for Crohn's disease. Awareness of IBD was found to be particularly low in young people, at the age that they are most likely to be diagnosed.

Crohn's and Colitis UK believes that a greater public understanding of IBD and what it means to live with the condition will help every person affected by IBD in their daily lives and influence policy decisions about services for people living with IBD.

Influencing health services

National IBD audits show considerable local variation in the resources, organisation and clinical care for people with IBD. Further information on the IBD National Audit can be found in Chapter 20. Crohn's and Colitis UK works with health professional groups and the IBD community at national and local level to implement an overall strategy for the improvement of IBD Services.

1. IBD Standards

NACC has played a pivotal role within the IBD community in the development of the IBD Audit and promotion of national standards of care. National service standards for the healthcare of people who have IBD have now been published, and the organisation continues to lead the ongoing campaign for implementation of these standards throughout the UK (see Chapter 20).

2. Patient representation

Crohn's and Colitis UK encourages and supports the involvement of volunteer patient representatives in the design and improvement of NHS services and IBD research projects, and the development of good practice for patient involvement.

2.1 Patient Panels

This is a huge leap forward for a patient group to have a meaningful voice in our Trust, which can only improve the service that is offered to people who have IBD (Local Crohn's and Colitis UK Group member)

Inflammatory bowel disease nursing

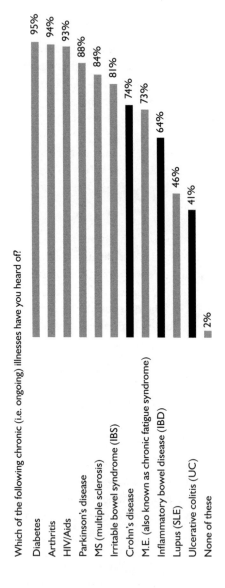

Figure 18.2 Awareness of chronic illnesses.

Crohn's and Colitis UK facilitates a programme of Patient Panels, set up to explore how patients and IBD health professionals can work together to improve services and patients' experiences of healthcare.

Lobbying

Crohn's and Colitis UK seeks opportunities to bring IBD and the needs of people living with IBD to the attention of politicians, organisations and the public within the four UK countries to promote understanding of the illness and highlight its impact on many different aspects of people's lives.

Supporting research

Funds raised by members, groups, volunteers and supporters have led to important advances in our understanding of IBD through a programme of NACC medical research awards. Funded projects continue to search for the cause and better treatments to manage the physical aspects of IBD, and also the social and psychological impact of the illness on patients and their families, the health and economic impact on society and the most effective ways of providing appropriate health services. Opportunities to work collaboratively with other researchers and organisations are sought to secure sources of external funding for IBD.

Fundraising

Fundraising provides the means for delivering services, campaigns and research, and has a value beyond the money raised by enabling patients and their families to participate as volunteers in positive activities. By supporting people to become involved in fundraising activities, Crohn's and Colitis UK helps them to develop skills and achieve goals that they might not otherwise have achieved.

Conclusion

Support for people affected by IBD can come from many sources: for example family, friends, healthcare professionals, community organisations. Patient support organisations can uniquely provide support for the individual and community groups, but also for professionals, multidisciplinary teams and local healthcare organisations, whilst also influencing strategic development within the speciality. This chapter has outlined the work of one such organisation, Crohn's and Colitis UK, to illustrate these activities. Encouraging patients to use support services, and to become involved can help their confidence, develop their understanding of the disease and enable them to manage their own condition. Fostering mutual understanding, using patient voices and feedback about the care they receive helps shape local and national services, and puts the needs of patients at the heart of IBD care.

References

Donnison, S. and Whitehead, H. (2007) *NACC Guide to Claiming Disability Living Allowance*. http://www.nacc.org.uk/downloads/disability/adultguide.pdf (accessed 8 September 2010).

Ipsos Mori (2009) *National Association for Colitis and Crohn's Disease – Public Awareness Survey*. http://www.nacc.org.uk/downloads/research/NACC_Ipsos_Mori_Awareness_Report_May_2009.pdf (accessed 8 September 2010)

Lancaster, H. (2007) *NACC Information and Support User Survey*. Unpublished observations.

NACC (2010) *NACC Plan 2010–2012: Meeting the Challenge of Colitis and Crohn's Disease*. http://www.nacc.org.uk/downloads/NACC_Strategy_Plan_2010-12.pdf (accessed 8 September 2010).

World Health Organization (2010) *Patient Support Groups*. http://www.who.int/genomics/public/patientsupport/en/ (accessed 30 November 2010).

CHAPTER 19

Supporting and educating patients

Kathy Whayman

Introduction

Patient education and support are now considered a vital part of the clinical management of IBD. Care for patients and families which assists their understanding and supports them to achieve the best possible quality of life has been highlighted in the ECCO statement of quality of healthcare (Elkjaer *et al.*, 2008) and comprises Standard D in the UK Service Standards for Healthcare for people with IBD (IBD Standards Group, 2009).

Management of these diseases is increasingly complex, and treatment options are varied, often involving a combination of pharmacological, surgical, dietary and psychological therapy. The symptoms and complications of IBD are unpleasant, unpredictable, embarrassing and painful, considerably affecting physical health (Walters, 2000; Forbes, 2000; Longobardi *et al.*, 2003). It has been suggested that, in addition, psychological morbidity inevitably accompanies the organic physical aspects of these diseases (Forbes, 2000). An integrated biopsychosocial approach to disease management is therefore required for total care of patients, incorporating the aspects of medical therapy, psychosocial assessment, support, information and education (Drossman, 1998; Waters *et al.*, 2005). The importance of employing a holistic approach when caring for a person with inflammatory bowel disease (IBD) cannot be overstated and it has been proposed that the two most significant interventions to dramatically improve quality of life and patient–physician relationships are good patient education and appropriate treatment of concurrent depression and anxiety (Husain and Triadafilopoulos, 2004).

Patients with IBD are considered eager to learn and want to participate in decision making about their treatment (Leahy, 2009). In combination with psychological support, patient education can increase the individual's insight and knowledge in IBD and help them understand the rationale for their medical therapy. This can enhance adherence to treatment and patient satisfaction whilst reducing hospital outpatient visits (Elkjaer *et al.*, 2008). A structured approach has been advocated (Kennedy *et al.*, 2004; Waters *et al.*, 2005), with a multidisciplinary team approach to care now seen as the gold standard: each team member educates patients about illness and the increasingly varied treatment options available (Elkjaer *et al.*, 2008; Carter *et al.* 2004). This keeps the patient at the centre of the decision-making process and importantly allows them to be the fully informed final arbiter of therapy (Rampton and Shanahan, 2008). The move to educating patients to self manage their condition is gathering speed, yet little is known so far on the long term effect of this intervention.

This chapter will provide an overview of the process of supporting and educating patients with IBD, using patient case studies to highlight issues which can significantly affect patients' quality of life. Current healthcare policy within chronic disease management and self-management will be explored, and its perceived effect on the individual's quality of life, disease status and healthcare usage. The importance of the nursing role in providing support and patient education will be discussed in relation to the issues raised by these studies.

Chronic disease management and current health policy

The incidence of chronic illness is rapidly increasing which presents a major challenge for contemporary healthcare systems to develop an effective response to the chronic disease burden (Busse *et al.*, 2010). Over 17 million people are estimated to be living with a chronic disease in the UK (Department of Health, 2004a). Approximately 240,000 people in the UK and 2.2 million across Europe are estimated to be living with IBD (Loftus, 2004). As a long-term condition, IBD has a disproportional high impact on society, occurring often at a young age and with the potential to result in lifelong ill health (Carter *et al.*, 2004); hence it is classed as a long-term condition.

Managing long-term conditions – the UK perspective

Improving patient information and education for people with long-term conditions is a key priority for the Department of Health. Empowering people with a chronic illness to self-manage where possible, and providing access to specialist advice and personalised care when patients need it, are specified objectives for the NHS. In 2000, the Department of Health outlined its vision of a patient-centred service (*The NHS Plan – a Plan for Investment, a Plan for Reform*) with strategies to improve patient choice, information and access to specialist care. Patients are encouraged as users to become involved in their own care, participate in decisions about their treatment, and to help shape healthcare services as a whole for the future.

To achieve this vision, a number of frameworks and documents have since been published by the Department of Health. In *The Expert Patient Programme* (Department of Health, 2001) recommendations were given for the development of lay-led generic education programmes for patients to increase their knowledge of their condition, with the aim of improving symptom control, self-esteem and quality of life. These programmes are run by trained volunteers and are designed to improve confidence and self efficacy for individuals, fostering a positive attitude to living with their condition, and resulting in fewer visits to the GP or hospital.

Building on the Best Choice, Responsiveness and Equity in the NHS (Department of Health, 2003) focused on giving patients more choice in their healthcare, improving user experience and again developing a partnership between patients and their healthcare professionals. *Better Information, Better Choices, Better Health* (Department of Health, 2004b) put informational care at the forefront of healthcare to empower people to get the right information at the right time, making information more effective, and using information to drive up health outcomes. In respect of IBD care, poor quality information for patients has long been cited as a problem (Scholmerich *et al.*, 1987; Kennedy *et al.*, 2003; Carter *et al.*, 2004). This political restructuring has therefore assisted patient associations, such as Crohn's and Colitis UK, and bodies such as the IBD Standards Group to bring supportive care to the forefront, ensuring that standards are set and patients' experiences are being valued. The aim of empowering, educating and informing patients is to ultimately reduce the time spent in secondary care by individuals with chronic conditions, moving care closer to the individual, whether at home or in other community settings (Department of Health, 2005). The most recent paper (*Your Health, Your Way – a Guide to Long Term Conditions and Self Care*) outlines the concept of supported self-care and personalised support planning, continuing the theme of self-care planning, self-management plans and structured information – such as in the form of information prescriptions (Department of Health, 2010).

The nursing role

UK guideline recommendations
Since the development of IBD nursing as a speciality in the 1990s, the IBD nurse is now an emerging force within the IBD multidisciplinary team, whose role is seen as core to the provision of high quality holistic care (IBD Standards Group,

2009). According to the British Society of Gastroenterology (Carter *et al.*, 2004), support and education is a key function of nurses caring for patients with IBD. From a support and education perspective, they advocate that the role of the IBD Nurse may encompass:

- the development of programmes of education
- providing and interpreting often complex information for patients
- providing individualised support and advice for patients and families in coping with IBD
- providing resources such as helplines, rapid access and follow-up clinics

Case study 1

Marc is a 28-year-old man with ileocolonic Crohn's disease, diagnosed in 2008, who has been steroid-dependent on budesonide since this time.

He presented to the gastroenterological clinic for a second opinion with the above history. His symptoms included diarrhoea up to 5 times a day, significant urgency and erythema nodosum on his legs.

In terms of Marc's medical options, he was counselled regarding azathioprine and commenced on this. At this point he was introduced to the IBD CNS, to be followed up in her clinic two weeks later for the relevant blood tests.

Marc works for a large gas company and has done so for 11 years. He lives with his partner and their 2½-year-old child. On speaking with Marc it became apparent that he and his partner were keen to have another child and Marc's main worry was the effect that any new medication would have on his ability to father a child. Marc raised this concern with the IBD CNS and it was clear from speaking with him that currently, due to poor control of his disease, on steroids, he was unable to interact and play with his child as much as he wanted. When it was explained to Marc that the azathioprine therapy would offer him better control of his disease and therefore quality of life, he relaxed about the need to have another child. Marc was reviewed in the IBD CNS's clinic over a six-month period, during which time he tolerated azathioprine well and was able to reduce and appropriately stop his oral steroids.

During this time, Marc spoke with the IBD nurse regarding a number of issues. He complained of being anxious on leaving the house, but admitted that he believed this to be psychological. He explained that he had experienced one episode of incontinence at his local train station and this has had a significant impact on him and his confidence. It was necessary firstly to reassure Marc that the team now had much better control of his disease, as was evident from a recent colonoscopy and barium follow through which showed quiescent disease. The next step for Marc once he acknowledged that his disease was in remission was to re-build his confidence. The IBD CNS provided Marc with a RADAR Key (see below in useful resources) which gives access to all of the disabled toilets in the UK. Many patients find that having a RADAR key is a confidence booster, but importantly it provides access to more private toilet facilities. Once it was confirmed Marc had quiescent disease, the IBD CNS also spent a long time discussing techniques to help boost his confidence, such as the 'holding on technique' (Box 19.1). Marc was reviewed in the IBD CNS clinic recently and his disease is currently well controlled on azathioprine. He and his partner have deferred having another child at this time, as Marc is currently enjoying his improved quality of life. He is now managing to leave the house without worrying about needing to find a toilet.

Box 19.1 Holding on techniques (Case study 1)

Next time when you need to open your bowels – try the following (in the comfort of your own home to begin with):

■ Sit on the toilet and hold on for 1 minute (use a watch). Gradually increase this to 5 minutes. Don't worry if you cannot do this to begin with – keep practising.
■ When you have mastered this, repeat the above but hold on for 10 minutes before opening your bowels – it may help to take something to read with you to the toilet. Remember that you are safe as you're on the toilet.
■ Once you are able to delay opening your bowels for 10 minutes whilst sitting on the toilet, now it is time to begin to move away from the toilet. This stage is when you sit on a chair by the toilet or on the edge of the bath or just outside the toilet area. Now hold on for 5 minutes, and gradually increase the time to 10 minutes.
■ When you are able to delay opening your bowels for 10 minutes whilst off the toilet you should now gradually move further away. Maybe

sitting on your bed in the bedroom. As your muscles are now becoming stronger you should be able to hold on for 10 minutes and feel more confident; increase the distance between you and the toilet.

Gradually you will find that you will be able to increase the distance and the time away from the toilet, and therefore give confidence in managing your bowels better.

Case study 2

Andrew, a 26-year-old man with a two-year history of distal ulcerative colitis (UC), was diagnosed at flexible sigmoidoscopy following a change of bowel habit and rectal bleeding. A very motivated individual, he engaged in self-managing his disease. Soon after his diagnosis Andrew was seen in clinic by the IBD CNS for education purposes. During that appointment the anatomy and physiology of normal gastrointestinal function was explained along with the remitting, relapsing nature of UC and other clinical features. Ways of identifying potential flares were discussed and a management plan developed for both maintaining his UC and, importantly, what actions to take in the event of a flare, including contacting the IBD advice line. Andrew learned when he should increase his oral 5-ASA and when to use rectal 5-ASAs or steroid preparations. He worked well with his IBD team, using their services appropriately, but also took personal responsibility for his disease management to ensure, for example, that routine investigations such as blood monitoring took place in an appropriate time frame.

Discussion

IBD has an unpredictable course, often with rapid onset of symptoms. These symptoms can have substantial psychosocial implications and cause sufferers to limit their lifestyles, consequently affecting the individual's quality of life (Ghosh and Mitchell, 2007). In the first case study, Marc was referred to the IBD CNS for a programme of follow-up after commencing azathioprine. Over a period of six months, his medication regimen was reviewed and optimised. During this time he and the CNS were also able to talk about psychosocial problems he was experiencing as a result of the disease and its treatment.

In the second case study, Andrew was referred to the IBD CNS for education purposes. A young, motivated individual, he was able to learn about the function of the bowel, and about the nature of his condition, including how to recognise the symptoms of potential flares. Together, he and the IBD CNS were able to identify his particular needs and design a tailor made management plan. This action gave Andrew control of his disease and allowed him to carry on with his usual daily activities knowing what to expect from his symptoms and how to deal with them should they arise.

Both of these individuals could be considered the 'ideal' patient to undertake self-management – they demonstrate an eagerness to learn and self-efficacy to reach a desired goal. The rationale for selecting patients to participate in self-management of their disease will be discussed in more detail later in this chapter.

The IBD CNS had the time and skills to address these issues as part of Marc and Andrew's follow-up. By developing a therapeutic relationship over time, the nurse was able to provide information, education and overall support to help them as individuals toward improved psychosocial well-being (Further information on building therapeutic relationships can be found in Chapter 16.) Having this time enables patients to gain confidence in their relationship with professionals, allowing for more in-depth discussion to take place about matters of importance to that individual. With respect to the first case study, it is important to consider whether Marc would have felt comfortable to raise the issue of incontinence with a nurse or doctor he had not met before or whose time was limited. Having established a therapeutic relationship with him, the nurse had enabled Marc to discuss the difficult problems he was experiencing. This is appreciated and can come as a relief to many patients (Thomas, 2009) who may perceive doctors to be too busy for extensive discussions during a ten-minute consultation, or who may even find it difficult to talk openly with friends and family when time is limited. Patients have described specialist nurses as having good listening skills and have appreciated their ability to make time to discuss problems and provide a constant point of contact (Belling *et al.*, 2008).

Psychosocial issues are also often not the primary concerns of doctors, who, by nature of their 'medical model', may focus on diagnosis and treatment of disease and managing physical symptoms (Younge and Norton, 2007). Although nurses often perform tasks considered to be within the medical domain, they work differently from doctors (Norton and Kamm, 2002). By virtue of their training and models of care, nurses are in a good position to help people toward physical and psychological adaptation to living with the condition, adhering to treatment plans and in many cases self-management.

A study conducted by deRooy *et al.* (2001) to determine the concerns of patients with IBD, highlighted many physical, psychological and social concerns of patients. The highest ranking related to energy level, effects of medications, uncertainty of disease symptoms, having surgery and/or an ostomy bag, achieving full potential, loss of bowel control, being a burden on others and producing unpleasant odours (deRooy *et al.*, 2001). Nurses can address these concerns with patients in a supportive role, and it has been identified that nurses whose attributes are empathetic, caring, supportive and skilled communicators make a real difference to patient care (Belling *et al.*, 2008).

These two case studies highlight areas where nurses address the symptoms and effects of IBD that, although treatable by medications, can still have a significant impact on patients' day-to-day living with IBD. In particular, the issues of incontinence, fatigue, pain and adaptation to living with a chronic disease will be discussed to provide examples of how simple advice and practical support can make a difference. The following section is not designed to be a 'one stop' management for these aspects of IBD, but lists simple steps that can be helpful when managing the complexity of the illnesses, symptoms and treatment options: facts that might otherwise be overlooked.

Faecal incontinence

Faecal incontinence is something that potentially affects most people with IBD – not all experience actual loss of bowel control, but the fear of it can be equally debilitating. Symptoms of IBD, such as loose stool, urgency, fistula and diarrhoea can all result in incontinence. For some it may be inability to control wind or a small amount of leakage; for others it may be a lot more. Thomas (2009) conducted a comprehensive phenomenological study, constructing reflexive research around counselling for individuals with IBD, and amongst many findings, she established that one episode of incontinence was sufficient to sensitise participants to an immense fear of recurrence. Participants often experienced a feeling of urgency and were sometimes unable to reach a toilet in time (Thomas, 2009). This kind of occurrence can result in feelings of shame and distress, with individuals experiencing a disabling lack of confidence, and even a fear of actually leaving their house, as in Marc's case described above.

What can help?

Supportive care and simple advice can complement the medical and surgical management of disease in helping promote continence:

- Ask! Often patients will not volunteer this information – actively and sensitively enquire about symptoms (National Institute of Clinical Excellence, 2010)

- Optimise medical management to reduce symptoms
- Provide information to patients about anal sphincter exercises (see http://www.stmarkshospital.org.uk/patient-information-leaflets)
- Educate patients (with quiescent disease) about urge resistance techniques (see 'holding on' programme shown in Box 19.1)
- Advise patients about perianal skin care (effective evidence-based skin care products for faecal incontinence are outlined from page 71 in the recent NICE Guidelines (National Institute for Clinical Excellence, 2010).
- Discuss dietary manipulation (as agreed with the multidisciplinary team). Page 6 of the NICE guidelines has a quick reference guide containing useful tips and information (see useful resources at the end of this chapter).
- Consider specialist management for dietary assessment and management, bowel habit retraining or behavioural therapy (biofeedback).
- Discuss practical coping strategies with patients (e.g. using pads, anal plugs if clinically indicated, giving information to employers)
- Be aware of the physical and emotional impact this condition can have on individuals and their carers and offer emotional and psychological support.
- Planning and establishing the location of toilets prior to going out can lessen anxiety when needing to find a toilet quickly.
- In the UK, patients can buy a 'RADAR' key giving them access to disabled toilets and also a directory of all the disabled toilets in the country. The EFFCA website Life and IBD contains information regarding similar schemes in other European countries (see useful resources at the end of the chapter for both websites).
- Both the Bowel and Bladder Foundation and Crohn's and Colitis UK provide a 'Can't Wait Card' for people with bowel problems to carry should they need quick access to toilets in a shop, garage or other setting which has staff toilets. This works on the premise that organisations have good customer care policies and enables the person carrying the card to confirm they have a genuine and urgent need to use a toilet.
- Planning for an emergency can help increase patients confidence in dealing with an episode of incontinence should it actually occur – e.g. taking a kit with them when going out including spare underwear, wipes and pads.
- Provide patients, families/carers information on relevant support groups and financial assistance such as (in the UK) psychosocial grants from Crohn's and Colitis UK or Disability Living Allowance.

Fatigue

Patients with IBD, in active as well as in quiescent disease, frequently cite fatigue or tiredness as a symptom present in their everyday life (Minderhoud *et al.*, 2003). Described as difficult to define and underappreciated, this is a common and disabling effect of chronic disease, and specifically in IBD care, there is little evidence on prevalence, correlation with disease activity or causes of fatigue (van Langenburg and Gibson, 2010). The IBD standards Group (2009) identified that, in conjunction with other symptoms of IBD, fatigue can severely affect work, social functioning and self-esteem, especially in the young and newly diagnosed. Assessing and managing fatigue needs to be a part of patient care from time of diagnosis onwards. In a recent systematic review, despite the lack of data so far, van Langenburg and Gibson (2010) propose useful assessment and management guidelines and an algorithm for fatigue which nurses can incorporate in consultations with patients.

What can help?

As before, simple and practical information can help patients manage this debilitating symptom, thus nurses might advise the following:

- Plan in advance as much as possible – with time set aside to recover from occasions (such as a long shift at work or special occasion).
- It may help during periods of fatigue to take naps during the day.
- Exercise regularly (such as starting off with gentle walk around the block and going from there) even if feeling tired, as this can help relieve the feeling of tiredness and encourage better sleep.
- Aim for a good night's sleep regularly (6–8 hrs).
- Eat a well-balanced diet as much as possible (as discussed and advised by the team) and keep well hydrated.
- Any underlying caused of fatigue should be established and treated as necessary (for example, if active disease or iron deficiency anaemia).

Pain management

Present for the majority of people with IBD during active disease, abdominal pain is a common symptom of Crohn's disease and UC. There are many possible mechanisms of pain involved in IBD. Carter *et al.* (2004) offer a comprehensive list, including obstructive episodes due to disease or adhesions, inflammation, visceral hypersensitivity and/or distension, secondary irritable bowel syndrome and proctalgia fugax, in addition to non-gut manifestations such as arthritis, iritis and painful skin complications. Analgesia may be ineffective, and treating the underlying cause can result in improved pain control (Carter *et al.*, 2004). For some patients, symptoms of pain often persist after improvement or even resolution of inflammation and continue to impair the quality of life (Bielefeldt *et al.*, 2009). Thomas (2009) found that sometimes physical pain can be under-recognised, which leads to psychological pain and is an individual experience – some patients in this study reported pain as their major concern, whereas others had learned to accept pain as 'normal', which disrupted or sometimes even controlled life at times. A comprehensive model of pain has been proposed by Bielefeldt *et al.* (2009) involving the physical effects of inflammation and also the emotional/cognitive processes of pain, where the inflammatory process sensitises afferent neurons, leading to increased central input and perception. They suggest that the affective dimension of pain triggers emotional responses, resulting in hypervigilance and worrying, decreasing inhibitory control and increasing sensory input, which in turn leads to more vigilance. Managing total pain requires continual input of the MDT and in-depth assessment (see Chapters 5 and 6) and often requires specialist pain management support.

What can help?

Nurses are ideally suited to this 'palliative' symptom-orientated model, as proposed by Bielefeldt *et al.* (2009), and following discussion with the MDT may offer advice such as the following:

- Treat the pain early rather than leaving it – many patients with IBD think it is part of their disease to simply put up with the pain.
- Take paracetamol up to four times a day – emphasis being on having a background analgesic.
- Use buscopan/spasmonal for spasmodic pain.
- Avoid NSAIDS.
- Topical analgesics can be used for muscular/joint pain.
- Employ the expertise of the pain team/family doctor as needed for ongoing pain management.

Adapting to living with IBD

One of many psychosocial therapies, developing adaptive coping strategies in order to manage symptoms and the effect of IBD on lifestyle, has been discussed in Chapter 16, where it was highlighted as a key psychosocial intervention between professionals and patients.

What can help?

Having developed a therapeutic relationship, nurses are in a good position to offer practical information in order to help patients adapt to their altered lifestyle:

- Explore ways with patients to talk to their family and friends about their disease and treatments. Anecdotally patients have reported that it is of most help to them when their family understand and help them overcome periods of active disease (for example by helping out with household chores, cooking etc). Equally important to some has been the support and encouragement of family and friends to return to usual daily living during periods of inactive disease.
- There are no explicit restrictions to living with IBD, in terms of travelling, work etc. Associations such as Crohn's and Colitis UK provide useful information sheets, for example regarding travel advice, information for employers, and how to discuss IBD with colleagues. The patient and professional education website 'Life and IBD' (see list of useful resources at the end of the chapter) is an excellent online resource in designed to help people to lead a life that is as normal as possible, managing day-to-day life with IBD.
- Advise patients to be honest with health professionals, especially regarding preference of and adherence to medications and treatments.
- Discuss with patients how learning about the disease process as well as how their own disease reacts is useful to allow for prompt contact with the team, initiation of treatments earlier and potentially subsequent restriction of flare.

Information for patients

Lack of quality information for patients with IBD was recognised as a problem 20 years ago (Scholmerich *et al.*, 1987) and still highlighted as poor 16 years later (Kennedy *et al.*, 2003). Patients were not routinely told about relevant supportive voluntary organisations like the National Association for Colitis and Crohn's Disease (NACC), there was a lack of consistency about the information available, and crucially little information on how to prevent relapse. However, guidelines on the management of IBD strongly highlight a need for information and patient education as an essential approach to care (Carter *et al.*, 2004).

The two case studies in this chapter illustrate the value of individualised, timely and relevant information for patients. In Marc's situation, for example, information about the effects of steroid therapy enabled him to understand why his disease was poorly controlled and how azathioprine could improve this and his feeling of well-being. He also received practical information from the IBD CNS, which improved his confidence when going out of the house.

Another increasing and very convenient source of information is the Internet, and many patients and their relatives are using this to provide themselves with disease-specific information – accurate or otherwise. The difficulty with information obtained from the Internet is that many patients are not able to judge its quality or accuracy. Indeed, a lack of structured and official informational materials risk patients receiving unregulated, skewed information from the Internet which can result in (among other effects) psychological instability and fear of treatment (Elkjaer *et al.*, 2008). Nurses need to anticipate questions and concerns of IBD patients, providing answers or at least clear direction for finding answers (Leahy, 2009). Nurses might find it helpful to work with patients to find web-based information together, for example during a consultation, which the nurse can assess for quality, or even provide a shortlist, as Leahy (2009) suggests, of useful websites and online support agencies.

The use of the Internet and other sources of information for patients with IBD was the subject of a very useful discussion during a focus group of patients, professionals and support group representatives within one NHS Trust facilitated by the IBD nursing team, a clinical psychologist and the author (Younge *et al.*, 2007). Due to the small size of this group (17: 9 patients, 3 representatives of support groups, 1 dietitian and 4 nurses), the results are not representative of the wider population of IBD patients or professionals. Nevertheless, the findings in Tables 19.1 and 19.2 are helpful when determining potential sources of information and what type of information patients value following diagnosis of IBD. So, in response to patient feedback about the quality of information for patients, the aim of this group was establish the effect and current state of information (Table 19.1), and to identify topics and content of information that patients want following diagnosis of their disease (Table 19.2).

Three occasions were identified by participants when information is essential: at time of diagnosis, when changing treatment and when starting a new medication. The participants also reported that good information can give patients confidence, remind patients what their doctor or nurse told them and allow people to make informed decisions. Information was felt to give people time to go away, read the literature/leaflets and think about the issues involved, helping to make sure that they are prepared for procedures or operations. Overall, provision of accurate information was identified to involve patients and their carers in decisions about their treatment and condition if they wish.

Table 19.1 Perceived current information provision in IBD.

What information is currently available?	How is it given?	By whom is it given?	Identified problems with current information
■ Descriptions of IBD ■ Treatment explanation ■ Some nutritional information ■ Cancer risk ■ How to access nursing support ■ How to access group support ■ Drug information	■ Verbally ■ Leaflets ■ Video/DVD ■ Internet ■ Information packs ■ Helplines ■ Business cards	■ Doctors (Hospital & GP) ■ Nurses ■ Dietitians ■ NACC ■ Family/friends ■ Pharmacists ■ Pharmaceutical firms	■ Wide variability in the quality of information ■ There is need for a type of 'kite marking' of information to ensure it is safe and reliable ■ Information can be difficult to understand or interpret ■ Information can be vague, ambiguous or contains jargon ■ Information is not relevant to the individual

Table 19.2 What information is required for IBD care and how should it be given?

What information is required	How should it be given?	Potential sources
■ Terminology ■ Definitions of IBD ■ Living with IBD ■ Diet ■ Travel ■ Pregnancy/fertility ■ Family history ■ Sexual relations ■ Dealing with incontinence ■ Planning for an emergency ■ Questions to ask your healthcare professional ■ Gender-specific information ■ 'Tailor-made' information	■ In plain, clear language for correct reading age ■ Free from jargon and should contain illustrations ■ Offered in a variety of modes – e.g. audio/visual/leaflets/web material/helplines ■ Offered over the telephone/face to face/online/discussion boards/chat rooms ■ Via open/information days	■ Healthcare agencies: Hospitals/PCTs ■ Patient organisations ■ GPs ■ Pharmacists ■ Pharmaceutical companies ■ Family members/friends ■ Online/chat rooms ■ Local support groups, working in partnership with specialist nurses ■ Befriending services ■ Patient education groups ■ NHS Direct ■ Carers' association

Evidence for practice

Studies investigating the varying methods of information provision, patient education and self management in IBD are evident, although there appears to be some contradiction in their findings on anxiety, level of knowledge and quality of life (Borgaonkar *et al.*, 2002; Probert and Mayberry 1991; Verma *et al.*, 2001). There does seem to be consensus, however, that education and information provision have had at least a qualitative impact on patient experience and can assist in developing the individual's ability to cope, adherence to treatment plans and improving long-term management of the disease (Scholmerich *et al.*, 1987; Mansfield *et al.*, 1997; Larsson *et al.*, 2003). In addition, there is at least a suggestion, if not evidence, that education and increase in knowledge can improve quality of life and psychological well-being for this patient group (Husian and Triadafilopoulos, 2004; Quan *et al.*, 2003). Indeed, Rakshit and Mayberry (2008) agree that until a large study is conducted to give conclusive data, evidence suggests that patients should be actively involved in decision making, and this requires that they are educated about their disease.

Self-management

What is self-management?

The Department of Health strategy for supporting people with long-term conditions (Department of Health, 2005) outlines self-care and self-management as increasingly important in improving wellbeing, maintaining independence and quality of life. These two terms are often interchangeable in papers and models for care, and the meaning of the two concepts can be unclear, which results in confusion, especially for patients. They are, however, different and Hall *et al.* (2007) make an important distinction between the two in respect to IBD.

- People with a chronic disease routinely carry out self-care as part of their daily life. These are the actions people employ to stay fit, maintain good physical and mental health, and care for ailments and long-term conditions.
- People with IBD routinely cope with symptoms and everyday IBD related problems, for example deciding what to eat, when to take medication, whether to attend out-patient appointments or ring the telephone helpline.
- Thus guided self-management incorporates these elements, developing the individual's skills in knowing when and how to take action should a problem occur (Hall *et al.*, 2007).

Self-management in chronic disease

Self-management education programmes are distinct from simple patient education, information-giving or skills training, in that they are designed to allow people with chronic conditions to take an active part in the management of their own condition (Foster *et al.*, 2007). Lorig *et al.* (2001) reported a cohort study on the effectiveness of generic self-management programmes in chronic disease, where improvements in health status and self-efficacy were found. Although these improvements were small, the recommendation was offered that health systems should now consider self-management programmes for the chronic disease patient group (Lorig *et al.*, 2001). Indeed, there is now an expectation that patient expertise is seen as central to care delivery for chronic disease (Department of Health, 2001).

Further evidence of the effectiveness of self-management approaches to chronic disease, including both generic and disease-specific education programmes, was appraised by Barlow *et al.* (2002). The results of this review showed a variation in approach to self-management and outcome measurements depending on the disease, and it was suggested that disease-specific approaches might have more relevance to particular patient groups. Although this evidence of generic chronic disease programmes is useful, no specific studies on gastrointestinal disease were included in the review.

Self management in IBD

Three studies focused on the implementation of self-management techniques in IBD, including the use of a guidebook, training consultations and/or education programmes (Robinson *et al.*, 2001; Kennedy *et al.*, 2004; Waters *et al.*, 2005). All demonstrated improvements in anxiety levels, disease activity, and self treatment prior to accessing healthcare resources. Quality of life scores in the main remained unchanged, although patients reported satisfaction with these interventions. The evidence is not conclusive as to the impact of such interventions on long-term quality of life and patient confidence in managing their own illness.

Stansfield and Robinson (2008) looked at nurse-led self-management clinics as part of a primary care trust (PCT) funded project. Patients in the intervention group agreed a self-management plan with the nurse in clinic following diagnosis, involving education and a guidebook (Kennedy *et al.*, 2004). All were given access to a helpline and clinic when required. They found that, on average, patients accessed the self-management clinic three times per year. Pressure on other gastroenterology clinics was alleviated, most patients reported satisfaction and there was a cost saving to the PCT. As before, no longer term outcomes or changes in quality of life were reported, but patient satisfaction was high, and information received was reported by participants as sufficient for their needs (Stansfield and Robinson, 2008).

What is interesting is that all the education interventions in these studies were led by healthcare professionals, in contrast to more generic programmes such as the Expert Patient Programme, which is lay-led by trained volunteers. A recent Cochrane Review (Foster *et al.*, 2007) looked at the outcomes for lay-led self-management programmes and the findings appear to correlate with the disease-specific interventions outlined previously. Small, short-term improvements in participants' self-efficacy, self rated health and cognitive symptom management were evident, but there is currently no evidence to suggest that such programmes improve psychological health, symptoms or health-related quality of life, or that they significantly alter healthcare use (Foster *et al.*, 2007). The effects of patient education in IBD are difficult to assess. This may be in part due to the unpredictability of the disease. Rakshit and Mayberry (2008) contend that this is also because of the variability in communication skills of the healthcare professionals and facilities available as well as the methods of information dissemination to a range of patient groups. All researchers seem to be in agreement, however, that studies now need to focus on longer term results to show significant improvements in clinical outcomes.

So, although the evidence is as yet inconclusive on education for patients, we are, according to Saibil *et al.* (2008), in the age of self-management. International evidence is said to be clear that this and self-efficacy are drivers for health policy on long-term conditions (Wilson, 2010). In IBD care specifically, nurses who are deemed responsible for setting up education programmes (Carter *et al.*, 2004), need to appraise such interventions in relation to their local patient population. In order to do this, it is important to consider what the challenges may be when informing and educating patients.

Which patients should participate in self-management?

Both the case studies in this chapter outline the experience and care of two young, motivated and educated patients, who appear to be receptive to education on how to deal with their symptoms and how to access the service should they need to. Self-management and in-depth information about their condition, however, is not for everyone. There has been criticism of the model of self-management such as the difficulty in involving people from ethnic minority groups and those with low health literacy: for example Lorig's work has been shown to involve mainly white, motivated, stable communities (Greenhalgh, 2009). Thus it is important to remember that not everyone wants to be or can be actively involved in managing their own condition. Individuals with complex disease (such as the case study discussed in Chapter 7) or multiple pathology may require in-depth professional care and thus may not be candidates for self-management programmes. For the growing number of people who do want to be involved, however, more support is needed from the professionals involved in their care (Corben and Rosen, 2005).

Each individual's experience of their condition is unique and so will be their information needs (Tables 19.1 and 19.2 illustrate the diversity of information which may be required at all stages of disease). Sensitive explanation and a good therapeutic relationship between patients and professionals are vital (see below). Documentation and communication within the IBD team about the information given and patients' wishes about information required are also important. If patients are encouraged to participate in an education programme or self-management plan and they opt for a more traditional follow-up, the team needs to assure them the care they receive will not be comprised due to this decision. Equally, if patients participate in such programmes, information needs to be clear as to the aim of the intervention, expectation of patients, and assurance that they will have access to hospital/community support when it is required. One issue raised by Stansfield and Robinson (2008) was the differing needs of the local patient population and those who were tertiary referrals to the hospital in relation to accessing the hospital. Assessing individual and local needs is paramount and ensuring rapid access will increase patient confidence.

What access to services do patients have?

An age of self-management has implications for the current models of care practised by clinicians caring for IBD patients. Most individuals with IBD are currently managed in secondary care, by specialist teams involving physicians, specialist nurses and relevant other professionals as required. Access is available in the event of a problem, and scheduled follow-ups ensure that the patient is monitored with regard to complicated medications, and any potential complications of the disease itself. Many patients find episodic follow-up reassuring, especially if all is well. Consequently, with the proposed changes to chronic healthcare delivery, focusing on patient initiated care in the primary healthcare setting, IBD patients may feel they are at risk of losing this open door approach. This may result in decreased perceptions of support and access when managing their condition. Again, clear information, good communication and a supportive professional– patient relationship are vital. Services provided by the IBD CNS become even more important to patients. Ensuring adequate and evidence-based protocols are in place for self-management programmes informs the MDT as a whole, ensuring that they understand the process.

Patient education groups

Corbett and Whayman (2007) reported on a meeting of IBD nurses held to consider ways of developing a patient education strategy with particular emphasis on running a group education programme. Specialist IBD knowledge, funding, group skills training and clinical supervision/support from a clinical psychologist were identified as necessary for facilitators of IBD education programmes. Skills and attributes of IBD nurses are considered very important to patients (Belling *et al.*, 2008). In fact, one of the major factors in successfully supporting and educating patients with IBD is the professional–patient relationship. Sensitivity and empathy from all healthcare professionals are highly valued by patients (DeRooy *et al.* 2001; Belling *et al.* 2008). Discussions with patients by professionals should include enquiries as to the impact of IBD symptoms on patients' well-being and quality of life (Ghosh and Mitchell, 2007), and clinicians need to engage with the challenges that face individuals trying to get on with life with a chronic disease (Greenhalgh, 2009).

The recent European consensus on the management of Crohn's disease, places education and informational care in the category of special situations (Van Assche *et al.*, 2010). Within this consensus, there is strong support for the doctor–patient relationship in helping people with IBD psychologically, as clinicians take psychosocial factors into account from diagnosis onward. The paper goes on to report that patient education programmes have limited influence on disease outcomes or psychological affects of patients. What is interesting, despite other evidence mentioned previously, is that there is no reference to the role of the IBD nurse anywhere in the paper. Therefore it would seem there is further work required on a European level to establish the evidence base for nursing, and their work in support, informing and educating patients.

Conclusion

The aim of this chapter was to give an overview of the role of the nurse in supporting and educating patients with IBD, with specific reference to patients' support needs, information giving and self-management. The role of the specialist nurse has been advocated as instrumental to establishing support and education packages in IBD practice (Carter *et al.*, 2004) and we are now said to be in an era of self-management (Saibil, 2008). There is some evidence to suggest the efficacy of self-management initiatives and education programmes for patients with IBD.

Other evidence and expert opinion is conflicting, however, and the effects on anxiety, patient confidence and long-term quality of life are not yet clear. Careful appraisal of the nature of all educational interventions, and of individual patient and service need is important. In respect to self-management programmes, further evidence on the patient's experience, the role of the facilitator, and ultimately their long-term outcome is also necessary. There is already an argument that it is time to move beyond the self-management approach to care and embrace richer, more holistic models which consider a person's family, social and political context (Greenhalgh, 2009). Nurses already do this. Often it is the simple practical support and advice, which nurses are best placed to offer, that makes a difference to the patient's experience. If the political agenda for chronic disease management is realised in IBD care, then nursing support services will be even more vital, and must have evidence, funding and team support behind them.

Useful resources

RADAR Disability Network
http://www.radar.org.uk/

Life and IBD (EFFCA)
http://www.lifeandibd.org/

Crohn's and Colitis UK
http://www.nacc.org.uk/

Bladder and Bowel Foundation
http://www.bladderandbowelfoundation.org/

Disability Living Allowance
http://www.direct.gov.uk/en/DisabledPeople/

Faecal Incontinence Quick Reference Guide (NICE)
http://guidance.nice.org.uk/CG49/QuickRefGuide/pdf/English

References

Barlow, J., Wright, C., Sheasby, J., Turner, A. and Hainsworth, J. (2002) Self-management approaches for people with chronic conditions: a review. *Patient Educ. Counseling*, **48**, 177–87.

Belling, R., Woods, L. and McLaren, S. (2008) Stakeholder perceptions of specialist Inflammatory Bowel Disease nurses' roles and personal attributes. *Int. J. Nurs. Practice*, **14**, 67–73.

Bielefeldt, K., Davis, B. and Binion, D. G. (2009) Pain and inflammatory bowel disease. *Inflamm. Bowel Dis.*, **15**, 778–88.

Borgaonkar, M. R., Townson, G., Donnelly, M. *et al.* (2002) Providing disease related information worsens health-related quality of life in inflammatory bowel disease. *Inflamm. Bowel Dis.*, **8**, 264–9.

Busse, R., Blumel, M., Scheller-Kreinsen, D. and Zentner, A. (2010) *Tackling Chronic Disease in Europe. Strategies, Interventions and Challenges.* http://www.euro.who.int/__data/assets/pdf_file/0008/96632/E93736.pdf (accessed 15 October 2010).

Carter, M. J., Lobo, A. J. and Travis, S. P. (2004) Guidelines for the management of inflammatory bowel disease in adults. *Gut*, **53**(suppl. V), V1–V6.

Corben, S. and Rosen, R. (2005) *Self-management for Long-term Conditions: Patients' Perspectives on the Way Ahead.* London: King's Fund.

Corbett, S. and Whayman, K. (2006) Delivering patient education programmes as part of an inflammatory bowel disease service – what is the way forward? *Gastrointest. Nurs.*, **4**(5), 10–11.

Department of Health (2000) *The NHS Plan – a Plan for Investment, a Plan for Reform.* London: Department of Health.

Department of Health (2001) *The Expert Patient: a New Approach to Chronic Disease Management for the 21st Century.* London: Department of Health.

Department of Health (2003) *Building on the Best Choice, Responsiveness and Equity in the NHS.* London: Department of Health.

Department of Health (2004a) *Improving Chronic Disease Management.* http://www.dh.gov.uk/prod_consum_dh/groups/dh_digitalassets/@dh/@en/documents/digitalasset/dh_4075213.pdf (accessed 9 October 2010).

Department of Health (2004b) *Better Information, Better Choices, Better Health: Putting Information at the Centre of Health.* London: Department of Health.

Department of Health (2005) *Supporting People with Long Term Conditions: Improving Care Improving Lives.* London: Department of Health.

Department of Health (2010) *Your Health, Your Way – A Guide to Long Term Conditions and Self Care.* London: Department of Health.

de Rooy, E. C., Toner, B. B., Maunder, R. G. *et al.* (2001) Concerns of patients with inflammatory bowel disease: results from a clinical population. *Am. J. Gastroenterol.*, **96**, 1816–21.

Drossman, D. A. (1998) Presidential address: Gastrointestinal illness and the biopsychosocial model. *Psychosomatic Medicine*, **60**, 258–67.

Foster, G., Taylor, S. J. C., Eldridge, S., Ramsay, J. and Griffiths, C. J. (2007) Self-management education programmes by lay leaders for people with chronic conditions. *Cochrane Database Syst. Rev.*, Issue 4. Art. No.: CD005108.

Ghosh, S. and Mitchell, R. (2007) Impact of inflammatory bowel disease on quality of life: results of the European Federation of Crohn's and Ulcerative Colitis Associations (EFCCA) patient survey. *J. Crohn's and Colitis*, 1, 10–20.

Hall, A., Porrett, T. and Cox, C. (2007) Self-management in the care of patients with inflammatory bowel disease. *Gastrointest. Nurs.*, 5(5), 34–8.

Husain, A. and Triadafilopoulos, G. (2004) Communicating with patients with inflammatory bowel disease. *Inflamm. Bowel Dis.*, 10, 444–50.

Elkjaer, M., Moser, G., Reinisch, W. *et al.* (2008) IBD patients need in health quality of care: ECCO consensus. *J. Crohn's and Colitis*, 2, 181–8.

Forbes, A. (2000) *A Clinician's Guide to Inflammatory Bowel Disease*. London: Arnold.

Greenhalgh, T. (2009) Chronic illness: beyond the expert patient. *Br. Med. J.*, 338, 629–31.

IBD Standards Group (2009) *Quality Care: Service Standards for the Healthcare of People Who Have Inflammatory Bowel Disease (IBD)*. http://www.ibdstandards.org.uk/uploaded_files/IBDstandards.pdf.

Kennedy, A., Robinson, A., Hann, M., Thompson, D. and Wilkin, D. (2003) Cluster-randomised controlled trial of a patient-centred guidebook for patients with ulcerative colitis: effect on knowledge, anxiety and quality of life. *Health and Social Care in the Community*, 11, 64–72.

Kennedy, A. P., Nelson, E., Reeves, D. *et al.* (2004) A randomised controlled trial to assess the effectiveness and cost of a patient orientated self management approach to chronic inflammatory bowel disease. *Gut*, 53, 1639–45.

Larsson, K., Sundberg Hjelm, M., Karlbom, U., Nordin, K., Anderberg, U. M. and Loof, L. (2003) A group-based patient education program for high-anxiety patients with Crohn's disease or ulcerative colitis. *Scand. J. Gastroenterol.*, 38, 763–9.

Leahy, Y. (2009) Inflammatory bowel disease: patient education using web based resources. *Gastroenterol. Nurs.*, 32, 415–18.

Loftus, E. V. Jr (2004) Clinical epidemiology of inflammatory bowel disease: Incidence, prevalence, and environmental influences. *Gastroenterology*, 126, 1504–17.

Longobardi, T., Jacobs, P. and Bernstein, C. N. (2003) Work losses related to inflammatory bowel disease in the United States: results from the National Health Interview Survey. *Am. J. Gastroenterol.*, 98, 1064–72.

Lorig, K. R., Sobel, D. S., Ritter, P. L., Laurent, D. and Hobbs, M. (2001) Effect of a self-management program on patients with chronic disease. *Effective Clinical Practice*, 4, 256–62.

Mansfield, J. C., Tanner, A. R. and Bramble, M. G. (1997) Information for patients about inflammatory bowel disease. *J. Roy. Coll. Physicians Lond.*, 31, 184–7.

Minderhoud, I. M., Oldenburg, B., van Dam, P. S. and van Berge Henegouwen, G. P. (2003) High prevalence of fatigue in quiescent inflammatory bowel disease is not related to adrenocortical insufficiency. *Am. J. Gastroenterol.*, **98**, 1088–93.

National Institute of Clinical Excellence (2010) *Faecal Incontinence: the Management of Faecal Incontinence in Adults.* http://www.nice.org.uk/CG049 (accessed 10 October 2010).

Norton, C. and Kamm, M. A. (2002) Specialist nurses in gastroenterology. *J. Roy. Soc. Med.*, **95**, 331–5.

Probert, C. S. J. and Mayberry, J. F. (1991) Inflammatory bowel disease: patients' expectations in the 1990s. *J. Roy. Soc. Med.*, **84**, 131–2.

Quan, H., Present, J. W. and Sutherland, L. R. (2003) Evaluation of educational programs in inflammatory bowel disease. *Inflamm. Bowel Dis.*, **9**, 356–62.

Rakshit, R. C. and Mayberry, J. F. (2008) What is the role of patient education in the care of IBD? *Inflamm. Bowel Dis.*, **14**(suppl. 2), S66–S7.

Rampton, D. S. and Shanahan, F. (2008) *Fast Facts: Inflammatory Bowel Disease*, 3rd edn. Oxford: Health Press.

Robinson, A., Wilkson, D., Thompson, D. G. and Roberts, C. (2001) Guided self-management and patient-directed follow-up of ulcerative colitis: a randomised trial. *Lancet*, **358**, 976–81.

Saibil, F., Lai, E., Hayward, A., Yip, J. and Gilbert, C. (2008) Self management for people with inflammatory bowel disease. *Can. J. Gastroenterol.*, **22**, 281–7.

Scholmerich, J., Sedlak, P., Hoppe-Seyler, P. and Gerok, W. (1987) The information needs and fears of patients with inflammatory bowel disease. *Hepato-gastroenterology*, **34**, 182–5.

Stansfield, C. and Robinson, A. (2008) Implementation of an IBD nurse-led self-management programme. *Gastrointest. Nurs.*, **6**(3), 12–18.

Thomas, G. (2009) *Counselling and Reflexive Research in Healthcare: Working therapeutically with Clients with Inflammatory Bowel Disease.* London: Jessica Kingsley.

Van Assche, G., Dignass, A., Reinisch, W. *et al.* (2010) The second European evidence-based consensus on the diagnosis and management of Crohn's disease: special situations. *J. Crohn's and Colitis*, **4**, 63–101.

van Langenburg, D. R. and Gibson, P. R. (2010) Systematic review: Fatigue in inflammatory bowel disease. *Aliment. Pharmacol. Ther.*, **32**, 131–43.

Verma, S., Tsai, H. H. and Giaffer, M. H. (2001) Does better disease-related education improve quality of life? A survey of IBD patients. *Dig. Dis. Sci.*, **46**, 865–9.

Walters, S. (2000) *NACC Audit of IBD.* Chichester: Aeneas Press.

Waters, B. M., Jensen, L. and Fedorak, R. N. (2005) Effects of formal education for patients with inflammatory bowel disease: a randomized controlled trial. *Can. J. Gastroenterol.*,

19, 235–44.

Wilson, J. H. (2010) Self-management is key for long-term conditions (editorial) *Br. J. Nurs.*, **19**, 73.

Younge, L. and Norton, C. (2007) Contribution of specialist nurses in managing patients with IBD. *Br. J. Nurs.*, **7**, 208–12.

Younge, L,. Whayman, K. and Corbett, S. (2007) Unpublished observations.

PART 3

Advancing practice

CHAPTER 20

Organisation of IBD care

Richard Driscoll

Introduction: the UK experience – an historical perspective

This chapter focuses initially on the UK experience and then draws out key issues that may well have relevance to IBD care in other countries.

Care for patients who have IBD has always tended to be provided more within secondary and tertiary centres than in primary care. With an individual GP (family doctor) in the UK having a list size on average of about 1,750 patients (Royal College of General Practitioners, 2004), their experience of IBD is inevitably limited to a handful of patients and many are reluctant to play more than a supporting role in IBD care. The variability between patients in the presentation and pattern of IBD required that the management of IBD developed as a consultant-led, hospital-based activity. Initially this was part of the general gastroenterology workload, but as more consultant posts were created and more treatment options developed, particularly in the 1990s, IBD developed as a sub-speciality, and some hospitals with larger numbers of IBD patients began to separate their clinic provision for IBD from general gastroenterology.

The natural next step for those hospitals with significant IBD workloads was to introduce a specialist nurse role. The first posts were created in the 1990s in the UK with quite varied operational roles and objectives – some developing as part of general Gastroenterology Nurse roles, others as part of Research Nurse roles. The first specifically recognised IBD Specialist Nurse Role in the UK was created by Sheila Phillips at Weymouth Hospital in the early 1990s. Sheila secured national recognition for the role she was playing in the outpatient management of the IBD patients, not only undertaking her own clinic each week but also an outreach and helpline role for patients. The number of IBD specialist nurses has grown significantly in the last decade and a national campaign to promote the role was undertaken by National Association of Colitis and Crohn's Disease (NACC), (now Crohn's and Colitis UK) in 2005.

Multidisciplinary working has always been essential in IBD care, which requires the involvement of physicians, radiologists, pathologists and surgeons as a minimum and will often require additional specialities or disciplines for individual patients. For many years this took place on an *ad hoc* referral or discussion basis, but increasingly hospitals have created time for multidisciplinary meetings to ensure effective collaboration.

Paediatric gastroenterology has followed a similar course of development since the 1980s. Most care was originally being provided by a paediatrician with support from adult gastroenterologists; then, as research fellows became available who had specialised in IBD at the few important centres of paediatric gastroenterology research, there was a gradual increase in the number of consultant paediatric gastroenterologists providing specialist IBD care. Over time these have developed into full multidisciplinary teams, though often this development began with a single-handed consultant role. One of the key concerns for these developing paediatric IBD teams has been to ensure that children and young people are referred to them quickly for diagnosis and early management rather than being managed initially in less specialist hospitals.

Patient organisations have played an important role in IBD – in the UK NACC and CICRA (Crohn's in Childhood Research Association), were founded in 1979 to support the care of adults and children respectively. Both organisations developed patient information materials initially, followed by local support activities and then raising funds for research. In recent years NACC has also developed a significant campaigning role and has recently rebranded as Crohn's and Colitis UK. The research funding proved an important factor in the development of IBD as a subspeciality, enabling interested clinicians to focus on IBD research at important early stages in their career and then move into the increased number of gastroenterology posts that became available.

By the mid-2000s IBD care had developed significantly: research had produced more understanding of the condition and improved treatments, notably the use of immunosuppressive and biological therapies together with wider availability of ileoanal pouch surgery, and clinical guidelines were in place to promote good practice in the UK and overseas. However, the provision and organisation of IBD care had developed according to local interest and available resources and was widely felt to be variable and often under-resourced. This contrasted with other diseases for which national plans and priorities had been developed in a series of National Service Frameworks (NSF) (for example cancer, diabetes and stroke), each of which had received additional national investment to develop services. One or two of these national initiatives may also have benefited IBD –

for example endoscopy and funding for specialist nursing within the cancer plan – but for the most part gastroenterology was somewhat neglected (British Society of Gastroenterology, 2006).

Similarly, other national health priorities were being established with targets that Trusts had to meet – Accident and Emergency (A&E) and surgery waiting times, referral waiting times, efficiency targets – some of which had unintended negative effects on IBD care. A useful example is the two-week cancer wait target, which prioritised patients with gastrointestinal symptoms that could be interpreted as indicating cancer over others whose symptoms could not, and also had the effect of increasing the number of IBD patients initially referred to surgeons for investigation rather than to gastroenterologists.

The UK experience – IBD audit and national service standards

The UK IBD Audit Project developed as a collaboration at national level between the Royal College of Physicians (RCP), the British Society of Gastroenterology (BSG), Association of Coloproctology of Great Britain and Ireland (ACPGBI) and NACC. The Audit Partners applied for £500,000 in charitable funding as part of a quality improvement initiative and this enabled the project to operate over four years, undertaking an audit in 2006, a programme of feedback and then repeating the audit in 2008. The audit was in two parts, the first focusing on organisation and service provision and the second a retrospective audit of clinical care. The 2008 audit also included paediatric gastroenterology for the first time.

The report of the 2006 audit was an important milestone in IBD care in the UK (UK IBD Audit Steering Group, 2006). The participation rate, entirely voluntary, was an impressive 75%, and for the first time there was a UK-wide picture of IBD services and of the quality of some important aspects of hospital care. It is probably reasonable to say that whilst the organisational findings were not on reflection very surprising, they provided the evidence to justify the development of UK-wide service standards for IBD.

Some of the findings are given in Table 20.1, along with some of the key findings on clinical quality. These were not good and probably did surprise many IBD professionals in the UK, who thought that their hospitals were delivering better standards of care. Possibly the most important message was the need for consistent delivery of good practice on the basics of inpatient and outpatient management.

In between the 2006 and 2008 audits there was a programme of feedback in regional meetings which enabled the IBD community, professionals and

Table 20.1 Selected findings from the UK IBD Audit First Round Report.

Organisation – number of sites with:	
No specialist nurse for IBD	44%
Dedicated gastroenterology ward	67%
Searchable IBD database	34%
Timetabled meetings between gastroenterologists and surgeons	74%
Joint or parallel medical–surgical clinics	47%
Dietitian time for gastroenterology	Median 2 sessions per week
Beds per toilet	4.5 (standard is 3)
Ileoanal pouch procedures	72% of hospitals offered this, but median number of operations was only 4 per year
Clinical care – ulcerative colitis inpatients	
Patients admitted and not transferred to specialist GI ward	31%
Stool culture done	59%
CDT done	47%
Prophylactic heparin given	60%
Clinical care – Crohn's disease inpatients	
Weight recorded	52%
Seen by dietitian	37%
Prophylactic heparin	62%
Patients on systemic steroids:	45% prescribed bone protection 18% had bone density measured
On immunosuppressive therapy	90% monitored every 3 months by full blood count

patient representatives to participate in discussions about how to improve services, together with the collation of examples of good practice that were made available online as a Model Action Plan (Royal College of Physicians, 2009). A collaborative working group, the IBD Standards Group, was established to agree and publish national standards, which it did alongside the results of the 2008 IBD audit, providing an opportunity for effective campaigning at government and local health authority level. The participation level in the 2008 audit was 93% of hospital Trusts or Boards in the UK and comparison of the results for hospitals who took

Table 20.2 Comparison of results for IBD hospitals participating in both rounds of the UK IBD audit.

	2006	2008
Organisation – number of sites with:		
No specialist nurse for IBD	41%	33%
Dedicated gastroenterology ward	70%	80%
Searchable IBD database	37%	47%
Timetabled meetings between gastroenterologists and surgeons	76%	73%
Joint or parallel medical-surgical clinics	47%	55%
Dietitian time for gastroenterology	Median 2 sessions per week	Median 2 sessions per week
Beds per toilet	4.5 (standard is 3)	4.2
Ileoanal pouch procedures:	76% of hospitals offered this, but median number of operations was 4 per year	77% of hospitals offered this, but median number of operations was 4 per year
Clinical care – ulcerative colitis and Crohn's inpatients combined		
Stool culture done	55%	63%
CDT done	44%	55%
Prophylactic heparin given	56%	73%
Clinical care – Crohn's disease inpatients		
Weight recorded	53%	58%
Seen by dietitian	37%	34%
Surgery done laparoscopically	10%	19%

part in both audits showed improvement in some areas, although the pressures on professional time were evident in that a key aspect of multidisciplinary working was less common in 2008 than in 2006.

The findings of the IBD Audit are powerful, but the limitations, particularly of the clinical care audit, also have to be recognised. The clinical audit was conducted as a retrospective review of the hospital notes of 40 successive inpatients (20 Crohn's and 20 UC) together with the last 12 months of outpatient care for the Crohn's patients. Whilst this ensured that patients admitted under non-specialist care would also be included, the focus of the audit had to be on aspects of care that should have been recorded in the hospital notes. Inevitably this meant that they were more process than outcome focused and also that they did not include measures of the patient's experience or outcomes. (This is being addressed in the third round of the UK IBD audit in which patients are being asked to complete a patient experience questionnaire.)

Previous clinical guidelines in the UK had identified the lack of any service standards, but had not attempted to create these (Carter *et al.*, 2004). Following the 2006 IBD Audit a working group of professional and patient organisations was established to produce UK-wide service standards (IBD Standards Group, 2009)

Key principles underpinning the IBD Standards were that they:

- should set the standards to be achieved rather than prescribe how the service should be delivered
- recognise the value of both specialised and local standard care
- be centred on the needs of patients
- be realistic and deliverable rather than 'gold standard'

Perhaps the most important conceptual change introduced by the IBD standards is that hospital teams should review and plan their IBD care as a distinct service within the gastroenterology department. Although this may seem a rather semantic distinction, it is an important one. It enables IBD care to be planned and provided in a way that meets the needs of IBD patients rather than a more generalised hospital service. It is embodied in the proposals for an IBD Clinical Lead to be appointed and to define the members of the core IBD team and the essential supporting staff.

An example of how this approach can lead to significant improvement in quality of service is one hospital that previously saw IBD patients in with other GI patients in clinic, but reorganised outpatient clinics so that all non-emergency IBD outpatients attended on the same morning at a clinic that had gastroenterologists, colorectal surgeons, IBD nurses and the dietitian all working alongside each other. The resulting ability to obtain multidisciplinary views on the same patient in the one clinic is a more efficient use of hospital staff and facilities and much better for the patient than a series of different appointments.

The IBD standards are set out under six headings:

Standard A:　High quality clinical care
Standard B:　Local delivery of care
Standard C:　Maintaining a patient-centred service
Standard D:　Patient education and support
Standard E:　Information technology and audit
Standard F:　Evidence-based practice and research

There are relatively few standards in the document that could be evidence-based, but from the widespread support that they have received in the UK it is evident that they represent a broad consensus of UK health professional opinion. Health managers at national and local levels have also not disputed their validity, even if the resources for full implementation are lacking, and in Wales the IBD Standards have been formally endorsed by the Health Minister of the Welsh Assembly in a letter to all Health Boards.

The IBD standards emphasise the need for IBD care to be delivered by staff with knowledge and experience of IBD working in a multidisciplinary system with access to designated GI inpatient facilities. Outpatient care should be delivered within a framework that provides professionals and patients with a choice of three models – hospital-based care, shared care with the GP or supported self-management by the patient. This approach integrates primary and secondary care involvement, putting the patient's needs and wishes at the centre of the system.

The IBD audit has been accepted into the UK government programme of National Health Service Audits and the IBD standards form the benchmark for organisation and service delivery. Whilst these may seem to be UK-specific developments, there are transferable messages for any country.

The UK audit revealed that whilst many hospitals believed they adhered to good practice, this was not achieved as consistently as they had thought. Their willingness to adopt good practice was not in question, but there was a lack of systematic processes to ensure consistent performance.

- Having the IBD audit results enabled hospitals to assess their performance for the first time against national averages – previously there was no real opportunity to benchmark.
- Subsequent to the audit the organisation of care has become a frequent topic for IBD professional meetings, with very beneficial exchanges of ideas and practice.
- An important step in improving the organisation of care for IBD is to change the conceptual standpoint away from the provision of good clinical care to individual IBD patients to thinking about how IBD care is provided as a service to all patients.
- Service delivery can often be improved by reorganisation without necessarily needing extra resources.

The UK experience – what do IBD patients want?
There have been a number of reports on what IBD patients want. A set of focus groups commissioned by NACC led to a report called *Improving Standards of*

Care for Colitis and Crohn's Disease (Gray, 2005). A more recent project called IMAGE (Improving Management in Gastroenterology in Primary Care) also ran focus groups of IBD patients asking what aspects of care they thought were most important (Jones *et al.*, 2009). The focus groups in both cases found that patients wanted better information; GPs who were more informed about IBD; access to hospital teams through a helpline or IBD nurse; structured, coordinated care; and health professionals to take a holistic view of their illness, care and their life with IBD. Their ideals rested more on the attitudes of professionals, good organisation, good communication and better awareness of IBD and its implications than on additional resources within the healthcare system.

A Cochrane Review of the evidence for specialist nursing in gastroenterology undertook a thematic analysis of nominations for a national IBD Specialist Nurse Award and found that whilst the importance of the in-depth knowledge of specialist nurses and their ability to help patients manage their disease, routinely or at times of flare-up, was acknowledged, it was the traditional nursing values and qualities such as empathy, support, continuity and closeness of contact, communication, time, individualism, advocacy and holism that patients frequently mentioned as important (Woods *et al.*, 2005).

Similar thoughts were echoed in a published version of a conversation between a UK patient and IBD consultant (Westwood and Travis, 2008). There is, however, no substitute for asking individual patients locally what they want from their hospital service, and often they can be much more specific about the changes that might benefit them. There are now a growing number of IBD patient panels in the UK, supported by Crohn's and Colitis UK (NACC), which enable a dialogue between the professionals and their patients about how services could be improved locally (Canham, 2008)

Current issues in the organisation of IBD care

Developing different care relationships – shared care and supported self-management

The traditional hospital outpatient clinic approach to the management of IBD patients should no longer be the single preferred mode of care offered to most patients. Ongoing hospital-based outpatient care is only cost-effective for those with more severe or active disease. For patients whose IBD is in remission, stable or causing relatively mild symptoms, the preferred approach should be a more flexible system of management in which the patient has sufficient information and understanding about their disease and its treatment to monitor their IBD and seek assistance when required, either from their family doctor or by contacting their hospital team.

Such approaches, best described as supported self-management, have been shown to be safe and effective in reducing use of hospital resources and to be preferred by a majority of eligible patients (Robinson *et al.*, 2001; Williams *et al.*, 2000). However, it is essential that such a system ensures that patients are well informed, takes patients' preferences and level of confidence into account and has effective arrangements for rapid access back into specialist care when needed.

Many IBD services now provide outreach care through their specialist nurses using telephone helplines and telephone, email or postal review systems. These approaches minimise both the patient's use of hospital outpatient services and the time the patient has to take off work or away from normal family roles. To be effective and safe these approaches to ongoing IBD care must include good information and education about IBD for the patient, have clearly defined parameters for which patients are safe to self-manage, be responsive to individual patient's preferences and have effective systems for regular review and rapid access back into specialist care. The arrangements should be agreed between the patient, family doctor and hospital team and should be properly documented.

One hospital reviewed the patients attending its IBD outpatient clinic and decided that a significant proportion could be placed on a postal review system. Each year the IBD nurse arranges for blood tests to be done locally and for the patient to complete a review form. She then reviews the patient's notes with these results and decides if the patient needs to attend clinic. There is a fast track back into hospital care when needed (Hunter *et al.*, 2010).

The role of the specialist nurse

The specialist nurse role is now being widely adopted in many countries as a key aspect of delivering a high quality IBD service. The role may be created with a different emphasis in different hospitals, but the contribution the nurse makes usually includes being the primary contact for IBD outpatients when they need advice or support, facilitating communication, coordinating patients' access to specialist care, ensuring patients have the information they need and at times being the patient's advocate within the multidisciplinary team.

An IBD specialist nurse can be cost-saving, preventing unnecessary admissions or clinic visits, or perhaps performing a clinic or endoscopy list previously undertaken by medical staff, but the greatest impact is probably upon consistent quality of care. There are a number of descriptive workload audits and patient satisfaction surveys for IBD nurse roles, but comparatively little evidence from controlled or health economic studies (Woods *et al.*, 2005). One study in Swansea demonstrated cost-effectiveness (Williams *et al.*, 2000) and a review of the UK IBD audit showed some association between presence of an IBD specialist nurse and higher standards of clinical care (Kemp, 2010).

The role of the primary care physician

Given the emphasis on hospital-delivered IBD care, most family doctors play only a supporting role for their IBD patients, prescribing the medicines initiated by the hospital team and perhaps being party to formal shared care arrangements. They also of course have an important role in identifying possible IBD in new patients and referring them quickly for investigation. However, family doctors need to recognise that they have another important role in checking the well-being of patients who have been diagnosed with IBD but who are no longer in active hospital follow-up. One published study in the UK found that 30% of patients identified as having IBD in GP practice records were not in active hospital follow-up (Rubin *et al.*, 2000). Although a proportion of these may have been wrongly coded as IBD, two other unpublished studies have produced estimates of 20–25% of such patients. It is important that family doctors review such patients at least annually and identify those patients who could benefit from more active management of their disease or who should be in a surveillance programme for colorectal cancer.

Managed clinical networks

There is always a tension between providing care close to home for patients whilst also giving them access to the best in more specialised care. In other disease areas managed clinical networks have proved to be a cost-effective way of organising services across a group of hospitals whilst also facilitating collaboration in education and research activities. The approach has been adopted in some UK counties as the preferred way of organising paediatric services that need to be provided on a regional basis. For more information, visit http://www.bspghan.org. uk/professional_groups/regional.shtml.

IBD care for adolescents

There is a growing recognition that the traditional split between paediatric and adult services is particularly unsatisfactory for IBD, given the number of adolescents who are diagnosed. These young people need specialist support care to ensure that the issues of growth and pubertal development are managed as well as possible, but they also need specialist support to assist them in adapting to the impact of IBD on their education, peer group interaction and family relationships. Investment in their emotional and psychological development at this crucial stage can make a significant difference to their capacity to lead a full and productive life in their twenties and afterwards. This requires an IBD staff capable of discussing all aspects of adolescent life as well as the disease, handling the often difficult balance of communication and responsibility between the parents and the young patient and able to prepare the young person for what is usually a very different style of care under an adult IBD team. Arbitrary ages for transfer to adult care are not helpful and should be challenged. Transition should be planned well in advance and take place at the age suitable for the particular individual (NACC and CICRA, 2008). Adolescence and transition services are covered in more detail in Chapter 15.

Psychological support

This is gradually coming to be seen as an important part of an IBD service, although in the UK the 2008 IBD audit found only 21% of hospitals said they had a defined pathway for direct access to psychological support (UK IBD Audit Steering Group, 2008). All patients need some recognition and affirmation of the feelings they experience as a result of their IBD and, at a basic level, this should be present in every encounter with a health professional. However, some patients find their IBD creates a level of psychological distress that can become disabling and that they cannot resolve on their own. This group of patients could benefit significantly from timely access to formal psychological support. It is important that such support is seen as a normal part of an IBD service, thus removing one of the barriers to patients seeking help, and that there is some guidance as to the most appropriate form of help for each patient. Cognitive behavioural therapy (CBT), for example, may assist some patients, but is not appropriate for all. As with adolescents, provision of good quality psychological support at important stages of the patients' life with IBD may be very beneficial to their longer term quality of life.

A recent UK workshop has gone some way towards describing a psychological support model for IBD based on that developed for cancer services in the UK. The aim is to continue developing these ideas within the IBD community and to produce guidelines for good practice that will be linked to the UK IBD standards referred to above. A description of the workshop can be found at http://www.crohnsandcolitis.org.uk/content/research/articles.asp.

Maintaining equity in countries with devolved healthcare systems

There is a natural wish on the part of professionals and patients to ensure that all IBD patients have access to the same quality of care – either in service provision or in access to expensive medicines. This becomes difficult when policy decisions and resource allocation are devolved to regional or local levels in countries. Health professionals can only minimise these inequities by formally adopting agreed standards and guidelines within their national bodies and then campaigning to implement these at the lower governmental levels. Sharing any examples of such documents and any evidence of cost-effectiveness internationally is potentially one of the best ways of tacking this issue.

Involving patients in service feedback and redesign

This has been shown in the UK to be very valuable in developing IBD services. Even quite basic patient experience surveys are useful in a generalised way, but there are ways of encouraging direct patient feedback. Recently a joint project between the BSG, NACC and an organisation called Patient Opinion experimented with a publicly available website on which patients were encouraged to report their opinions about their interaction with the IBD team. Evaluation of the projects suggests useful comments were made by the patients, very few entries needed moderating and some IBD teams engaged in dialogue by posting replies to the comments. Patient Opinion was founded by a GP who wanted to find a way to make the wisdom of patients available to the NHS. For further information visit http://www.patientopinion.org.uk/.

Also in the UK patients are increasingly being involved in service planning and redesign, particularly through the formation of IBD patient panels. The objective of these is to provide a safe framework in which patients and professionals can discuss how to improve IBD services and their development has been supported by NACC since a pilot study was completed in 2007. IBD patient panels have sometimes lobbied local management about particular service issues, for example the lack of a specialist dietitian or nurse, but political lobbying is not the prime objective of a panel (Canham, 2008).

Examples of how patient involvement has changed services include: provision of a refrigerator and microwave on a ward so patients could prepare their own preferred food, following a patient's journey through an emergency admission to highlight how this could be improved, highlighting the need for improved toilet facilities, looking at the information needs of patients, and exploring whether the needs of an ethnic minority group were being adequately met.

Developing electronic care records in IBD

This is an essential development for all IBD teams if they are to be able to monitor their patients effectively and plan their services. IBD patients accumulate huge sets of paper records which are often not helpful for current management. The key requirement for progress in this area is for the data gathered to be useful both in the individual management of patients and in audit and service development. Only then will the majority of clinical staff feel that entering data at the point of contact with the patient is worthwhile. Perhaps one of the best examples of the benefits arising would be for all data relating to patients on biologic therapies to be accessible electronically, enabling review to be undertaken easily – even more important as a greater number of patients undertake self-administration of biologic therapy at home.

Once up-to-date data is available, then it should be possible to provide access for patients to a selected summary of their clinical records, including recent test results and possibly medicine and appointment reminders. Such access might also make real shared care with GPs a realistic option.

Developing local and national audit and patient registers

Once the hurdle of electronic data capture has been overcome, then local and national audit can become much more meaningful. As mentioned above, one limitation of the UK IBD audit has been that the questions must be answerable from the patients' notes, and capturing this information takes many hours of work. If the data is recorded electronically then review of patient data individually and collectively becomes much simpler and the focus can be on the questions and analysis rather than on the data collection.

Within a unit the potential exists for a clinical dashboard showing numbers of patients undergoing various therapies and the relevant monitoring protocols, with easy access to identify those patients who fall outside the safety limits. Of equal value is the opportunity to benchmark one hospital against another and both against the national standards, thus providing an incentive if one were needed to improve IBD care locally to meet the expected standards. Collating anonymised data for national audit and the creation of a national register of patients is a logical next step offering significant benefits in being able to assess the effectiveness of treatments in a normal (non-trial) and much bigger population. Reporting on patient outcomes and health economic data becomes more viable and more useful.

The value of international links

The value of collaboration or sharing of information and ideas internationally is intuitively recognised by most health professionals in relation to research and clinical management of IBD, but is much less well developed in terms of the organisation of care. Perhaps understandably, given that the health systems and economies differ so much between countries, there has been a tendency not to focus on issues of the organisation of care because superficially the provision of healthcare seems to operate in such different ways.

Yet the principles underlying what constitutes good practice and safe, cost-effective care for IBD patients must transcend national boundaries. The key domains adopted for the UK IBD standards are surely important in every country – high quality clinical care, local delivery of care, maintaining a patient-centred service, patient education and support, information technology and audit, and evidence-based practice and research. There is a need for early referral and investigation, for multidisciplinary working, for a balance of local ongoing care and access to more specialised services.

Exchanging ideas and experiences on the organisation of care is one of the benefits for European patient organisations of being a member of the European Federation for Crohn's and Ulcerative Colitis Associations (EFCCA). This organisation brings together over 20 independent national associations to increase public awareness of colitis and Crohn's disease; to encourage interaction amongst existing colitis and Crohn's disease groups within a widening Europe and to assist in the establishment of new associations where they do not exist; to campaign for improvement in the quality of life and quality of care for those with IBD; to encourage patients and their families to travel and to meet with people who have IBD from other countries; and to promote both medical and social research related to IBD. For further information visit http://www.efcca.org/.

Increasingly the links between IBD patient associations are extending globally, and 2010 saw the first World IBD Day, organised collaboratively by the associations. This mirrors the IBD and gastroenterology professional associations and these international links could usefully be applied more extensively to the organisation of IBD care, enabling the exchange of different perspectives and experiences.

Conclusion

Inflammatory bowel disease will always have to compete with other more prevalent or more dramatic conditions for health resources and management attention, but within that constraint there is much that can be done to improve the organisation of IBD care. The professional disciplines of evidence-based practice, clinical guidelines, audit and quality improvement all contribute to a better service for the patient, but these can be helpfully supplemented by bringing in the patients' experiences and perspectives on what changes would make most difference to the quality of care in their eyes. Perhaps the key message for this whole issue is that whilst the objectives and principles underlying good care should be similar across all IBD services, how that care is delivered and organised can be adapted to suit local circumstances and needs.

References

British Society of Gastroenterology (2006) *Care of Patients with Gastrointestinal Disorders. A Strategy for the Future.* http://www.bsg.org.uk/bsgdisp1.php?id=e03c8e070f26 b05ff275&m=00023 (accessed 25 August 2010).

Canham, P. (2008) Patient consultation – ask the panel. *Health Serv. J.*, 3 April, 26. http://www.crohnsandcolitis.org.uk/patientpanels (accessed 2 August 2010).

Carter, M. J., Lobo, A. J. and Travis, S. P. L. (2004) British Society of Gastroenterology guidelines for inflammatory bowel disease. *Gut*, **53**(suppl. V) v1–v16.

Gray, J. (2005) Improving standards of care for colitis and Crohn's Disease http://www.crohnsandcolitis.org.uk/content/research/articles.asp (accessed 2 August 2010).

Hunter, J., James, S., Chan, D., Stacey, B., Stroud, M., Patel, P., Cummings, F. and Fine, D. (2009) *Virtual Inflammatory Bowel Disease Clinics in the Real World.* http://gut.bmj.com/site/abstractbooks/A1b.pdf (accessed 2 October 2010).

IBD Standards Group (2009) *Quality Care – Service Standards for the Healthcare of People Who Have Inflammatory Bowel Disease 2009.* http://www.ibdstandards.org.uk/ (accessed 2 August 2010).

Jones, R., Hunt, C., Stevens, R. *et al.* (2009) Management of common gastrointestinal disorders: quality criteria based on patients' views and practice guidelines. *Br. J. General Practice*, June, 199–208.

Kemp, K. (2010) UK inflammatory bowel disease audit: nurse correlations between 2006 and 2008. *Gut*, **59**, A39; Abstract No OC-094.

NACC and CICRA (2008) *Transition in IBD: Transition to Adult Health Care – Guidance for Health Professionals.* http://www.ibdtransition.org.uk/ (accessed 25 August 2010).

Robinson, A., Thompson, D. G., Wilkin, D. *et al.* (2001) Guided self-management and practice-directed follow-up of ulcerative colitis: a randomised trial. *Lancet*, **358**, 976–81.

Royal College of General Practitioners (2004) *General Practitioner Workload.* http://www.rcgp.org.uk/pdf/ISS_INFO_03_APRIL04.pdf (accessed 25 August 2010).

Royal College of Physicians (2009) *The Model Action Plan for IBD Services.* http://www.rcplondon.ac.uk/clinical-standards/ceeu/Current-work/IBD/Pages/Driving-Change.aspx (accessed 2 August 2010).

Rubin, G. P., Hungin, A. P. S., Kelly, P. J. and Ling, J. (2000) Inflammatory Bowel Disease: epidemiology and management in an English general practice population. *Aliment.*

Pharmacol. Ther., **14**, 1553–9.

UK IBD Audit Steering Group (2006) *UK IBD Audit 2006*. http://www.rcplondon.ac.uk/ clinical-standards/ceeu/Current-work/IBD/Pages/1st-Round.aspx (accessed 24 August 2010).

UK IBD Audit Steering Group (2008) *UK IBD Audit Second Round Report*. http://www.rcplondon.ac.uk/clinical-standards/ceeu/Current-work/IBD/Documents/UK-IBD-Audit-2nd-Round-Full-National-Report-(2008).pdf (accessed 2 August 2010).

Westwood, N. and Travis, S. (2008) What do IBD patients want? *Aliment. Pharmacol. Ther.*, **27**(suppl. 1), 1–8.

Williams, J. G., Cheung, W. Y., Russell, I. T., Cohen, D. R., Longo, M. and Lervy, B. (2000) Open access follow-up for inflammatory bowel disease: a pragmatic randomised trial and cost-effectiveness study. *Br. Med. J.*, **320**, 544–8.

Woods, L., Belling, R. and Maclaren, S. (2005) *Systematic Review of the Published Evidence for Specialist Nursing in IBD and a Thematic Analysis of the Nominations for the NACC IBD Nursing Award in 2005 (LSBU)*. http://www.crohnsandcolitis.org.uk/ content/research/articles.asp (accessed 24 August 2010).

CHAPTER 21

Developing the role of the Clinical Nurse Specialist in IBD

Cath Stansfield, Julie Duncan, Marian O'Connor and Kathy Whayman

Introduction

Over recent years nursing practice has advanced rapidly in response to local and national needs. In the UK healthcare provision has changed, with nurses becoming central to these changes. We have seen the development of roles such as Clinical Nurse Specialist (CNS), Advanced Nurse Practitioner (ANP) and Nurse Consultant (NC). The advent of non-medical prescribing (Department of Health, 2004a) and advanced practice has seen patients, in some organisations, receive care by nurses independent of medics. Skills that these advanced practitioners use include advanced assessment, clinical examination, procedures that were previously the remit of medical practitioners (such as endoscopy), and prescribing treatment independently. Despite first attempts by the Royal College of Nursing (RCN) at defining nurse practitioner roles and their educational requirements in 1996, there still remains a lack of an explicit description of advanced nursing practice which is now limiting its development (Royal College of Nursing, 2010a).

Almost two decades have passed since the role of CNS in Inflammatory Bowel Disease (IBD) was first recognised and developed in response to the enthusiasm of nurses and other clinicians to improve the quality of care, education and support to patients with IBD (Phillips, 1995). The role of IBD CNS is now pivotal within the team supporting and treating patients with IBD. The UK national IBD standards (IBD Standards Group, 2009), in combination with the RCN role descriptives document (Royal College of Nursing, 2007), have resulted in greater clarity of IBD CNS roles and responsibilities. This chapter explores the remit of the role of IBD CNS in relation to wider definitions of advanced nursing practice, drawing upon personal experiences, along with those of colleagues who have established and deliver specialist nursing services for people with IBD.

Case study 1

A local district hospital decided to implement the role of IBD Nurse Specialist to reduce the demand for follow-up appointments with the consultant gastroenterologists in outpatient clinics. A business case was developed, and it was proposed that the use of a specialist nurse to undertake routine reviews of patients with IBD would release consultant time to review new patients and meet the demands of the 18 week pathway (Department of Health, 2006a). Once the nurse was appointed, she undertook a six-month period of supervision and education with a nominated gastroenterologist. In addition, she completed degree-level modules in IBD Nursing and non-medical prescribing.

Over the two years that followed it became evident that the role of the IBD Nurse Specialist encompassed far more than outpatient clinic reviews. A database was developed to record IBD patient activity and a local population of 800 patients was identified. The nurse supported IBD patients on immunosuppression and biological therapies. All patients with a new diagnosis of IBD were seen by the specialist nurse and educated about their diagnosis, helping them adapt to life with a chronic disease. A telephone helpline was established, the aim being to provide easy access to the IBD team for patients when unwell, and in addition to provide general advice and support at all stages of their condition.

Defining advanced/specialist practice roles

Posts such as CNS, ANP and NC became possible following publication by the United Kingdom Central Council for Nursing, Midwifery and Health Visiting (UKCC; then UK nursing's governing body) of the document *Scope of Professional Practice* (United Kingdom Central Council for Nursing, Midwifery and Health Visiting, 1992) which introduced the concept of extended practice: that is, nursing roles which went beyond the traditional scope of nursing practice, including the development of skills which had previously been in the domain of medical practice. Further national agendas followed, such as the European initiative to reduce junior doctor hours, and the UK's Department of Health encouraging a blurring of the boundaries of healthcare professionals' individual roles and responsibilities (Department of Health, 2006b). Key components of advanced or specialist nursing practice include:

- Clinical (caseload) management
- Education
- Management
- Consultation
- Research
- Service development

According to Raja Jones (2002), a specialist nurse can only term him or herself as such if involved in all of these activities. A survey of nurses in advanced practice or specialist roles within the UK found that the majority of their activity was in direct clinical practice (60% on average). Their remaining time was spent in education (17%), management (14%) and research (4%) (Royal College of Nursing, 2005).

These roles are normally undertaken by senior nurses educated to at least honours degree or masters level (Royal College of Nursing, 2010a). This is thought to enable them to practice autonomously, accepting accountability for a caseload of patients. The parameters of advanced practice are yet to be clearly defined and regulated by the UK's Nursing and Midwifery Council (NMC). The RCN is now calling on the NMC to define these parameters and set standards as a matter of priority for the development of advanced nursing practice (Royal College of Nursing, 2010a). To this end, the RCN has published a list of suggested characteristics of the Advanced Nurse Practitioner (see Table 21.1).

Table 21.1 Characteristics of Advanced Nurse Practitioners (Royal College of Nursing, 2007, 2010a).

- Makes professionally autonomous decisions, for which he or she is accountable
- Receives patients with undifferentiated and undiagnosed problems and makes an assessment of their healthcare needs, based on highly developed nursing knowledge and skills, including skills not usually exercised by nurses, such as physical examination.
- Screens patients for disease risk factors and early signs of disease
- Makes differential diagnoses using decision making and problem solving skills
- Develops, with the patient, an ongoing nursing care plan for health, with an emphasis on preventative measures
- Orders necessary investigations, and provides treatment and care both individually, as part of a team; referral to other agencies.

The role of the Nurse Consultant

In the UK, one of the more recent developments in advancing nursing practice has been the development of the Nurse Consultant role. Nurse Consultant posts were introduced by the Department of Health as part of the *Making a Difference* strategy (Department of Health, 1999) to provide better outcomes for patients by improving services and quality, to strengthen leadership and to provide a new career framework for nurses. This strategy was designed to help retain experienced and expert nurses, midwives and health visitors in clinical practice. Currently within IBD practice there are four Nurse Consultant posts across the UK, though these are commonly integrated within the wider scope of gastroenterology rather than focused specifically on IBD alone. Nurse Consultants have five essential domains within their practice. The Department of Health (1999) describes these as:

- expert practice
- practice and service development
- research and evaluation
- professional leadership and consultancy
- education and training

The key differences between this role and other specialist and advanced practice roles are the leadership and strategic components. Nurse Consultants are considered to influence the development of specialist practice and IBD patient care, and post holders are considered to be national leaders within their speciality.

Case study 2

The IBD CNS received a call on the telephone advice line from Derek, a 31-year-old male well known to the IBD team. He reports a severe flare of his colonic Crohn's disease with a bowel frequency of approximately 30 times per 24 hours, diarrhoea and fresh rectal bleeding. Unsurprisingly he feels fatigued and systemically unwell. He is advised to attend the hospital's accident and emergency (A+E) department. Following clinical assessment in A+E by the gastroenterology registrar, he is admitted to an acute admissions ward. There he is reviewed by his consultant gastroenterologist and IBD CNS. Due to the severity of his flare, and the refractory nature of his IBD, it is discussed with him that should he not respond to medical therapy on this occasion he may need surgical intervention, and that this would be a colectomy with permanent ileostomy.

Derek expressed a feeling of devastation at this news. Although he has known for a long time that if medical management failed he would require surgery, he had not previously understood the implications of this. He was shocked at the speed and severity of this flare, as previous exacerbations had been managed fairly quickly and he had never considered living with a stoma. The IBD CNS spent a significant amount of time with Derek discussing his fears and concerns and identifying educational needs. She clarified the proposed medical plan and what events would prompt escalation to surgical intervention. His case was discussed that day in the IBD multidisciplinary meeting with his consultant gastroenterologist, colorectal surgeon, radiologist, IBD CNS and other members of the treatment team. Derek asked the IBD CNS to meet his parents to explain the current clinical situation to them and answer their questions.

The IBD CNS also liaised with the ward nursing team to ensure that aspects of his clinical and psychological care plan were understood. She also referred him to the stoma care CNS for pre-operative counselling, and discussed the possibility of arranging a meeting between an established stoma patient and Derek to enable him to discuss his concerns with a patient expert.

Role definitions of IBD CNS

Despite a lack of clarity on role definitions for advanced nursing practice as a whole, significant progress has been made in IBD nursing practice. The role of the IBD CNS was first developed in response to a belief that local healthcare provision did not meet the needs of patients with IBD (Phillips, 1995). Since then the IBD CNS has been an emerging force and the role seen as core to the provision of high quality healthcare to patients with IBD (IBD Standards Group, 2009). The RCN Crohn's and Colitis specialist interest group developed role descriptors which outline the key skills and attributes an IBD CNS should possess or attain to (Royal College of Nursing, 2007). Castledine (2002) suggests that specialist nurses should possess personal characteristics including:

- Motivation and enthusiasm
- Excellent interpersonal skills
- Confidence
- Sensitivity to patients' needs
- Assertiveness

- Approachability
- Flexibility

The Royal College of Nursing (2007) adds that the following are central to the IBD CNS role:

- Holistic care provision
- Health promotion
- Patient advocacy
- Innovation and change
- Expert role modelling
- Working in a complementary role to the multidisciplinary team (MDT)

It is important to remember that, although IBD CNSs are often involved in advanced and autonomous practice, they do not practice independently of the wider IBD team, but rather use their skills to complement and enhance those of the other team members (gastroenterologists, surgeons, dietitians, pharmacists, etc.). Rather than a simple reallocation of tasks between doctors and nurses, Norton and Kamm (2002) advocate that collaborative working is essential to establish new ways of working for the benefit of patient care. Patients often see the CNS as a supportive link between patients and doctors, a reliable and consistent person to contact with time to listen (Belling *et al.*, 2008). This is an important function of the IBD CNS to work as part of the MDT to enhance patient care and the patient experience, providing efficient, holistic and accessible care.

Demonstrating the worth of the IBD CNS

Since the proliferation of advanced practice roles there has been a body of literature reviewing the benefits of these posts. Although there is a paucity of literature examining the worth of the IBD CNS post specifically, there is much evidence that nurses can effectively undertake advanced practice roles in areas traditionally led by doctors, such as case management. Most of these studies are unable to demonstrate that the nurse achieves better health outcomes (doctors and nurses achieving similar outcomes), but, consistently, nurse-led intervention is associated with an increase in patient satisfaction and reduction in cost (Faithfull *et al.*, 2001; Moore *et al.*, 2002; Laurant *et al.*, 2005; Woods *et al.*, 2006; Knowles *et al.*, 2007). In the UK, within the context of global financial restraints, many CNS roles have been under threat with posts lost or redefined. In response to this the Royal College of Nursing (2010b) has pressed for the continued support of CNS posts due to their important contribution to patient-centred high quality care.

A systematic review of the impact of IBD nurses on patient care found the benefits of an IBD nurse service included improved access to specialist services, particularly at times of disease exacerbation, provision of both physical and emotional support, self-management programmes, education and advice, and reduction in the need for outpatient attendances and waiting times (Woods *et al.*, 2006). This concurs with the findings from the IBD Standards Group (2009) that the presence of a CNS within the IBD team is associated with improved patient outcomes. Belling *et al.* (2009) failed to demonstrate the cost effectiveness of the role, however, identified a pressing need for more extensive research to evaluate the role nationally. This has reinforced anecdotal evidence that had previously emerged (Pearson, 2005; Nightingale *et al.*, 2000).

Preparation for practice

According to the Royal College of Nursing (2010a), there is a danger that, due to the current lack of role clarity and defined preparation for practice, some nurse practitioners and CNSs may be practising under the label of advanced practitioners although they are not educated to the expected level. Despite pressure on CNSs to gain specialist education and training, educational opportunities in the current financial climate are increasingly difficult for nurses to maximise. Gaining funding for courses and obtaining time away from clinical practice are often not given a high priority by departments struggling to meet financial targets. Many nurses therefore fund themselves on expensive educational courses such as degree or masters programmes. This has the potential for unfairness, where only the very motivated or financially well-off can obtain the appropriate qualifications. There are often other avenues a CNS can explore in order to obtain funding. Applications to organisations in the voluntary sector, private sector or nursing bodies (for example national patient support groups, pharmaceutical companies, or RCN) often result in full grants, or at least part funding for courses. Listing education and training costs in the business case for a new IBD CNS post is one very useful method of ensuring that a postholder will be able to maximise educational opportunities in the longer term, and keeps the issue of adequate preparation for practice as part of the IBD team vision (see Chapter 22). It is not always easy at the outset to identify training needs, as there is no clearly defined route to prepare nurses to undertake the role of IBD nurse. McGee and Castledine (2003) acknowledge this in the wider context of specialist nursing. Another way of meeting training/educational requirements is through portfolio development. McGee and Castledine (2003) contend that by doing so:

The nurse is able to demonstrate their ability to fulfil the role effectively and expertly. Standards of competence are evidence of the ability to demonstrate knowledge, skills and attitude to undertake the role.

In relation to IBD Nurse Specialists, this is usually a combination of work-based learning and academic courses. In terms of academic preparation, the completion of at least a degree-level module in IBD is considered a benchmark on which to base practice (Royal College of Nursing, 2007). This should give the nurse a good grounding in areas such as pathophysiology of IBD, treatment and the holistic impact of diagnosis. Advanced assessment skills, including clinical examination and non-medical prescribing qualifications are often beneficial in promoting the smooth running of clinic and optimising patient care. Degree and masters-level courses in generic advanced practice skills such as these, along with more specialised modules in IBD and other related areas of gastroenterology, are available in various academic institutes in the UK.

Additionally, a strong relationship with a supervising medical gastroenterologist is essential. Often nurses new in post will spend a considerable amount of time observing the care of the IBD patient, learning clinical assessment skills and approaches to treatment pathways. It is often the consultant who will identify when the nurse is competent to undertake clinics independently. Even after this point, the IBD nurse is likely to work closely with the consultant(s), frequently discussing patient care and receiving clinical supervision. This collaborative way of working is essential for the benefit of patient care and for the success of the IBD CNS role in the long term (Norton and Kamm 2002). It also meets the requirements of the National Health Service Knowledge and Skills Framework (Department of Health, 2004b). This was part of the Agenda for Change strategy for pay restructuring and progression, where 'on the job learning' is now seen as a fundamental part of training and career development. Evidence of fitness to practice can be consolidated in a comprehensive portfolio, demonstrating the nurse's ability to undertake the role of IBD nurse specialist (Royal College of Nursing 2007). This type of portfolio can integrate both experience with academic preparation. Many specialist clinical programmes of education also recognise this and offer this as a clinical option in degree and masters programmes.

The scope of practice of the IBD CNS

As can be seen in Figure 21.1, the IBD CNS is responsible for a wide variety of clinical and non-clinical activity (Royal College of Nursing, 2007). Clearly each institution will have its own needs, and these activities are not exhaustive, nor

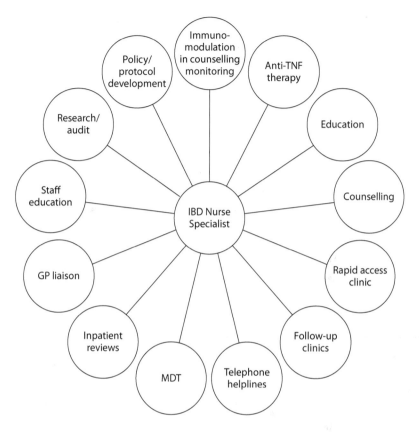

Figure 21.1 Role descriptors of the IBD CNS (RCN, 2007).

universal. However, the following activities and services are common to many IBD nurses:

- IBD advice service (or helplines)
- Psychological and social support (see Chapter 16)
- Nurse-led clinics
- Immunosuppressant management
- Rapid access clinics
- Biologics service
- Inpatient advice and support
- Education (patients and staff)
- Research and audit

- Service development
- Networking

IBD advice service (or helplines)

The provision of IBD advice lines is common to most IBD CNS roles and is clearly advocated in the literature amongst specialist nurses caring for patients with IBD (Phillips, 1995; Nightingale *et al.*, 2000; Pearson, 2006). The very nature of IBD as a chronic, unpredictable disease means that services need to provide access to open and flexible approaches to management, and providing telephone (and email) services is a key method of improving patient access (Younge and Norton, 2007). It is recommended by the Department of Health as a mainstay of chronic disease management in preventing a crisis or deterioration in the patients' condition, and IBD patients are encouraged to actively use telephone services in the event of increased symptoms, in order that they can be effectively and appropriately managed (Department of Health, 2004c).

For the most part, patients who access the IBD advice lines can be appropriately managed over the telephone, and in the authors' practice (O'Connor, 2010) this was demonstrated in a recent audit (Table 21.2). Chapter 22 provides further information on setting up an advice service.

Table 21.2 Audit of advice line 2009–2010 (O'Connor, 2010).

Advice line calls April 2009–March 2010	
Total	3441
Number of calls dealt with by advice alone	2761 (80%)
Number of calls which resulted in outpatient appointments	680 (19%)
Number admitted to hospital	12(< 1%)

Nurse-led clinics

The following clinical activities are often the remit of the IBD CNS within nurse-led outpatient services:

- Routine review
- Rapid access clinics
- Immunosuppressant management
- Health promotion
- Education

- Promoting adherence
- Smoking cessation advice

Routine review

Regular review of patients with IBD is often a driver behind the IBD nursing role. The review of patients in remission by an IBD CNS frees capacity in consultants' clinics to review more new patients and meet strategic challenges or national targets such as the UK's 18 week pathway (Department of Health, 2006a). CNS outpatient clinic appointments normally vary between 20 and 30 minutes in duration, allowing the assessment and review to be more holistic than is realistically managed in busy medical clinics. During such reviews, the IBD CNS is likely to assess the patient's current health status (see Chapter 5 for a comprehensive guide to patient assessment) and the control of the patient's condition since the last review. Recurrent relapses may indicate poor disease control and identify the need for repeat endoscopic evaluation and discussions around adherence with treatment plans. Other roles the IBD CNS may perform during routine follow-up appointments include education; health promotion such as smoking cessation; and colorectal cancer and osteoporosis surveillance, as will be later discussed. More recently, some IBD teams are offering alternatives to traditional outpatient review appointments (normally to stable, well patients), such as telephone clinics and email or postal reviews.

Rapid access clinics

The IBD Standards (IBD Standards Group, 2009) outline that rapid access to services when patients are unwell is fundamental to operating a quality service to patients with IBD. The literature also supports the development of rapid access clinics suggesting that early review of patients who are experiencing disease exacerbation reduces the duration of flare and the risk of hospitalisation (Nightingale *et al.*, 2000). Models of rapid access clinics vary: in some centres patients are added to an already full clinic; in other areas there are dedicated rapid access/drop in clinics for patients who are unwell, or in some cases two or three non-routine appointment slots are added to existing clinics accessed under control of the IBD team.

During these clinics the IBD nurse will assess the patient and arrange any necessary investigations (refer to Chapters 4 and 5). During this process, the nurse collects data to provide an objective assessment of the flare and subsequent monitoring, enabling treatment interventions to be evaluated. In some cases the IBD Nurse Specialist may, as appropriate, arrange admission for patients or referral onwards to other specialist services such as surgical, dietetic or psychological review. If the nurse is a non-medical prescriber treatment may be prescribed by the specialist nurse, or if not, following discussion with medical colleagues. Prescribing should be undertaken in line with local and national guidelines. Clinical imaging requests can be made by the IBD CNS, provided local training and policy is adhered to (Royal College of Nursing, 2006).

Immunosuppressant management

Azathioprine (AZA), 6-mercaptopurine (6MP) and methotrexate (MTX) are common treatments in refractory IBD. Once the decision to commence immunosuppressant therapy has been made, the patient is often referred to the IBD Nurse Specialist for counselling and onward follow-up. In preparation for commencing immunosuppressant therapy, the CNS and patient will ideally engage in a process of education and counselling, to ensure that the patient understands the rationale for treatment. Key areas for discussion include:

- Identification of pre-existing health problems apart from IBD (see contraindications to therapy in the British National Formulary 2010: http://www.bnf.org/).
- Exploration of key life events, such as pregnancy (see Chapter 13). Although some issues may not be of immediate concern to patients, if treatments are likely to be used long term, life priorities may subsequently change.
- The nurse should explain to the patient the role of immunosuppressant therapy in replacing steroids and promoting remission, the potential response and remission rates and outline possible side-effects related to taking immunosuppressants (see Chapter 6.)
- Signs and symptoms of adverse events should be clearly outlined, including monitoring for common side-effects of the individual drugs (such as flu-like symptoms, headaches, nausea, vomiting and abdominal pain) which may indicate complications like neutropaenia and pancreatitis.
- Potentially serious side-effects such as the risk of lymphoma should be openly discussed (see Chapter 6). However, patients can be reassured that the relative risk is low, and the necessity of therapy should be reviewed regularly (Holbrook, 2007).

In some centres the IBD nurse assumes responsibility for undertaking the haematological monitoring of patients on AZA, 6MP and MTX. The British Society of Gastroenterology (2005) guidelines advocate that full blood count, liver and renal profiles are completed weekly for the first month, fortnightly for months

2 and 3, monthly for months 4 and 5, and three-monthly thereafter. However, local protocols or guidelines may vary. With reference to National Patient Safety Agency (2007) guidelines for the administration of methotrexate, blood results should be recorded in a disease-modifying antirheumatic drug (DMARD) blood monitoring book. Although not universal, ideally the same approach would be adopted for all immunosuppressants and biological therapies in IBD.

Increasingly, Primary Care Trusts are undertaking the blood monitoring for this group of patients. In such scenarios, any shared care arrangements should be clearly defined, acknowledging the role and responsibilities of each of the healthcare professionals involved in delivering care. The patient is the ideal candidate for ensuring that these tests are completed as necessary and thus should be encouraged to take responsibility for ensuring this happens. Further information on immunosuppression monitoring can be found in Chapter 22.

Health promotion

Health promotion is a key component of follow-up care. Common subjects include:

- smoking cessation
- colorectal cancer surveillance
- osteoporosis screening
- lifestyle changes, e.g. healthy eating and stress management

Smoking cessation

In Crohn's disease smoking cessation is seen as one of the biggest contributors to refractory disease. Smoking cessation in patients with Crohn's disease sees remission rates of 60% occur (Johnson *et al.*, 2005), the highest therapeutic remission rates of any treatment for the condition. In the UK there is a big drive to encourage patients to engage with smoking cessation services. To that end some IBD nurses may have undertaken smoking cessation courses, or will refer patients on to local smoking cessation programmes.

Colorectal cancer surveillance

Colorectal cancer surveillance should be undertaken in accordance with local and national guidelines. In the UK, British Society of Gastroenterology (BSG) guidance is normally utilised (Cairns *et al.*, 2010). The IBD Nurse should discuss with the patient the risk and prevalence of colorectal cancer in IBD and the importance of screening at each review. A clear audit trail to ensure patients are recalled in line with BSG guidelines should be established.

Osteoporosis

The diagnosis of IBD, combined with reduced nutritional intake and possible malabsorption, active inflammation, and the use of corticosteroids increases the patient's risk of osteoporosis. Both the BSG guidelines (Lewis and Scott, 2007) for osteoporosis and UK National Osteoporosis Guidelines (National Osteoporosis Guideline Group, 2000) provide a clear framework for specialist nurses to develop practice upon. This includes:

■ Development of protocols to outline practice.
■ Osteoporosis risk assessment (National Osteoporosis Guideline Group (2010).
■ Written information from the National Osteoporosis Society on how to reduce the risk of osteopaenia, including sufficient Vitamin D and calcium intake in their diet, increasing exercise, stopping smoking and the importance of supplemental calcium and vitamin D in patients taking steroids.
■ Patients who are identified as having osteopaenia or osteoporosis should be referred by the IBD nurse to osteoporosis services for assessment.
■ Dexa (bone) scanning should be undertaken every three years to observe for any deterioration.

Education and promoting self-management

Patients will have educational needs at different stages of their disease process. The IBD CNS is well placed to provide this due to his or her expert knowledge, communication skills and time made to listen. Possibly the key time for this type of intervention is at diagnosis, at which point the CNS can explain the implications of the diagnosis, supported by patient information literature, along with engaging the patient to work with the IBD team to manage their disease. A crucial aspect of controlling any chronic disease is learning to self-manage (Department of Health, 2006c). The IBD CNS, through education and advanced knowledge of IBD care, is ideally placed to promote self-management techniques. This will be further explored in Chapter 19.

Biologics service

The IBD CNS is often focal to coordinating biological services, including pre-treatment assessment and counselling, administration and monitoring of therapies. Chapters 6 and 7 explore the indications for biological therapies and special considerations, including pre-treatment screening. Some important factors to consider in promoting consistency and safety are:

■ Baseline assessment (including routine bloods and symptom scores
■ Vaccination history and exposure to opportunistic infection

- Assessment of tuberculosis risk (British Thoracic Society Standards of Care Committee, 2005)
- Pre-treatment counselling (including risks and benefits)
- Evaluation of efficacy and complications

Some centres have dedicated multidisciplinary meetings (MDMs) to justify initiation of biological therapy along with monitoring efficacy and potential complications. Although labour-intensive, it could be argued that these drugs are expensive and associated with significant potential risk, and therefore warrant such input (Duncan *et al.*, 2010).

Inpatient management

Relatively few patients require admission to hospital as a result of IBD. When they do, however, the experience can be frightening, as fears around the need for surgery can become intense. The IBD nurse will often visit inpatients to provide support and education during this difficult time, and perhaps liaising or facilitating referrals to other members of the MDT including dietitians, stoma care CNSs and the medical team as in the case study of Derek described earlier in the chapter.

The IBD nurse is also important in facilitating ward nurses' support and education to care for their patients. Prompting specific care, such as the daily weighing of patients, completion of stool charts and ensuring medication is delivered in a timely manner, is commonly done by the IBD Nurse (UK IBD Audit Steering Group, 2007). The IBD nurse may also provide a role in supporting ward staff administering adjuvant immunosuppressant therapies such as ciclosporin and biologicals, ensuring that protocols are available to ward staff and the patient is appropriately prepared for therapy.

Staff education

The IBD CNS is often engaged in providing education to the healthcare team regarding management of patients with IBD. Education sessions regarding aetiology and pathogenesis of IBD, diagnosing IBD, the treatment of IBD and psychosocial aspects of diagnosis are fundamental. This helps rationalise the importance of basic elements of care which enable objective assessment of the progress of the patient. In UK wards CNSs often develop 'link nurses'; a ward nurse who, with the support and education of the CNS, becomes an expert within their clinical area, thus supporting and educating his or her peers. Supporting the medical team is also an important function, such as undertaking junior doctor training to ensure that they have adequate knowledge to care for patients with IBD.

IBD multidisciplinary meetings (MDM)

The IBD Audit (UK IBD Audit Steering Group, 2007) identified that 74% of those who participated had a timetabled and functioning MDM with gastroenterologists and surgeons. Other members of the IBD team are also considered essential to these meetings, such as the IBD CNS, radiologists, dieticians and histopathologist. This allows for a forum in which to discuss any difficult clinical cases, review of medical and surgical history with real time review of investigations (if radiology present) and consensus on the clinical management.

The IBD Standards Group (2009) has suggested the following regarding multidisciplinary IBD meetings:

- The IBD team should have regular timetabled meetings, preferably weekly, to discuss IBD patients with complex needs.
- The outcome of the discussions should be formally recorded.
- The team should agree who will discuss the decision with the patient.
- The patients to be discussed will be identified by the team. They may include patients with complex needs; patients with perianal Crohn's; patients with aggressive Crohn's at risk of needing further resections; new fistula patients; and patients unable to achieve steroid-free remission, but criteria for inclusion to be agreed locally.

There is a need for stronger evidence of the effectiveness of MDM, especially in terms of improving patient/disease outcomes in IBD. However, it has been demonstrated that MDM can be beneficial to the well-being of team members and improve job satisfaction (Taylor *et al.*, 2010). The role of the IBD CNS can be vital in playing the role of patient advocate, as the treatment recommendations made by the MDT may not always take into account the patients' preference highlighting that there is no consensus about how best to involve patients in the clinical decision making process in team meetings (Taylor *et al.*, 2010). The IBD CNS is likely to have a key role to play in communicating the decision made at the MDM to the patients.

Service development

Often nurses are a fundamental driving force in the development of IBD services and centres with IBD nurses have been shown to deliver services of a higher quality (IBD Standards Group, 2009). The recent development of the IBD standards is driving the way that services are developed nationally in the UK. In particular, the standards demand the development of evidence-based guidelines or protocols to inform practice and the establishment of patient panels. Both responsibilities are likely to be led by IBD Nurse Specialists.

Patient panels were instigated by Crohn's and Colitis UK (http://www.crohnsandcolitis.org.uk/) to promote the development of patient-centered services. They often take the form of open meetings, where single topics are discussed and service development plans formulated. They have been shown to be useful in improving access to dietitian services and increased specialist nurse input (for further information see http://www.nacc.org.uk/content/about/patientPanels.asp).

Research and audit

As discussed in Chapter 23, research is an activity that many nurses feel less confident in undertaking, despite it being an essential role descriptor. The IBD CNS is in a strong position to identify and initiate research priorities, particularly from a quality of life or living with IBD perspective.

However, auditing service provision, including clinical activity and patient satisfaction surveys are more commonly undertaken and are useful to include in annual service reports. A good information technology infrastructure is vital for healthcare research and audit activities. The development of IBD databases is now an expected service standard (IBD Standards Group, 2009). Not only does ready electronic access to patient records improve efficiency in the clinical management of patients, but if set up well they can improve access to evaluate patient outcomes.

Networking

IBD specialist nurses are often asked to develop services beyond their previous experience and expertise. In addition, new or lone post holders may feel vulnerable or unsure as to the expectations, opportunities, boundaries and limits of their role (also explored in Chapter 22). In such scenarios, networking is essential. Networking is best described as a supportive system of sharing information, knowledge and services among individuals and/or groups who have a common interest. Such networks can exist at a local, national and international level. Table 21.3 provides some examples of networks available to nurses working in IBD care.

The RCN Crohn's and Colitis special interest group (www.ibdnurses.com) is an example of a well-established IBD nursing network active throughout the UK. Originally initiated in September 2005, this network aims to provide support to relevant nurses through regional groups, disseminating information on role development and best practice, and giving IBD nurses a formal, recognised national voice. Meetings usually take the format of an educational update and the chance to discuss key issues of nursing practice.

More recently, the Nurses European Crohn's and Colitis network (NECCO) has been activated. The development of international IBD nursing networks

Table 21.3 Local, national and international networks.

Level of networking	Examples
Local	■ Immediate management ■ Colleagues/MDT ■ Local groups (e.g. specialist interest groups) ■ Pharmaceutical representatives
National (UK)	■ RCN Gastroenterology Forum ■ BSG endoscopy associates
European	■ European Crohn's and Colitis Organisation (ECCO) ■ Nursing European Crohn's and Colitis Organisation (NECCO) ■ United European Gastroenterology Federation (UEGF)
International	■ World Congress of Enterostomal Therapists (WCET)
Partnership with patients	■ Educational groups ■ Patient panels ■ Charity support groups

such as this (http://www.ecco-ibd.eu/) enables practice development from many countries to be discussed, and best practice to be shared. As part of NECCO's work, educational programmes throughout Europe have now been instigated to support both specialist nurses and general nurses caring for patients with IBD.

Conclusion

The role of the IBD CNS has developed rapidly over the last 20 years, and is now seen as pivotal to the development and delivery of high quality IBD services. Although there are many challenges to setting up and developing an IBD nursing service, defining specialist practice, role descriptors, protocol development and professional networking have all contributed to its success. According to anecdotal evidence, patients' views, and research and audit findings there is no doubt that an IBD specialist nursing service provides important contributions to the quality of care, improved patient experiences and rapid access to IBD healthcare services. There is still, however, an urgent need to provide larger scale research evidence to quantify the impact of the IBD nursing service, especially in terms of cost-effectiveness and quality of patient care. This will provide clearer definitions for service, but also career development. Such evidence will cement the work done so far on development of this role and assist its progress in the future.

References

Belling, R., Woods, L. and McLaren, S. (2008) Stakeholder perceptions of specialist Inflammatory Bowel Disease nurses' roles and personal attributes. *Int. J. Nurs. Practice,* **14**, 67–73.

Belling, R., McLaren, S. and Woods, L. (2009) Specialist nursing interventions for inflammatory bowel disease. *Cochrane Database Syst. Rev.* 2009, Issue 4.

British Society of Gastroenterology (2005) *Azathioprine Guidelines.* http://www.bsg.org.uk/pdf_word_docs/aza_ibd_dr.doc (accessed 10 October 2010).

British Thoracic Society Standards of Care Committee (2005) BTS recommendations for assessing risk, and for managing *M. tuberculosis* infection and disease, in patients due to start anti TNF treatment. *Thorax,* **60**, 800–5.

Cairns, S. R., Scholefield, J. H., Steele, R. J. *et al.* (2010) Guidelines for colorectal cancer screening and surveillance in moderate and high risk groups (update from 2002). *Gut,* **59**, 666–89.

Castledine, G. (2002) The development of the role of the clinical nurse specialist in the UK. *Br. J. Nurs.,* **11**, 506–8.

Department of Health (1999) *Making a Difference – Strengthening the Nursing, Midwifery and Health Visiting Contribution to Health and Health Care.* London: Department of Health.

Department of Health (2004a) *Extending Independent Nurse Prescribing Within the NHS in England.* http://webarchive.nationalarchives.gov.uk/20040216034425/http://doh.gov.uk/nurseprescribing/implementationguide.pdf (accessed 10 October 2010).

Department of Health (2004b) *The NHS Knowledge and Skills Framework and Development Review Process.* London: Department of Health.

Department of Health (2004c) *Improving Chronic Disease Management.* London: Department of Health.

Department of Health (2006a) *Tackling Hospital Waiting: the 18 Week Patient Pathway. An Implementation Framework.* London: Department of Health.

Department of Health (2006b) *Modernising Nursing Careers – Setting the Direction.* London: Department of Health.

Department of Health (2006c) *Supporting People with Long Term Conditions to Self Care. A Guide to Developing Local Strategies and Good Practice.* London: Department of Health.

Duncan, J., Caulfield, S., Clark, A., Anderson, A., Sanderson, J. and Irving, P. (2010) A multidisciplinary virtual biologic clinic: is it worthwhile? *ECCO abstract p143n* http://www.ecco-ibd.eu/publications/abstracts/abstract_detail.php?presentationNo=P143n&year=2010&referer=abstract_search_result.php&navId=31 (accessed 10 October 2010).

Faithfull, S., Corner, J., Meyer, L., Huddart, R. and Dearnaley, D. P. (2001) Evaluation of nurse-led follow up for patients undergoing pelvic radiotherapy. *Br. J. Cancer*, **85**, 1853–64.

Holbrook, K. (2007) A triangulation study of the clinician and patient experiences of the use of immunosuppressant drugs azathioprine and 6 mercaptopurine for the management of inflammatory bowel disease. *J. Clin. Nurs.*, **16**, 1427–34.

IBD Standards Group (2009) *Quality Care. Service Standards for the Healthcare of People Who Have Inflammatory Bowel Disease (IBD)*. http://www.ibdstandards.org.uk/ (accessed 10 October 2010).

Johnson, J. G., Cosnes, J. and Mansfield, J. (2005) Review article: smoking cessation as primary therapy to modify the course of Crohn's disease. *Aliment. Pharmacol. Ther.*, **21**, 921–31.

Knowles, G., Sherwood, L., Dunlop, M. G., Dean, G., Jodrell, D., McLean, C. and Preston, E. (2007) Developing and piloting a nurse-led model of follow-up in the multidisciplinary management of colorectal cancer. *Eur. J. Oncol. Nurs.*, **11**, 212–23.

Laurant, M., Reeves, D., Hermens, R., Braspenning, J., Grol, R. and Sibbald, B. (2005) Substitution of doctors by nurses in primary care. *Cochrane Database Syst. Rev.* Issue 2.

Lewis, N. R. and Scott, B. B. (2007) *Guidelines for Osteoporosis in Inflammatory Bowel Disease and Coeliac Disease.* http://www.bsg.org.uk/images/stories/clinical/ost_coe_ibd.pdf (accessed 10 October 2010).

McGee, P. and Castledine, G. (2003) *Advanced Nursing Practice*, 2nd edn. Oxford: Blackwell Publishing.

Moore, S., Corner, J., Haviland, J., Wells, M., Salmon, E., Normand, C., Brada, M., O'Brien, M. and Smith, I. (2002) Nurse-led follow up and conventional medical follow up in management of patients with lung cancer: randomised trial. *Br. Med. J.*, **325**, 1145–52.

National Osteoporosis Guideline Group (2000) *Osteoporosis – Clinical Guideline for Prevention and Treatment.* http://www.shef.ac.uk/NOGG/NOGG_Executive_Summary.pdf (accessed 10 October 2010).

National Osteoporosis Guideline Group (2010) *Osteoporosis – Guideline for Diagnosis and Management of Osteoporosis.* http://www.sheffield.ac.uk/NOGG/NOGG_Pocket_Guide_for_Healthcare_Professionals.pdf (accessed 10 October 2010).

National Patient Safety Agency (2007). *Improving Compliance with Oral Methotrexate.* http://www.nrls.npsa.nhs.uk/resources/?entryid45=59800 (accessed 16 October 2010).

Nightingale, A., Middleton, W., Middleton, S. and Hunter, J. (2000) Evaluation of the effectiveness of a specialist nurse in the management of inflammatory bowel disease. *Eur. J. Gastroenterol. Hepatol.*, **12**, 967–73.

Norton, C. and Kamm, M. (2002) Specialist nurses in gastroenterology. *J. Roy. Soc. Med.*,

95, 331–5.

O'Connor, M. (2010) Audit of advice line 2009–10. *Unpublished observations* (September).

Pearson, C. (2005) A nurse led IBD service in a district general hospital. *Gastrointest. Nurs.*, **3**(1), 33–9.

Pearson, C. (2006) Establishing an inflammatory bowel disease service. *Nurs. Times*, **102**(23), 27–30.

Phillips, S. (1995) Gut reaction. *Nurs. Times*, **91**(1), 44–5.

Raja Jones, H. (2002) Role boundaries – research nurse or clinical nurse specialist. A literature review. *J. Clin. Nurs.*, **11**, 415–20.

Royal College of Nursing (2005) *Maxi Nurses: Advanced and Specialist Roles*. London: Royal College of Nursing.

Royal College of Nursing (2006) *Clinical Imaging Requests From Non-medically Qualified Professionals*. http://www.rcn.org.uk/__data/assets/pdf_file/0003/78726/003101. pdf (accessed 10 October 2010).

Royal College of Nursing (2007) *Role Descriptives for Inflammatory Bowel Disease Nurse Specialists. Rcn Guidance*. London: Royal College of Nursing.

Royal College of Nursing (2010a) *Advanced Nurse Practitioners – an RCN Guide to the Advanced Practioner Role, Competencies and Programme Accreditation*. http://www.rcn. org.uk/__data/assets/pdf_file/0003/146478/003207.pdf (accessed 10 October 2010).

Royal College of Nursing (2010b) *Clinical Nurse Specialists: Adding Value to Care – an Executive Summary*. London: Royal College of Nursing.

Taylor, C., Munro, A. J., Glynne-Jones, R. *et al.* (2010) Multidisciplinary team working in cancer; what is the evidence? *Br. Med. J.*, **340**, c951.

UK IBD Audit Steering Group (2007) *UK IBD Audit 2006 National Results for the Organisation & Process of IBD Care in the UK*. http://www.rcplondon.ac.uk/clinical-standards/ceeu/Current-work/IBD/Pages/1st-Round.aspx (accessed 25 September 2010).

United Kingdom Central Council for Nursing, Midwifery and Health Visiting (1992) *The Scope of Professional Practice*. London: UKCC.

Woods, L., Belling, R. and McLaren, S. (2006) *Systematic Review of the Effectiveness of Inflammatory Bowel Disease Specialist Nurses*. http://www.rcplondon.ac.uk/clinical-standards/ceeu/Documents/ibd-review-specialist-nurses.pdf (accessed 30 September 2010).

Younge, L. and Norton, C. (2007) Contribution of specialist nurses in managing patients with IBD. *Br. J. Nurs.*, **16**, 208–12.

CHAPTER 22

Setting up specialist nursing services

Marian O'Connor

Introduction

This chapter represents a major driving force behind the creation of this book: i.e. the consideration of setting up specialist nursing services for people with IBD. Therefore the aims of the chapter are to identify and provide a guide to the processes which are involved in laying down the foundations for a robust specialist nursing service. Following these processes ensures the establishment of thorough policies and protocols for practice, engagement with healthcare management and collaboration with all the relevant team members (including patients). This helps to shape an effective service built around patient need.

The role of developing this type of service is likely to be assumed by the specialist nurse, but not exclusively, and should include members of the multidisciplinary team, ideally the consultant gastroenterologist, lead nurse and senior management. The context of setting up specialist nursing services in this chapter is within secondary care (based in a hospital setting), which is the predominant base for the majority of IBD nursing services in the UK. The following case study is a typical example of an IBD nursing service.

Case study

A nurse is employed into a new role as an IBD Clinical Nurse Specialist (CNS). An established Gastroenterology CNS, she has not worked directly in IBD care since ward nursing 10 years previously. The service in which she is employed originally had an IBD nurse in post, but the service had collapsed following her departure almost a year before. One of the consultant gastroenterologists had attempted to continue the IBD telephone helpline, but in the main, callers left unreturned messages on an answering machine. The IBD team relied on an external company to run the biologics service but there was a clinical incident which led management to discontinue this service. Patients receiving infliximab then had to be admitted as inpatients to receive their infusion, which led to delays in their maintenance regime. New patients starting on immunomodulators were inconsistently monitored, which caused concern amongst the IBD team. Overall patients were expressing dissatisfaction with the service and the IBD team felt the service lacked cohesion. They had been unable to obtain secure funding via the NHS to continue the post, but had recently obtained a grant from a pharmaceutical company to fund an IBD nurse for one year. The senior nursing management for the directorate had no experience in IBD and so was unable to provide directional leadership. The new post holder was given free rein to set up the IBD nursing service with the only directions being to re-establish the helpline, the biologics infusion service and monitoring for immunosuppressant drugs.

Despite having little leadership, support and direction within the service, the nurse drew on her previous experience as a CNS, and of the expected role of a CNS, supplemented by the IBD nurse role descriptors (Royal College of Nursing, 2007) and IBD Standards (IBD Standards Group, 2009) to ascertain what the aims of a modern IBD nursing service should be. Additionally, she spoke with patients about their recent experiences and future expectations. She joined established networks of IBD nurses via the Nursing European Colitis and Crohn's Organisation (NECCO) and the Royal College of Nursing (RCN). A telephone and email advice service was quickly established with clear expectations of the service outlined to patients on the answer machine message and by patient information literature. A suitable clinical area for biological infusions was identified with the support of nursing management. The infusion service was then re-developed as a day-case service managed by the CNS, supported by an external company. This was popular with the patients receiving biologics, as they felt confident in the nursing support, the efficiency of the service and that they would receive their infusions in a timely fashion. An outpatient nurse-led clinic was established to run alongside the IBD medical clinic to offer immunosuppressant monitoring, patient support and education as well as case management. Additionally, the IBD CNS engaged with the relevant clinical areas to offer a staff teaching programme. She audited her service development and activity to build a business case for a permanent post in addition to a second IBD CNS. She brought cohesion to the IBD team with the introduction of regular service reviews, and arising from these has progressed to leading overall service development.

Getting started

For an IBD CNS new into post it can be a daunting task to begin setting up a specialist nursing service. As a nurse, whose previous role is likely to have been predominantly direct nursing care, a new IBD CNS will find themselves having to become rapidly familiar with service planning, forging links with senior management and considering the interface with primary and secondary care in addition to income generation for their service. The first stage of setting up a specialist nursing service begins with an understanding of the driving forces behind it, in order to define its purpose.

Driving forces behind service development

The specialist nursing role

The development of any IBD nursing service cannot begin without the IBD CNS. It is important to appreciate that there were several key changes which led to the development of the CNS role (not least in IBD) in the UK over the past decade. The New Deal for junior doctors clearly stated the maximum working hours per week, shift patterns and rest requirements for all junior doctors and became a contractual obligation for all hospital trusts to comply with in 2003 (Department of Health, 1999a). As a result nurses were required to take on more responsibilities, which were identified in the document: *Making a Difference* (Department of Health, 1999b). This outlined the strategic intention for strengthening the contribution of nurses, midwives and health visitors in the delivery of healthcare. Furthermore, the National Health Service (NHS) plan outlined a vision for health services designed around the patient (Department of Health, 2000). In 2002 the Chief Nursing Officer published the details of the extended roles of nurses, paving the way for nurses to increase their skills and autonomy within specific aspects of healthcare delivery (Department of Health, 2002). Agenda for Change was a radical reorganisation of the (NHS) pay system to ensure 'equal pay for work of equal value' and, this in particular, allowed nurses to gain recognition for their extended roles (Department of Health, 2004a).

Within the specialty of IBD, the British Society of Gastroenterology (BSG) identified the need for patients to have access to the following (Carter *et al.*, 2004):

- continuity of care
- direct telephone access
- attention to physical, emotional and quality of life issues
- opportunity to meet non-medical staff including a nurse specialist

This strengthened the case for the development of the IBD nursing role and subsequent expansion of IBD services.

Defining the role

A systematic review of the effectiveness of IBD specialist nurses (Belling *et al.*, 2006) demonstrated:

- Nurses are instrumental in developing new services.
- Patient satisfaction was generally reported as high.
- Explicit models of IBD Specialist nursing practice were largely absent in the published literature.

The need, therefore, for a formal definition and evaluation of the role of IBD nurse specialists was highlighted. This subsequently led to the RCN document *Role Descriptives for Inflammatory Bowel Disease Nurse Specialists*, which provides a guide to the development of best practice and the creation of specialist nursing roles within local organisations (Royal College of Nursing, 2007).

Understanding patients' needs

IBD services ultimately should be set up with the patient needs at the centre. The need for greater access to IBD nurses as key to the management of IBD patients' care was identified in 2005, with only 26% of National Association for Colitis & Crohn's Disease (NACC) members at that time having access to an IBD nurse (Crohn's and Colitis UK, 2005). Following a campaign by NACC to raise awareness and support for IBD nurses, and also owing to the above changes within healthcare in the UK, the number of IBD nurses has risen to 62% in acute hospital trusts (UK IBD Audit Steering Group, 2008). Understanding the needs of the local IBD patient population when setting up IBD services is therefore vitally important, as what the patients want and what the team *thinks* they want, may be two very different things. An example of this is shown in Box 22.1.

There are several methods of gaining the patients' views, such as requesting that patients complete a survey or by engaging the local patient panel (if one exists).

> ## Box 22.1 Understanding patients' needs
> There is a review of the waiting times within an outpatient department. An IBD team is working on reducing the time that patients and relatives have to wait to be seen, as they identify this as the most important factor for patient satisfaction. On discussion with a patient panel however, the CNS finds that patients understand that they may have to wait to be seen, but they state that having adequate time once in the consulting room is the most important part of their outpatient visit, in addition to having more comfortable seating in the waiting area.

Since 2005, NACC (now Crohn's and Colitis UK), has provided support to patient panels as a primary means for patients and professionals involved in their care to exchange ideas on how local IBD services can be best developed. This forum provides a safe and constructive means by which patient can provide feedback on already existing services and provide suggestions for improvements. When considering setting up a patient panel, it is worth determining whether the patient panel is to be patient-led or team-led, as this will need defining from the outset. Early input from Crohn's and Colitis UK is invaluable: for more information, go to: http://www.nacc.org.uk/content/about/patientPanels.asp.

IBD standards
The publication of the IBD standards document has provided a nationally agreed structure by which to plan and/or further develop IBD services. The aim of the IBD standards is to ensure that patients who have IBD receive healthcare that is safe, effective and of a consistently high quality (IBD Standards Group, 2009). This document sets about defining what is required in terms of staffing, support services, organisation, patients' education and audit to provide integrated, high quality IBD services. To this end, the document provides an essential text for building an IBD service. Presenting this to the management within an institution is a starting point, and provides a template of minimum standards to achieve within an IBD service.

Purpose of the service
There are two distinct yet connected factors to consider when setting up services; the team's vision and the organisation's vision or needs.

Team vision

This is normally the starting point for most services. Establishing a team vision involves the identification by the gastroenterology team of a need to set up a service to better meet the needs of their patients. In the case study, patient safety regarding the biologics service and immunosuppressants as well as patient and team dissatisfaction with the service were the key drivers of the redevelopment of that particular IBD nursing service.

When setting up any service, it is vital to consider the purpose. The following questions provide a focus for planning of any service:

- Who is the service intended for?
- What is the rationale behind it?
- How it will function?
- How will it be used?

In addition, it is important to consider the skill set and training needs of the IBD CNS, to ensure there is adequate supervision and training in order to safely provide the necessary services (Royal College of Nursing, 2007). Establishing this type of support at the outset is fundamental so that it is incorporated into the team's vision and remains part of service development. CNSs with a lack of support and educational/training opportunities may in the longer term find it more difficult to provide effective specialist services (Reid *et al.*, 2009). Anecdotally, many IBD CNSs report that they can struggle to gain training/educational opportunities and supervision if they are not incorporated into the original business case for the post. Training and support needs of the CNS should also form part of the appraisal process and is important for ongoing career development.

Organisational needs

When making any change, such as setting up new services, especially within large organisations such as hospitals, it is important to also consider the organisation's needs. An IBD team might ask the following questions:

- How do the services being planned fit in and complement the overall aims and targets of the organisation?
- Is the service in line with the organisational and corporate objectives?

The Trust board normally sets the organisational or corporate objectives, on an annual/biannual basis, in line with the local and national directives (such as from the Department of Health), which provide direction for service development within the organisation.

Within the organisational needs, it is also necessary to recognise the local departmental (Gastroenterology or IBD department) needs, as in the case study earlier in this chapter. The department needed an adequate biologics, immunosuppressant and helpline service in order to alleviate concerns regarding patient safety and ensure an effective, safe service for patients.

Collaboration

For the effective establishment of the IBD nursing service, most commence with dialogue amongst the main MDT members. As in the case study, for many this begins with the acquisition of appropriate funding for the IBD nursing post. The initial funding for many IBD nursing posts within the UK is acquired from industry (such as pharmaceutical companies) or clinical research funding. Over time, most are then substantiated by the organisation (e.g. hospital trust) once the value and worth of the role and IBD nursing service has been demonstrated.

Once funding is secured, involvement of the following members of the team is ideal (this is not an exclusive list and may involve other team members):

- Consultant gastroenterologist
- IBD specialist nurse
- Local patient group/panel
- Nursing manager
- Divisional general manager

A valuable collaborative activity involves networking with other specialist nurses, such as CNSs working within other specialities within the organisation and IBD nurses working within other hospitals. This allows for a greater understanding of the initial barriers and also sharing of best practice (such as relevant policies and protocols). See Chapter 21 for further information on networking.

Protocols, policies and guidelines

Development

For any service a protocol/policy or guideline ought to be in place and agreed by your institution. The development of these clinical documents forms the foundation for an effective IBD nursing service. The reasons for this are as follows:

- To provide protection to the nurse practising at an advanced level.
- To set locally agreed standards of care, which provides cohesion and consensus.
- To provide a consistent, structured and safe approach to care of all patients.

Inflammatory bowel disease nursing

- To provide a benchmark and ensure a sound evidence base to care being provided.
- To ensure care is delivered in a systematic and appropriate way.
- To allow for audit of care.

Definitions

Table 22.1 provides definitions for the mainstream documents used to describe and define clinical practice or an aspect of clinical service.

Table 22.1 Definitions.

Protocol	'In science and medicine, a formal set of rules and procedures to be followed during a particular research experiment, course of treatment etc.' (http://www.yourdictionary.com/protocol accessed 4 October 2010)
Policy	'... A plan for the conduct of a clinical trial or a course of treatment' (Youngson, 1999)
Guidelines	A medical guideline is a document with the aim of guiding decisions and criteria in specific areas of healthcare, as defined by an authoritative examination of current evidence (evidence-based medicine) – definition obtained from Wikipedia: http://en.wikipedia.org/wiki/Medical_guideline (accessed 4 October 2010)

Development and approval

Any policies, protocols or guidelines used in clinical practice are normally subject to a formal format or procedure for development and approval, within your local institution (e.g. hospital setting). Guidance should be sought from a direct line manager regarding this process.

Once drawn up, these clinical documents are usually subject to approval and ratification by the appropriate director/directorate before application to clinical practice. Figure 22.1 is an example of the likely process which is necessary to ratify clinical documents within the hospital environment (based on the author's experience within the UK). This may not be universal, as many documents are deemed adequate if agreed within the immediate multidisciplinary team, such as the IBD or Gastroenterology team, and local processes will differ.

It is essential that any clinical document should be reviewed and updated as specified on approval by the relevant department, or as evidence changes.

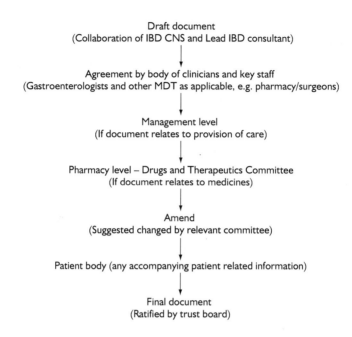

Draft document
(Collaboration of IBD CNS and Lead IBD consultant)

Agreement by body of clinicians and key staff
(Gastroenterologists and other MDT as applicable, e.g. pharmacy/surgeons)

Management level
(If document relates to provision of care)

Pharmacy level – Drugs and Therapeutics Committee
(If document relates to medicines)

Amend
(Suggested changed by relevant committee)

Patient body (any accompanying patient related information)

Final document
(Ratified by trust board)

Figure 22.1 The ratification process.

Setting out IBD services

The core IBD nursing services are listed below:

- Telephone advice line
- Nurse-led clinics
- Immunosuppressant monitoring/clinics
- Biological services

For these services the following is intended as a guide by which a service can begin to be described and established, with reference to the available literature. Key aspects of developing policies/protocols or guidelines will be considered to define these services adequately. Administrative support for any IBD nursing services should also be set up, in relation to the services described below.

Telephone advice line

The RCN document *Telephone Advice Lines for People with Long Term Conditions (Guidance for Nursing Practitioners)* provides an overview of the issues involved in setting up and safely running a telephone service (Royal College of Nursing,

2006). At the very least a protocol for the telephone advice line (telephone services) should be produced to clarify the following:

- Aim of the service (to provide a point of access, support and/or rapid access to clinic if patients are unwell)
- Scope of the service (define whether there will be voicemail, a direct line, and the opening hours)
- Consideration of alternative access for patients outside of opening hours
- Personnel undertaking the main service provision (e.g. CNS and/or specialist registrars)
- Scope of practice of personnel (e.g. to provide access to general advice, information giving, and/or medication advice)

As mentioned above, it is important to consider the scope of practice of the personnel undertaking the role of telephone nursing, as is the case for the advice line. PGDs (Patient Group Directions) and PSDs (Patient-Specific Directions) can be incorporated, with input from the pharmacy department, if deemed necessary to alter patients' medications.

PGDs
A PGD is a specific written instruction for the supply or administration of named medicines in an identified clinical situation by named nurses or other health professionals (i.e. nurses, midwives, health visitors, optometrists, pharmacists, chiropodists, radiographers, orthoptists, physiotherapists, ambulance paramedics, dietitians, occupational therapists, speech and language therapists, prosthetists and orthotists). A PGD should only be used in exceptional circumstances, where its use will lead to an improvement in patient care. It is important to note that PGDs cannot be used for unlicensed medications.

PSDs
A PSD outlines the supply of medication for the medicine to be signed by a prescriber for an individual patient.

Nurse-led clinics
Nurse-led clinics can take many different forms to provide nursing follow-up to IBD patients in the outpatient setting. They can occur face to face with the patients in clinic, over the telephone as in the case of the telephone follow-up clinic, or more recently via virtual clinics (VC), whereby the patient is sent a health questionnaire to complete with instructions for the necessary investigations

(such as bloods) to be carried out at their family doctor's surgery (Hunter *et al.*, 2010). It is worth noting that the recent advent of this model of virtual clinics was mainly in response to the organisational needs of hospitals to reduce their ratio of follow-up patients to new patients in the outpatient departments (Department of Health, 2010a). To this end, a defined protocol should be drawn up to identify the following:

- Aim of service (e.g. review of stable patient or rapid access clinic for unwell patients)
- Identify suitable and unsuitable patients in relation to the aim of the service
- Referral process for patients to be seen (e.g. will a letter from a consultant or GP be adequate? Managerial input may be needed here)
- Clinic code – collaborate with outpatient management to allocate a specified clinic code. This will ensure that the service is remunerated appropriately and will make service audit easier

Immunosuppressant monitoring

Collaboration with primary care (such as the family doctor) is essential for effective and safe monitoring of patients taking immunosuppressants (such as azathioprine, mercaptopurine, methotrexate, ciclosporin and tacrolimus). Ideally, although not always possible, shared care guidelines should be drawn up and agreed with primary care.

Shared care guidelines

The term 'Effective Shared Care Agreement' (ESCA) is now being used (Department of Health, 2004b). Effective shared care agreements are developed when sophisticated or complex treatments (such as those detailed above) that are initiated in secondary care (hospital setting) are then prescribed by a family doctor. The guidelines set out the process that needs to be followed for the family doctor to take on prescribing and monitoring responsibility.

For IBD CNSs undertaking the role of immunosuppressant monitoring, there should be locally agreed policies or guidelines to clarify the following:

- Identify the parameters that are acceptable for blood results including full blood count (fbc), renal and liver function and trough levels (necessary in the case of ciclosporin and tacrolimus). This ensures consistency and patient safety.
- State the appropriate action, when abnormal results are identified, and the personnel responsible for communicating this to the patient and/or GP.

- Agree the expected frequency of follow-up of patients on immunosuppressants and regularity of blood test monitoring.
- Consider the arrangement if patients do not comply with follow-up/appropriate regularity of monitoring.
- Consider whether renumeration of the service is appropriate and possible (it is worth noting that when this is undertaken by GPs in the UK they are renumerated appropriately – liaison with management may be needed).

Biological service

Protocols for patients on biologicals (such as infliximab and adalimumab) can allow for the identification of the following:

- Personnel permitted to administer biologicals (e.g. only CNS and/or specialist registrar). This may need clarification and agreement with the pharmacy department.
- Level of training necessary according to local policy (e.g. drug administration, basic life support and/or advanced life support training).
- Agreed local screening guidance of patients prior to therapy (e.g. infections and contraindications to treatment).
- Parameters for treatment response and long-term follow-up and monitoring.
- Special considerations (such as in pregnancy).
- Actions to be taken if a patient experiences an allergic or adverse reaction to treatment.
- The setting in which these treatments are to be given safely (e.g. day unit or ward) with adequate access to emergency equipment.

Other aspects of IBD services

Promotion of services

Within the organisation in which the CNS works, it may be necessary to promote the service adequately in order to fully meet its aims/purpose. To achieve this it may be useful to identify and meet prominent staff such as those working within the immediate departments (e.g. endoscopy, inpatient ward(s) and outpatient department). Word of mouth from these staff members will ensure that the appropriate patients are aware of the services provided by the IBD CNS. Collaboration and regular meetings with key staff (such as those identified above), and/or senior management within the institution may be useful and necessary to continually raise awareness of the service and allow for development.

Additional promotion of the IBD nursing services can be facilitated by means of service business cards, displaying posters within relevant departments and networking with local contacts, such as GPs. Information technology has also helped in this regard, with many services having a generic email account. Furthermore, as in the case of the author's IBD nursing service, an internal (or intranet) web page may be set up, providing access to all the relevant patient information sheets, algorithms, protocols and guidelines for all staff members within the institution. This has been revolutionary, within the authors' service, in allowing ease of access to information for all relevant staff. IBD nurses may also need to become familiar with presenting their services within appropriate forums or departmental meetings as another means of promoting the services.

Education and research
Within the remit of an IBD specialist nursing role, it is expected that nurses practising at this level are involved in both education and research (see Chapter 21). Providing access for staff to education on IBD is essential in preparing staff and promoting awareness of the disease and its management. Providing education to patients with IBD is considered fully in Chapter 19. The importance of undertaking research in relation to IBD nursing services is covered in Chapter 23. As discussed earlier, the training and education needs of the IBD CNS need to be considered regularly as part of the regular review or appraisal process.

Income generation
In the UK, in an era in which services provided within the hospital (secondary care) have to be properly funded, interaction and agreement for the local health authority to fund any services provided by the IBD nurse may be necessary. This may be an aspect of the service's development which can be taken on by the general manager. The income generation of IBD nursing services has only been exploited recently. An example of this is the recent introduction of an applicable tariff of £27.00 for the IBD advice line (Department of Health, 2010b).

Ongoing development of the IBD services

Audit
This aspect of service development often gets forgotten, especially once the service is running and clinical work takes over. It is necessary to consider how to record activity of the IBD nurse(s) to ensure that there is adequate recognition and payment for the service. General management should provide guidance on this.

Audit of any aspect of a service is useful to answer a specific question in relation to that service or patient care (such as survey and patient satisfaction audits.) If available, the Research and Development Department (R&D) will be able to provide further guidance and support with this. In the case of already established IBD services, it is valuable to identify how local IBD services compare with the National IBD Standards (IBD Standards Group, 2009) as a means of constructive review of the service.

Annual reports

An annual report is a valuable tool, not least as it will provide a rudimentary breakdown of the usage of the IBD nursing services. It also offers a useful outline of the services provided, summarising the rationale of the services, and can allow for appraisal of the efficacy of each service. This can also provide a means for identification and eliciting support for expansion of the service, in terms of resources (e.g. administrative support and additional IBD specialist nurses), and can be a useful tool for persuasion of management to support this. The annual report can also help to emphasise needs for development in line with the local and national requirements and draw attention to any difficulties encountered in improving these services (e.g. how services compare with that specified in the National IBD Standards). The annual report may also provide a means of highlighting other aspects of the IBD nursing service, such as how the IBD nurse raised the profile of the IBD nursing service and the hospital (for example, if they were involved in activities of other organisations such as in the authors case with Nurses European Colitis and Crohn's Organisation (NECCO)).

Allocating adequate time and the necessary resources (including meeting with the necessary departments/management to obtain figures on service usage) is crucial in order to construct and produce an annual report. In the author's practice, it is deemed necessary to allocate one week of non-clinical time (therefore cancelling clinical commitments) to compile and draft the annual report, and this is supported by direct management.

Engaging with management

Regular meetings with management can be constructive, ideally including both the nursing lead and the divisional general manager for the department. These meetings can provide a regular opportunity for update on the services that are being provided by the specialist nurse, and can allow for early planning for expansion of further services, ensuring adequate resources and training needs. Early planning is essential, as most nurses who enter these posts become busy very quickly and, by nature of the role, are unable to find sufficient time to write the necessary business cases to develop the service further. In the author's practice, a monthly meeting with nursing management and a quarterly review with general management occurs.

Conclusion

The ultimate goal of the IBD nursing is to provide an efficient, holistic, accessible and acceptable service for patients with IBD. Therefore collaboration with IBD team members when starting out, securing funding and engaging with management are central to the development of IBD nursing services. Equally important is the essential involvement of patients to ensure that the services remain patient-centred. Establishing rigorous policies, protocols or guidelines for these services ensures, above all, safety and consistently high quality care. Networking with management and other specialist nurses can allow for sharing of best practice, promotion of services and early planning for further development.

Key points

- Team work is important – involve the essential members of the MDT.
- Patient involvement in developing and reviewing of IBD nursing services is invaluable.
- When writing protocols/policies or guidelines it is important to keep them short and succinct as otherwise they are unlikely to be applied easily to practice.
- Follow local format/procedure for approval.
- Review any clinical documents regularly.
- Networking with management especially can allow for early service development, which is likely to be needed as service usage increases.
- Annual reports provide a good means of breakdown of service usage and appraisal.

References

Belling, R., Woods, L. and McLaren, S. (2006) *A Systematic Review of the Effectiveness of Inflammatory Bowel Disease Specialist Nurses*. London: South Bank University.

Carter, M. J., Lobo, A. J. and Travis, S. P. (2004) Guidelines for the management of Inflammatory Bowel Disease in adults. *Gut*, **53**(suppl. V), v1–v6.

Crohn's and Colitis UK (2005) *Survey Exposing the Shortage of IBD Nurses*. http://www.

nacc.org.uk/downloads/media/NACCSurveyRelease.pdf (accessed 1 October 2010).

Department of Health (1999a) *New Deal for Junior Doctors*. http://www.dhsspsni.gov.uk/scujuniordoc-2 (accessed 25 September 2010).

Department of Health (1999b) *Making a Difference*. http://www.dh.gov.uk/en/Publicationsandstatistics/Publications/PublicationsPolicyAndGuidance/DH_4007977 (accessed 25 September 2010).

Department of Health (2000) *The National Health Service Plan*. http://www.dh.gov.uk/en/Publicationsandstatistics/Publications/PublicationsPolicyAndGuidance/DH_4010198 (accessed 25 September 2010).

Department of Health (2002) Chief Nursing Officers 10 Key Roles for Nurses http://www.dh.gov.uk/prod_consum_dh/groups/dh_digitalassets/@dh/@en/documents/digitalasset/dh_4101739.pdf (accessed 25 September 2010).

Department of Health (2004a) *Agenda for Change*. http://www.dh.gov.uk/en/Publicationsandstatistics/Publications/PublicationsPolicyAndGuidance/DH_4090842 (accessed 25 September 2010).

Department of Health (2004b) *Management of Medicines: A resource to support implementation of the wider aspects of medicines management for the National Service Frameworks for Diabetes, Renal Services and Long-Term Conditions*. London: Department of Health.

Department of Health (2010a) *Revision to the Operating Framework for the NHS in England 2010/11*. http://www.dh.gov.uk/en/Publicationsandstatistics/Publications/PublicationsPolicyAndGuidance/DH_110107 (accessed 2 October 2010).

Department of Health (2010b) *Confirmation of Payment by results (PrB)*. http://www.dh.gov.uk/en/Publicationsandstatistics/Publications/PublicationsPolicyAndGuidance/DH_112284 (accessed 8 June 2010).

Hunter, J., James, S., Chan, D., Stacey, B., Stroud, M., Patel, P., Cummings, F. and Fine, D. (2010) *Virtual Inflammatory Bowel Disease Clinics in the Real World*. http://gut.bmj.com/site/abstractbooks/A1b.pdf (accessed 2 October 2010)

IBD Standards Group (2009). *Quality Care: Service Standards for the Healthcare of People Who Have Inflammatory Bowel Disease* (IBD). http://www.ibdstandards.org.uk/uploaded_files/IBDstandards.pdf (accessed 25 September 2010).

Reid, L., Chivers, S., Plummer, V. *et al.* (2009) Inflammatory bowel disease management : a review of nurses' roles in Australia and the United Kingdom. *Austral. J. Adv. Nurs.*, **27**(2), 19–26.

Royal College of Nursing (2006) *Telephone Advice Lines for People with Long Term Conditions (Guidance for Nursing Practitioners)*. London: Royal College of Nursing.

Royal College of Nursing (2007) *Role Descriptives for Inflammatory Bowel Disease Nurse Specialists*. London: Royal College of Nursing.

UK IBD Audit Steering Group (2008). *National Results for the Organisation and Process of IBD Care in the UK.* http://www.rcplondon.ac.uk/clinical-standards/ceeu/Current-work/Documents/UK-IBD-Audit-2nd-Round-Full-National-Report-Appendices.pdf (accessed 25 September 2010).

Youngson, R. M. (1999) *Collins Dictionary of Medicine.* London: Collins.

CHAPTER 23

Getting research into practice

Christine Norton

Introduction

There is nothing unique to IBD nursing in the problems of getting research implemented in clinical practice. The 'theory–practice gap' is well known in all areas of healthcare, not just nursing. There is known to be a very long time lag between when an intervention has been shown to be beneficial in clinical trials and when it reaches the textbooks or becomes routinely used in clinical practice.

Evidence-based healthcare has been a holy grail for decades, and more recently evidence-based nursing has become an aspiration (Callum *et al.*, 1997). However, for our care to be based on the best evidence requires firstly generation of the evidence (someone has to do the research); secondly publication and dissemination of the evidence; and thirdly practitioners to access the evidence and have the skills to interpret the relevance of the findings to their own clinical practice. The process can fall down at any or all of these stages. This chapter aims to give a broad overview of each of these stages of the use and generation of evidence, offering a straightforward discussion of the practical steps that can be taken by nurses caring for people with IBD to incorporate evidence more fully into their practice.

Accessing, interpreting and implementing the evidence

It is usually considered that there is a hierarchy of evidence, with the strongest evidence coming from the combination of several large, well conducted randomised controlled trials (meta-analysis, as performed in Cochrane reviews), less strong evidence from individual controlled trials, down to case series and, at the lowest level of evidence, narrative description and expert opinion.

Reviewing the literature

This can be really daunting at first. Using the Internet, if you enter almost any search term in MEDLINE, Google Scholar or PubMed you will get back an unmanageable number of results. How can you select the best articles? Where do you even start?

The good news is that often you don't have to – someone else has done it for you! The place to search for evidence on common clinical question is *not* to do an original search yourself. It is much more fruitful to see what others have already done for you. Most of the major clinical dilemmas in routine practice have already been subject to a systematic review.

Cochrane reviews

Cochrane reviews are often considered the 'best evidence' for treatments in healthcare. The reviews are undertaken by international groups of experts who systematically search the world literature for studies (randomised controlled trials – RCTs) and then, where possible, sum the results into a meta-analysis of evidence. For example, if there are four small studies of a certain intervention, each may have insufficient participants to show a definitive result. But if the studies have recruited similar patients and used comparable outcome measures it may be possible to pool the results and draw more definitive conclusions. While many of the reviews cover drug treatments, others cover psychological and nutrition interventions and surgery. All studies are rated for their quality and key features are summarised.

To access the Cochrane library go to: http://mrw.intrscience.wiley.com/cochrane. You can enter search terms or browse all reviews by entering 'inflammatory bowel disease'. In mid-2010 over 200 reviews were either directly about IBD or had findings directly relevant to IBD. Access to the Cochrane library is free and the plain language summary is often a good place to start for a quick overview of a topic. Most reviews are updated every few years, but it is worth checking the publication date if you know that there have been recent developments in an area.

As Cochrane reviews only include RCT evidence, however, they do not often cover many of the aspects of care which primarily concern nurses, such as different care pathways, either because there have not been RCTs, or the interventions are less amenable to RCTs. This can also mean that the reviews ignore good studies which have not used RCT methods.

Other reviews

Another good place to start to look for evidence is NHS Evidence: http://www.library.nhs.uk/evidence. Again, search terms can be entered and combined and many different published reviews are accessed via this central search point.

The National Institute for Health and Clinical Evidence (NICE) produces both overview clinical guidelines on clinical conditions as well as reviews of specific interventions (such as drugs or polyp surveillance). A clinical guideline on Crohn's disease is expected in 2012.

If your clinical problem or question is not covered by the above reviews, most databases such as MEDLINE or PubMed will allow you to search for review articles only. For example, if your question is about osteoporosis in IBD, you might use the search terms 'inflammatory bowel disease' combined with 'osteoporosis' and then restrict your findings to 'review articles only'. Although you will still get some irrelevant hits, it should be a lot more manageable than just using the two search terms.

In the age of the Internet, information sources are truly global, so always broaden your search for systematic reviews and evidence syntheses from countries other than your own. In the USA the National Institute for Diabetes and Digestive and Kidney Disease (NIDDK) has excellent information for both professionals and the public and can be found at http://digestive.niddk.nih.gov/.

If there really is no good review on your chosen question, then if you are inexperienced with searching, again enlist some help. Many librarians are delighted to use their extensive skills to help answer genuine clinical dilemmas. And remember not just to accept all research as high quality evidence, but learn to read critically (Greenhalgh, 1999) and keep in mind 'How does the research I am reading relate to my clinical group?'.

Interpreting the evidence

If you are using a systematic review or expert guideline, some interpretation will most likely already have been done for you – the 'so what for clinical practice?'. However, if you are conducting your own review, it can be difficult to draw out the implications for your own patient population, especially if the evidence seems to be conflicting in different papers. It can be difficult to know how good the research methodology was and if you can really trust the results, especially as many research reports tend to present their findings in rather impenetrable language, tables and statistics. There are some excellent guides (Greenhalgh 1999, 2006) to get you started with critiquing literature rather than simply accepting the results you are presented with.

It is usually wise to firstly read a paper and think about whether it makes sense to you and fits the patient population/clinical problem that you are trying to tackle. Enlist the opinions of others, either in your multidisciplinary team or via your network of contacts among other nurses with an interest in IBD. You might take the paper to a journal club for discussion, or start an email discussion with your peers. Look carefully at the results and the authors' interpretation of these. A statistically significant difference reported in a paper does not always equate to a clinically important difference for your patients. For example, if a study has included a large number of participants it can quote a statistically significant difference between two groups, but in practice you may decide that a few points difference on an IBD score is really not very meaningful or useful. Conversely, many studies are too small (underpowered) to demonstrate a difference that is really there and may be important. So do not always just accept the papers you read at face value.

Implementing research in practice

Once you have found relevant research, implementation in practice is not always straightforward. People are notoriously conservative and like to stick with what they know and trust. It can be very frustrating if you feel that you have identified new evidence which would improve patient care, but meet resistance from colleagues or your patients. It can take all your negotiating and change management skills to get all stakeholders on board and implement changes, even when evidence of benefit is really strong. The trick is to be persistent, gain support from wherever you can and not to give up if you feel that patients could be helped. The IBD nurse should at all times be the patient advocate for best care.

Generating the evidence – conducting research

It is important for IBD nurses to engage with the research process. Not that there should be any great divide between 'medical research' and 'nursing research', but in practice nurses do tend to ask research questions that have a different focus or emphasis from our medical colleagues. This may mean incorporating an additional element (for example on patients' views or effect on quality of life) into an existing or planned multidisciplinary research project, or conducting an independent study, alone or with colleagues. Conducting research and audit is likely to be in the role descriptors for most nurse specialist roles, but often it appears to be tacked on at the end, almost as an afterthought, and may not even make it into your job plan or appraisal objectives.

Barriers and some possible solutions to nursing research in IBD

Lack of time

Lack of time is almost always the number one reason nurses give for not engaging in research activities. There will always be more patients with more needs than any IBD nurse can possibly see individually. Yet many clinical nurse specialists (CNSs) spend over 90% of their time in direct clinical care and related activities, feeling that they have no time for other activities such as research or audit. This is contrary to recommendations that CNSs should spend about 60% of their time in direct patient contact (Royal College of Nursing, 2007). Clinical care is often the part of the job that is most comfortable and most rewarding – the reason why most nurse specialists like their job – but they should not ignore other equally important aspects of the role which will allow the service to develop into new areas.

It seldom happens that someone else will recognise the importance of allowing time for research in your job plan. It will usually be up to the individual nurse to make the time by ring-fencing sessions. This is not easy, but it would be irresponsible of any practitioner to be so busy that any time for nonclinical work becomes impossible. Allowing time for research is just as important for patient care as seeing individual patients – maybe more so in the long term. If you are serious about conducting research you will need to plan some time – and stick to your plan! Blocking out some time in your diary to think, read, meet with others or plan your research is an equally legitimate use of your time as providing direct clinical care. This may involve negotiating some objectives and time with your manager and building research time into your job plan and role profile.

Lack of skills
Although good textbooks on research methods abound (see, for example, Gerrish and Lacey (2010), Polit *et al.* (2001) and Bowling (2002) if you are new to research), it can be very difficult to learn 'how to do it' from a book. Participating in a research project being conducted by more experienced colleagues is often a good way to get started. Offer to help, but in exchange participate in research team meetings to learn from observation (and ask lots of questions). This can enable you to feel a lot more confident to later start to plan your own research. Ask others for help or advice and discuss any research plans widely before you get started. Many hospitals have a Research and Development team or a clinical trials unit who will give advice, or you may find support from colleagues at a local university. In England, there are Research Design Services which cover the whole country and are funded to give clinicians support in designing good research and suggesting possible sources of funding.

Probably one of the most structured ways to gain research skills is doing a supervised research thesis as part of a Masters qualification. There are many to choose from and it is very important to pick a course that suits both your interests and your learning style. Some nurses are clinicians through and through and will

419

thrive best if learning advanced clinical skills. Others are more theoretical in outlook. If your primary purpose in doing a Masters is to gain research skills and experience, make sure what the attitude of your chosen institution is to empirical research for your Masters thesis (some try to discourage doing actual research). While it can be challenging to get everything in place in time (such as Ethics and R&D approvals), if you are organised and determined from the start it is achievable.

If your primary motivation for undertaking a Masters is research skills and experience, you should look at Masters in Research (MRes) courses. These will have a much larger emphasis on your research project than most MSc courses, usually enabling you to complete a more ambitious study. Many of the courses are offered are multidisciplinary, giving a rich mix of fellow students and perspectives from a variety of backgrounds and clinical areas.

Multidisciplinary research

Starting research or even audit on your own can be very daunting and lack of experience can lead to much time and effort being wasted on projects that are never completed. If you are a novice researcher, don't struggle alone – find someone more experienced to mentor or even partner you. The best way to start is often to join in as part of the team with an existing funded project. If you work with medical colleagues who conduct research, use every opportunity to learn from them.

To start with, this might mean recruiting patients by explaining studies to potential participants. To do this you will need to be familiar with the research protocol and the patient information sheet, in order to be able to identify suitable people and answer any questions. If you show interest, colleagues may invite you to be part of the research team and attend team meetings.

Patient involvement in research teams is becoming increasingly recognised as important, particularly for obtaining external funding. Your initial participation in the research team may be conducting an audit or focus group among patients to clarify what are the important issues for them in any proposed research. Offering to help in this way can be a useful introduction to survey techniques and make a genuinely patient-focused contribution to the research team.

Alternatively, you might consider whether there are aspects of a planned research project which would be stronger if you added an element. An example might be a qualitative study on patient experience of taking a new medication that is the subject of a drug trial. Questions might include what is the patient experience of the new drug (positive and negative), is the dosing regimen acceptable, and are any side-effects tolerable? After all, there is no point developing a really effective new product if patients are unlikely to take it in the way intended. Spotting opportunities for 'piggy-backing' your research questions into existing or planned studies (obviously with appropriate Ethics approval) is an excellent way to learn research skills.

Or you might start by attending a journal club and listening to the way research papers are discussed and critiqued. Try reading Trish Greenhalgh's short book (Greenhalgh, 2006), or start with her classic paper (Greenhalgh, 1999). Attending conferences and listening to research presentations is also an excellent way of becoming familiar with research-minded thinking.

With experience comes confidence. It is amazing how the terminology and concepts of research become less daunting once you are familiar and comfortable with them. Language and methods which seemed impenetrable will gradually become as easy as clinical terms which were once difficult.

Nurse-led research

There is a need for research on almost every aspect of IBD nursing. At the simplest level, this could be the introduction of a new service or care pathway, with an audit of patient feedback, experience or waiting times before and after. We have very limited evidence that what we do makes a real difference to patients, yet we all believe that it does. But without evidence it is very hard to argue for scarce resources being devoted to IBD care rather than other equally compelling areas of health. For this reason, those in specialist services really do have a responsibility to demonstrate their worth and protect, if not expand, their service. How much harder will it be for administrators to think of cutting back a service which has published excellent results?

We also need evidence for nursing interventions for all aspects of IBD care. Symptom management in IBD has until recently been much neglected compared to drug and surgical interventions. Yet ongoing symptoms often have a tremendous impact on work and social life as well as psychological coping. Once you have the skills and confidence, there are numerous questions that need answering. One productive way to get started is to work with other IBD nurses and develop both the idea and the plan, then collect and pool data so that you have a much bigger study than you could ever do on your own, as well as sharing ideas and workload.

Funding for research

Not all research needs specific funding. Your manager may agree to some time and local consumables (some photocopying or phone calls) within existing resources if you are starting with an audit. You may find that you have access to help from your local audit department, who will often offer advice and even give help with analysing questionnaires or conducting focus groups.

Small grants of a few hundred or a few thousand pounds are also available from national bodies such as the Foundation for Nursing Studies or the Royal College of Nursing. Sometimes it may be appropriate to approach a commercial company such as a drug company for help or funding with conducting research, although if you are inexperienced with this, seeking advice from a senior colleague is prudent.

Once you become more ambitious, there are numerous local and national sources of funding. Have a look at the National Institutes of Health Research (NIHR) website (http://www.nihr.ac.uk/research/Pages/default.aspx). The Research for Patient Benefit funding stream is often appropriate for the research questions that nurses ask and the Research Design Service (RDS) locally is there to help you formulate your research question and protocol (see http://www.nihr.ac.uk/infrastructure/Pages/infrastructure_research_design_services.aspx to find your local contact). To apply for one of these grants you will need a credible team for the application and it often takes several months of hard work to develop the application. The rewards are also big – for example you can obtain funding for a research assistant to help with conducting your study and collecting the data.

Disseminating the evidence

Many times you will read an article or listen to a presentation and think 'I could have said that'. So why didn't you? Many IBD nurses conduct projects or audits, or write a Masters thesis, but very few complete the process by publishing the results to share with others. This is a great pity, as the body of knowledge is weak at present and some would say it is not ethical to ask patients to participate in a project and then not disseminate the results.

It really is not as difficult as you might imagine to have an article published or a conference paper or poster accepted. Obviously, you need to have something to say, and a target audience in mind. Who do you want to reach? This will tell you where to try to get published. Is your message for general nurses, specialist nurses or a multidisciplinary audience? Primary or secondary care or both? Which journals does your target audience read, or which conferences do they go to?

For a journal article, look at the instructions for authors and the type of articles that have been published recently. Don't be shy about phoning or emailing the editor and discussing your idea – this can give you valuable feedback and save you wasting a lot of time. It will also give you encouragement if the journal is positive about your idea.

If you don't know where to start when writing, it can help to start with the section you find easiest and build around that. Or imagine that you are giving a teaching session on your topic and write the PowerPoint slides – this will give you a basic structure to work with. Divide your presentation into background (what is the problem, how many people does it affect, what are the consequences and implications for the patient and/or the service?). Then describe what you did and how (a literature review will need a search strategy and how you decided what to include or exclude; an audit or research project will need a description of how the information was gathered). The discussion section should relate what you have found to other previous work and put it into context and a conclusion should summarise and draw out implications for your audience.

For a conference abstract, take careful note of the submission deadline and word limit. Posters can be a gentle start if you lack the confidence to present a paper. Although constructing a poster takes some time and thought, the facilities to produce these relatively cheaply are available in every commercial print shop. If you do not have access to professional designers, producing a simple design on a single PowerPoint slide can enable you to cut and paste text diagrams and photographs and position them as you wish. The poster will raise the profile of both your service and your organisation (and should be added to your curriculum vitae!).

With either a publication or a conference submission, get other people to be 'critical friends' by reading and giving you feedback on drafts. Use clear plain language, avoid too many abbreviations and don't use jargon. Wiley produce a free online resource which is useful if you are new to writing: see http://www.nurseauthoreditor.com/.

Conclusion

Despite increasing numbers of IBD nurses, IBD nursing is still in its early stages of development. For the speciality to become established and secure there is a need to develop the research base and to be seen to be leading implementation of research. The impetus for this will not come from others – IBD nurses will need to do this for themselves. Others may help, but ultimately IBD nurses will bear the responsibility if this does not happen. Collaborating with helpful colleagues and making patients' needs the focus of your research and writing will ultimately benefit your patients, helping to secure the future of your service and enhance your own career progression.

References

Bowling, A. (2002) *Research Methods in Health: Investigating Health and Health Services*, 2nd edn. Maidenhead: Open University Press.

Callum, N., DiCenso, A. and Chiliska, D. (1997). Evidence-based nursing: an introduction. *Evidence-Based Nursing*, Pre-release mini-issue, iv–v.

Gerrish, K. and Lacey, A. (2010) *The Research Process in Nursing*, 6th edn. Oxford: Wiley-Blackwell.

Greenhalgh, T. (1999) How to read a paper. *Br. Med. J.*, **315**, 672–4.

Greenhalgh, T. (2006) *How to Read a Paper: the Basics of Evidence-based Medicine*, 3rd edn. Oxford: BMJ Books, Blackwell Publishing.

Royal College of Nursing (2007) *Role Descriptives for Inflammatory Bowel Disease Nurse Specialists – RCN Guidance*. London: Royal College of Nursing.

Polit, D. F., Beck, C. T. and Hungler, B. P. (2001) *Essentials of Nursing Research*, 5th edn. Philadelphia: Lippincott.

CHAPTER 24

A vision of the future: celebrating the increasing sphere of influence

Isobel Mason

Introduction

Within the UK, inflammatory bowel disease (IBD) nursing has proliferated over the last ten years. Specialist nursing roles within secondary care are increasing. The last national audit of IBD care showed that 62% of acute Trusts have specialist IBD nurses in post (UK IBD Audit Steering Group, 2009) compared to 26% in 2005 (Crohn's and Colitis UK, 2005a). This proliferation reflects the acknowledgement by patients and patient groups, the nursing and medical community, acute Trusts and workforce planners of the essential role that IBD nursing provides within the patient experience.

The most recent government white paper on the future of the National Health Service (NHS) (Department of Health, 2010) sets the political vision and principles for patient care in the coming years. Putting patients at the heart of services, focusing on clinical outcomes and empowering healthcare professionals are the underpinning themes.

Undoubtedly, within IBD services and the care of those with long-term illnesses, the nurse specialist role will be fundamental in meeting these objectives. As services and nurses look to the future, important questions are raised: what can they expect to be the key influences on IBD nursing? How will nurses' sphere of influence clinically, locally, regionally, nationally and even internationally continue to increase? This chapter will celebrate the increasing influence IBD nurses have within the speciality, including a discussion around the likely changes to this influence within the coming years.

Case study

An IBD team in an acute trust met to discuss the implications of new national guidance on biologic treatments in Crohn's disease on the service and how to change the team's approach to include patient choice in these treatments. The IBD nurse within the team already had a good working knowledge of the guidance after contributing to its development by providing comments throughout via the Royal College of Nursing (RCN) Crohn's and colitis special interest group. The nurse was also able to feed back the patient's perspective, following a patient satisfaction survey of the current biologic service and discussion of the new guidance with the Trust IBD patient panel. The nurse had coordinated the panel meetings every three months which included several patients who were receiving biologic treatment at the time.

After the team agreed the necessary changes to practice arising from the new guidance the IBD nurse then reviewed the written patient information on treatment, the departmental guideline on its use, and the shared care guideline used to facilitate monitoring in primary care. The team agreed that patients, where appropriate, should be offered the choice between the available biologic treatments and that they should all be offered a review by the IBD nurse to discuss the practicalities of the treatments and to answer questions, whilst screening tests are carried out and funding for treatment is obtained.

This case study illustrates an example of an IBD nurse's central role within an IBD multidisciplinary team and reflects the increasing influence of the IBD nurse on patient involvement, evidence based care and care organisation. Ten years ago in the UK this nursing role existed in only a few specialist centres, whereas nurses are now commonly available to improve service planning and delivery and therefore influence clinical outcomes and patient experience.

Putting patients first

Clinically, increasing numbers of patients are finding that the nurse is their first point of contact with the specialist IBD team. IBD nurses provide ever-expanding nursing services to give patients more information and support and effective access to care. Many IBD nurses also provide advanced nursing services, including advanced assessment, diagnosis, treatment initiation, prescribing and evaluation. At a local level IBD nurses spearhead service development, increasing user involvement, making services more robust through the development and implementation of local guidelines and audit, keeping services patient focused and meeting individuals' needs.

IBD patients encounter nurses at all stages of their care pathway, in both hospital (secondary care) and the community (primary) care. In secondary care, some of these nurses become more familiar to them. It has often been these regular contacts that have led to the development of specialist nursing roles. As the nurse–patient relationship develops, so both parties identify the value that regular contact with an expert nurse can give to the patients' experience. Nurses are also increasingly aware of the effects of IBD on patients' quality of life and have identified a real need for effective nursing information and support. This, in turn, means that patients and other healthcare professionals have expectations that these expert nursing contacts address more than the physical clinical need.

Nurse specialist roles to provide this care have developed significantly in the UK, but geographically remain patchy. The value to patients has been documented and is universally accepted and published in seminal papers such as the British Society of Gastroenterology (BSG) Strategy Document (British Society of Gastroenterology, 2006), the National Standards for IBD care (IBD Standards Group, 2009), national patient-led campaigns (Crohn's and Colitis UK, 2005b) and the RCN role descriptives document (Royal College of Nursing, 2007).

There is an expectation that nurse specialist roles in IBD in the UK will continue to increase, and this may be reflected in similar role developments internationally. Certainly, there has been the political will to do so. The National Standards for IBD care (IBD Standards Group 2009) identify the nurse specialist role as fundamental and now state that there needs to be more than one nurse per department, so services are not closed when that nurse is away. These standards do have some influence and have facilitated some new nursing posts, but gaining funding can often be a struggle. Increasing financial pressures on public services is only going to increase the difficulty in finding money and may even lead to the withdrawal of funding for some posts.

It is clear that, currently, more patients than previously have contact with an IBD nurse specialist. The nature of that individual nurse's role does change from centre to centre. Previously, IBD nurse specialists often combined their role with other aspects of GI specialist care (e.g. nurse endoscopy, stoma care, outpatient nursing). However, over recent years they appear to have become increasingly specialised, focusing on IBD care only. Whether this trend will continue in the current financial climate remains to be seen.

The development of biologic treatments have meant that many nurses have a significant role in the administration of these therapies. Until now, and the recent NICE guidance on biological therapy in Crohn's disease (National Institute for Health and Clinical Excellence, 2010), nurses have focused on day case infusion services. Home self-administered biologics are becoming increasingly available and have, at last, enabled patient choice. This will change many nurse specialist roles considerably. Nurses will have to help patients make important treatment decisions and then support more of them at home, whilst continuing to provide a considerable day case service.

Many nurse specialists in the UK develop their roles to include advanced nursing practice. This may include physical assessment skills, the ability to request investigation, carrying out an endoscopy procedure, making treatment decisions under local guidelines and prescribing. Advanced nursing roles are not fundamental to a specialist nurse's role, but do complement it. Taking a call from a distressed patient requires skilled assessment and clinical judgement. Allowing nurses to complete the patient's treatment cycle without breaking continuity of care can improve the quality of the patient's journey.

Advanced nursing in the UK has been championed for many years and is now commonplace in both primary and secondary care. Patients are used to meeting nurses who carry out roles that previously were seen as being in the medical domain, in all aspects of their healthcare provision. IBD care is no different and these advanced roles will continue to proliferate. This is supported, with some reservations about the financial climate (Longley *et al.*, 2007).

Putting patients at the heart of the NHS is a fundamental aim of the UK government (Department of Health, 2010). This government white paper requests 'an information revolution and greater choice and control' for those who use our services. Continuing this theme, the NMC acknowledges that it will give a high priority to supporting self-care of growing numbers of patients living with long-term conditions (Longley *et al.*, 2007). Models of self-care facilitation have been well evaluated within IBD care (Barlow *et al.*, 2010). Providing information, support and patient education reduces the burden on services and allows patients to take more control of their disease process and management. Specialist nursing roles are central to this. The expert patient requires support, information and effective contact with the specialist team. The IBD nursing service provides this facility, with telephone and email advice lines central to patient empowerment.

Patients in the UK will have the choice of any provider of specialist care, choice of consultant-led team, choice of community care and choice of treatment (Department of Health, 2010). The IBD nursing role will continue to be an essential part of this patient empowerment, often providing support to patients whilst negotiating their care and choosing treatment options.

Also committed to supporting and empowering patients, Crohn's and Colitis UK is a powerful patient association that works closely with healthcare professionals across the UK to improve standards of IBD care. This association is dedicated to increasing user involvement in service delivery and actively supports the development of patient panels. These are initiatives through which people affected by colitis and Crohn's disease and the professionals involved in their care can exchange ideas on how local services for IBD are best developed (Crohn's and Colitis UK, 2005b). The most recent national audit of IBD care showed that user involvement is actively encouraged in only 28% of UK acute Trusts (UK IBD Audit Steering Group, 2009). The IBD nursing role is seen as a key relationship within the functioning of panels. Where those panels exist, IBD nurse specialists are often central in their planning, organisation and effectiveness. This type of nursing activity will have to increase to meet the demands of increasing user involvement.

Empowering healthcare professionals

Advanced and specialist practice must be underpinned by formalised education as well as close supervision and assessment locally. Whether through specialist IBD nursing modules or through generic advanced nursing courses, those nurse specialists must have the underpinning nursing theories and clinical knowledge to support practice. The NMC has acknowledged that 'there is a debate concerning the appropriate level of education for advanced level practice and this is linked to pre-registration educational requirements' (Longley *et al.*, 2007). As UK nursing moves towards the goal of becoming a graduate profession (Nursing and Midwifery Council, 2008), the pressure for advanced nurses to have Masters level education, relevant to their area of expertise, is going to increase. However, funding and study time are decreasing in the current financial climate. External education and qualifications are fundamental, but must be combined with in-house supervision, through formal departmental meetings and case reviews and through mentorship and supervision from other specialists in IBD care, whether medical or from other more experienced nurses. It may be that portfolio development and the ability to gain qualifications using competence in practice will become more common as the ability to fund and release nurses for study reduces and financial pressures on educational establishments increase.

Showing competence in practice is central to patient safety. In 2007, the UK government asked for the development of standards for higher level practice in particular for advanced practice in nursing (Department of Health, 2007). It accepted that the formal regulation of advanced practice is not required (Council for Healthcare Regulatory Excellence, 2009). Recommendations suggest that governance arrangements for advanced practice should be the responsibility of the employer. The NMC has acknowledged the need for greater structure and guidance and are currently planning a project group to develop national standards for higher level practice.

The delivery of IBD nurses' educational and professional development needs will change. As multimedia education becomes more commonplace, traditional lecture based, face-to-face traditional teaching methods will decrease. Already, online distance learning is a recognised methodology and this will expand. Nurses also have far more access to professional information and up-to-date evidence for care through all sorts of Internet applications, including free electronic libraries.

Just as post-qualification nursing education develops, so does the educational role of the nurse specialist in teaching and developing other healthcare professionals. As nurses' influence within local care increases, so they will have more teaching responsibilities within the multidisciplinary team. Whether teaching nurses, junior doctors, trainee gastroenterologists, pharmacists or dietitians, the fact that IBD nurse specialists are increasingly running clinical services means that they will be required to teach others about clinical and organisational aspects of the care they provide. The roles of ward, endoscopy and outpatient nurses are fundamental within the patient experience. Specialist nurses need to develop these nurses, using their clinical knowledge (understanding assessment and care planning and treatment strategies). National audit (UK IBD Steering Group, 2009) has shown how poor some standards of care can be: for example, inpatient nutritional assessment and weighing, taking stool cultures and providing good access to toilets. Nurses need to expand their influence beyond the direct face-to-face contact they have with patients to improve care at all points of the patient's journey.

There are many ways of doing this, but fundamentally, contact between the nurse specialist and other nurses within the specialty is key. Nurse specialists provide an important role model in nursing care to others and can have great influence. Facilitating IBD nursing, teaching nurses and providing them with a rationale for their care is an essential role of the nurse specialist. Projects such as documentation review, core care planning, care pathways that focus on bowel care, or the development of link nursing roles are all formal ways of doing this. As the number of nurse specialists increases and their time in post lengthens, these are vital local developments they must facilitate.

Whilst developing roles, nurses also need to remain aware of what makes them different from medical colleagues. The holistic view, the complementary, empathetic relationship and the caring role – all these aspects must underpin the patient–nurse contact.

IBD nurse specialists are almost entirely based in secondary care. The role has developed with support and guidance from gastroenterologists and is a central part of the hospital team. However, nursing services often bridge the gap between primary and secondary care. Primary care practitioners will call on the nurse specialist as their first source of advice. Nurses will often facilitate shared care guidelines to help patients keep their care local.

The coalition Government white paper *Equity and Excellence: Liberating the NHS* (Department of Health, 2010) will bring about the greatest change in the relationships between GPs and specialist services in the UK seen in a generation. The plan to devolve power and responsibility to healthcare professionals (through GPs and their practice teams) will significantly change service commissioning. Patients, particularly when in remission, will be able to request to have their routine reviews locally, and primary care services will be developed to provide this. The NMC, too, has acknowledged the change in hospital/community relationships with 'blurring of primary and secondary roles' in the next five years (Longley *et al.*, 2007).

IBD nurses are ideally placed to work in these services. The national standards call for all patients to have an annual review (IBD Standards Group, 2009), but acknowledge that this may not be in the traditional hospital outpatient setting; however, it must be undertaken by a member of the specialist IBD team working in primary care (this could easily be a nurse).

Improving clinical outcomes

Again, the white paper *Equity and Excellence: Liberating the NHS* (Department of Health, 2010) gives a clear message about the importance of showing effective working in terms of good clinical outcomes. 'The NHS will be held to account against clinically credible and evidence-based outcome measures, not process targets' (page 4). This is a fundamental shift in the evaluation of service provision. The national standards for IBD care (IBD Standards Group, 2009) are a good example of such evidence-based outcome measures, and importantly IBD nurses have been involved at all stages of their development. Indeed, national audit has shown that in those acute Trusts where IBD nurses are in post, standards of clinical care in all areas are higher than those without a dedicated nursing post (UK IBD Audit Steering Group, 2009).

Looking beyond the basics of clinical care, psychological pathways are now acknowledged to be a core standard of IBD care (IBD Standards Group, 2009). Providing information and support, listening to patients and their carers, whether through face-to-face contact, or through telephone advice lines, is the first point of such a pathway. As standard, IBD nurse specialists provide this level of support (Royal College of Nursing, 2007). However, nurses will need to develop the confidence and skill to supplement this basic support with the ability to identify patients at greater need of professional psychological input. National audit has shown that currently very few Trusts have a pathway for this area of care (UK IBD Audit Steering Group, 2009). Crohn's and Colitis UK is in the process of facilitating multidisciplinary guidelines on psychological care. Anecdotally, nurses often feel that whilst their role of support and information is clear, they cannot and should not provide more formal methods of counselling or psychological assessment. However, nurses may be the first healthcare professional that patients share their inner thoughts with, and they need the confidence and skills to open the discussion about how patients feel about living with their illness and the impact it is having on all aspects of their lives.

Psychological pathways must include training and supervision to encourage this. The development of similar pathways in other specialties show they must also identify clear services (whether through counsellors or psychology services) and routes of referral for those patients that nurses feel need professional psychological support once they have identified that need (National Institute for Health and Clinical Excellence, 2004). Psychosocial pathways of care are explored in depth in Chapter 16.

Whilst the impact of IBD nursing is often reiterated in anecdotes and narrative, it is clear that an underpinning evidence base for the role is severely lacking. (as discussed in detail in Chapter 23). A Cochrane review of the IBD nursing role highlighted this in 2006 (Woods *et al.*, 2006), identifying the lack of good quality research and audit into the role. IBD nurses, often locally, collect data on the impact of their role, but publications are scarce and the quality is low. Woods *et al.* (2006) make two main recommendations: there is a need for the development of nationally accepted descriptors of the IBD nursing role, whilst effective audit and review of national practice and its impact on patient care is also required. The seminal work published in the RCN role descriptors (Royal College of Nursing, 2007) document meets the first of these recommendations. National audit of IBD nursing, providing evidence of current practice and mapping it against outcomes and the descriptors document will be fundamental to meet the second, and strengthen the evidence base demanded by patients, commissioners and managers.

Only through effective national working will the real value of the IBD nursing role be measured and shown both to local providers and on the national platform. Individual nurses have a responsibility to increase the evidence base, and this can be achieved as Masters level education expands, with nurses completing dissertations and practice development portfolios to gain the required qualifications. The publication of this type of nursing audit and research will show the real impact that IBD nursing has on clinical outcomes.

National and international influence

The RCN gastroenterology and stoma care forum provides a strong national voice and influence for IBD nursing. Nine regional groups across the UK have developed over the last decade, allowing nurses to network and support each other. These regional groups are supported by a central committee. Members of the forum now represent IBD nurses in many influential positions with other agencies, including the BSG, RCN, Crohn's and Colitis UK, and with pharmaceutical companies. This emerging national working has allowed IBD nurses to influence many drivers for change within the speciality including the National Standards for IBD care, NICE appraisals of technologies and treatments, the national audit plan and research development.

This national influence is now beginning to be repeated within the European arena, with UK IBD nurses leading and representing IBD nursing issues through the European Crohn's and Colitis Organisation (ECCO). The RCN forum has created the ability for any IBD nurse specialist, with support from their peers, to influence national and European policy and clinical guidelines. This is an outstanding achievement. This level of influence can only increase as the body of IBD nurses in the UK expands in number, experience and confidence.

In summary

There are many reasons to celebrate the achievements of IBD nursing as a specialist area of practice over recent years:

- Greater numbers of patients have contact with IBD specialist nurses and benefit from the role.
- Nurses now have a positive influence on more patients' experience of IBD care.
- Nurses are spearheading local service development and driving up clinical standards.
- National standards and frameworks for IBD care include and have been influenced by IBD nurses.

- Nurses are influencing patients' treatment choice through the provision of information and support. This facilitates the ability to self-care.
- IBD nurses are developing advanced skill, critical thinking and nursing expertise.
- Where services involve users and their groups, this is often facilitated by nurses.
- Nurses are increasingly highly educated with formal qualifications to underpin their clinical competence.
- There is more nursing influence over the development of other nurses and healthcare professionals.
- Across the UK there is a productive, well-developed national network available for all IBD nurses, and a strong European wide network is developing.

Conclusion

There is so much good work to celebrate, but certainly in the UK and many other countries the provision of IBD nursing services is still patchy. Although now formally defined, roles vary greatly and there is limited publication of nurses' roles or their impact. As part of this celebratory process, perhaps IBD nurses should gain more confidence. By advertising and promoting the vital work they do in changing patients' experiences, not only will numbers continue to increase, but those currently working will feel more secure.

IBD nursing is complex: professionals must call upon their theoretical knowledge, clinical expertise and experience to effectively manage patient care. Specialist roles such as this are, however, difficult to standardise: the individual nature of IBD nursing posts should be driven by local need whilst adhering to national standards and role descriptives. Nurses who are able to provide holistic care – supporting patients, acting as their advocate and facilitating their care, working (and acknowledged) as key members of the IBD team – will feel more confident and supported to develop their role. Greater confidence and security, combined with a robust career framework, effective national and international working, and an underpinning evidence base are all factors which will ultimately shape the future success of this nursing speciality.

References

Barlow, C., Cook, D., Mulligan, K., Beck, E. and Newman, S. (2010) A critical review of self-management and educational interventions in inflammatory bowel disease. *Gastroenterol. Nurs.*, **33**, 11–18.

British Society of Gastroenterology (2006) *Care of Patients with Gastrointestinal Disor-*

ders in the United Kingdom: A Strategy for the Future. http://www.bsg.org.uk/clinical/ publications/index.html (accessed 1 August 2010)

Council for Healthcare Regulatory Excellence (2009) *Advanced Practice: Report to the Four UK Health Departments.* http://www.aanpe.org/LinkClick.aspx?fileticket=FU% 2B5JnHM1aw%3D&tabid=1386&mid=2768&language=en-US (accessed 22 September 2010).

Crohn's and Colitis UK (2005a) *Survey Exposing the Shortage of IBD Nurses.* http://www. nacc.org.uk/downloads/media/NACCSurveyRelease.pdf (accessed 1 August 2010).

Crohn's and Colitis UK (2005b) *NACC Plan 2005-8.* http://www.nacc.org.uk/content/ about/patientPanels.asp (accessed 1 August 2010).

Department of Health (2007) *Trust Assurance and Safety – the Regulation of Health Professionals in the 21st Century.* http://www.dh.gov.uk/en/Publicationsandstatistics/Publications/PublicationsPolicyAndGuidance/DH_065946 (accessed 1 August 2010).

Department of Health (2010) *Equity and Excellence: Liberating the NHS.* http://www. dh.gov.uk/en/Publicationsandstatistics/Publications/PublicationsPolicyAndGuidance/ DH_117353 (accessed 1 August 2010).

IBD Standards Group (2009) *Quality Care Service Standards for the Healthcare of People Who Have IBD.* http://www.ibdstandards.org.uk (accessed 1 August 2010)

Longley, M., Shaw, C. and Dolan, G. (2007) *Nursing: Towards 2015: Alternative Scenarios for Healthcare, Nursing and Nurse Education in the UK in 2015.* http://www.nmc-uk.org/Documents/Research%20papers/Nursing%20towards%202015%20full%20report%20.pdf (accessed 22 September 2010).

National Institute for Health and Clinical Excellence (2004) *Guidance on Cancer Services. Improving Supportive and Palliative Care for Adults with Cancer.* http://www.nice.org. uk/csgsp (accessed 22 September 2010).

National Institute for Health and Clinical Excellence (2010) *Infliximab (Review) and Adalimumab for the Treatment of Crohn's Disease.* http://guidance.nice.org.uk/TA/ Wave13/78 (accessed 22 September 2010).

Nursing and Midwifery Council (2008) *Nurse Education: Now and in the Future.* http:// www.nmc-uk.org/Get-involved/Consultations/Past-consultations/By-year/Pre-registration-nursing-education-Phase-2/Nurse-education-Now-and-in-the-future-/ (accessed 1 August 10).

Royal College of Nursing (2007) *Role Descriptives for Inflammatory Bowel Disease Nurse Specialists – RCN guidance.* London: Royal College of Nursing.

UK IBD Audit Steering Group (2009) *UK IBD Audit Second Round (2008) Report.* http:// www.rcplondon.ac.uk/clinical-standards/ceeu/Current-work/IBD/Documents/UK-IBD-Audit-2nd-Round-Full-National-Report-(2008).pdf (accessed 22 September 2010).

Woods, L., Belling, R. and McLaren, S. (2006) A systematic review of the effectiveness of inflammatory bowel disease nurse specialists. *Int. J. Nurs. Pract.*, **14**, 67–73.

Index

5-aminosalicylates   247–9, 271
6-mercaptopurine   271

abdominal pain   47
abscess   68
adalimumab   123, 250
adolescents   259–75, 281–91, 368–9
Advanced Nurse Practitioner   375, 377
advice service   384
aetiology   13
alcohol   141, 150
anaemia   142, 143–4
anal sphincter, incompetent   182
anastomosis   115–16
   anal   180
anastomotic leakage   172
anorexia   142
antibiotics   129, 251
antidepressants   305
anxiety   302
appendix   23–4, 34–5
arthritis   52
ASCT see autologous stem cell transplant
assessment   81–93
   holistic   307
      objective measurements   33–4
   physical   92–3
   proforma   86–7
audit   371, 391, 409–10
autologous stem cell transplant   130
autophagy   16–17
azathioprine   125, 271

B_{12} deficiency   144
baby care   253
bacteria   7
barium follow-through   66–7
biologicals   213–14, 250
biological service   388–9, 408

blood tests   71–2
bone mineral density   145
bowel obstruction   236
brain–gut axis   300
breastfeeding   17, 253–4

cancer   164–5
carbohydrates, refined   140
CD see Crohn's disease
cereals   148
childbirth   253
children   259–75
   different healthcare from adults   282
   family focused care   282
   growth assessment   263–4
   investigations   74
   paediatric services   273–4
   psychosocial impact   273
   schooling   274, 318
   Sneha Wadhwani   317
chronic disease management   334–5
chronic illness   295–6
ciclosporin   320
Ciclosporin A   251
clinical features   47–55
clinical guidelines   364
clinical networks   368
Clinical Nurse Specialist   375, 379–92, 397
   role of   399–400
   scope of practice   382–92
   see also specialist nurses
Clostridium difficile   72
cobblestoning   12
Cochrane reviews   416
colectomy
   segmental   174
   subtotal   162
   total   167

colitis, indeterminate   182
colon   227
colorectal cancer   54
  surveillance   387
colostomates   207
colostomy   203
  diet   207
  irrigation   207
communication skills   85, 90–1
complementary therapies   305
computed tomography   67–8
constipation   48
contraception   21, 35, 245
contrast studies   66
corticosteroids   249–50, 270
counselling   183–5
C-reactive protein   72
Crohn's and Colitis UK   267–74, 360,
    401
Crohn's disease   9–10
  active extensive   236
  clinical course   51
  clinical features in children   267
  clinical presentation   50–1
  colonic   172, 174–5
  dietary treatment   145–6
  histopathology   12
  intestinal   172
  intestinal failure   223–38
  Montreal classification   50
  oral   128
  pathology   12
  perianal   176–7
  perianal fistulising   73–4
  small bowel   172
  smoking   33–4
  surgery   171–7
  time trends   30–1
  treatment failure   130
Crohn's in Childhood Research
    Association   360
CRP *see* C-reactive protein
CT *see* computed tomography
cytokine profiles   6–7, 22–3

Department of Health   334–5
depression   302
devolved healthcare   370–1
diagnostic algorithm   75

diarrhoea   47, 142, 318
  bloody   63
diet   36, 139
  fibre   229
  ileoanal pouch   186–7
  oral nutrition   232
  reduced oral intake   230
  research   151–7
differential diagnosis   62–3
digestion   5
disability benefit   327–8
Disability Discrimination Act   299
dyspepsia   142
dysplasia   164–5

eating disorders   303
ECM locus   17
elderly patients, investigations in   74
electronic care records   371
employment   298
empowering healthcare
    professionals   429–31
endoscopy   62–5
enteral nutrition   87–8
enteric microflora   22
enterocutaneous fistula   69
environmental risk factors   17–21, 32–9
epidemiology   29–39
erectile dysfunction   184, 244
erythema nodosum   52–4
erythrocyte sedimentation rate   72
Escherichia coli   20
ESR *see* erythrocyte sedimentation rate
European Federation for Crohn's
    and Ulcerative Colitis
    Associations   372
eye conditions   54

faecal incontinence   282–3
fatigue   342
fats   141
FDA drug categories   248
fecundity   184
fertility   184–5, 241–54
  men   244
  typical problems   243
  women   244
fibre   18, 147, 187, 229
fibrostenotic disease   121–2

fish   148
fistulae   10, 213–19
   anal   177
   appliances   216
   discharge   217–18
   enterocutaneous   155–9, 232–5
      management   233
      nutrition   233–6
   general advice   218
   mucous   203–4
   pain control   219
   perforation site   234
   perianal   214, 217, 219
   rectovaginal   214, 217
   sexual intercourse   219
   skin care   217
   spontaneous closure   235
   tract development   176–7
   types of   214
fistula-in-ano   176
FODMAP   149
folate deficiency   144
food aversions and intolerances   147–9
fructan   149
fruit   148
fundraising   331
future of IBD nursing   425–36

Gastrointestinal Quality of Life
   Index   297
gastrointestinal strictures   148
genetics   260–1
genetic testing   73
geographical distribution   29–30
glucose–saline solution   230
GQLI *see* Gastrointestinal Quality of Life
   Index
grains   148
grief, stages of   315–16
growth failure   261–4
   aetiology   262–3
   incidence   262
gut   3–7
   absorptive properties   226–7
   anatomy   4
   cross-section   6
   malfunction   5–7
   pathology   11–13
   physiology   5–7

handover clinic   284
HEADS acronym   230–1
healthcare worker   283–4
health promotion   387–8
health-related quality of life   296–8
helplines   194
histology   73
history taking   84–5, 120
holding on techniques   337–8
Hospital and Depression Scale   308
HRQOL *see* health-related quality of life
hydration   150
hygiene theory   19

IBDQ *see* Inflammatory Bowel Disease
   Questionnaire
IBD Standards Group   362, 401
IBD-U *see* IBD (unclassified)
IBD (unclassified)   13, 51
identical twins   15
IF *see* intestinal failure
ileal thickening   69
ileoanal pouch   165, 168–9, 175
   absorption   186–7
   care of   179–94
   children   192
   compliance   185–6
   Crohn's disease reclassification   191
   diet   186–7
   dysfunction   187–91
   elderly people   192
   failure   191
   fistulation   190
   formation   181
   functional outflow obstruction   191
   patient selection   181–2
   retained rectal cuff   191
   urge resistance   185–6
ileoanal surgery, contraindications   182
ileocolonoscopy   62–4
ileo pouch anal anastomosis   180–1
ileorectal anastomosis   167
ileostomate   202
ileostomy   162, 202
   complications   164
   diet   208
   everted spout   179
   loop   179
immune deficiency   23

immunomodulator therapy   271
immunosuppressants   386–7, 407
immunosuppression   123, 131
  risks   127
infection   36–9
inflammatory bowel disease
  aetiology   13–17
  age trends   31
  children
    diagnosis and investigation   266–9
    clinical features in   264–5
  classification   3
  complex   117–33
  dietary causes   82–3
  epidemiology   261
  extra-intestinal manifestations   52–4
  in further education   318
  genetic factors   14–17
  geographical incidence   29–30
  growth failure   261–4
  heritability   245–6
  living with   315–23, 343–4
  Montreal classification   265
  nurse's role   132
  psychosocial aspects   295
  public awareness   329–30
  sex trends   31
  socioeconomic class   32
  time trends   30–1
  treatment in children   269
  triggers   13
  urban–rural differences   32
  work   298–9
Inflammatory Bowel Disease
    Questionnaire   297, 304
infliximab   123, 272, 320, 321
  pregnancy   250
information   344–5
inpatient management   389
interleukin-23 receptor   17
international links   371–2, 433
Internet   328, 345
intestinal barrier function   21–2
intestinal failure   223–38
  nursing   236–8
  psychological implications   237–8
  types of   224
investigations   61–76

jejunostomy   169–71
jejunum-colon anastomosis   232

key worker   285
Kock continent ileostomy *see* Kock pouch
Kock pouch   167–8, 179

lactose intolerance   148
leukocyte scintigraphy   70
liver   54
liver function tests   72
loperamide   231

magnesium deficiency   143, 231
magnetic resonance imaging   9–10, 69–70
malnutrition   142, 228
margarine   18–20
MDT *see* multidisciplinary team
measles   20, 38
meat   141, 148
MEDLINE   416
mental health   296
mesalazine   318
methotrexate   124, 250, 319
milk   141, 148
Montreal classification   48, 50, 265
mood   303
motility   226
MRI *see* magnetic resonance imaging
MTX *see* methotrexate
mucosal immune system   6–7
  dysregulation   22–3
multidisciplinary meetings   390
multidisciplinary team   193–4, 360
Mycobacterium paratuberculosis   20–1,
    37–8
mycophenolate mofetil   125

NACC *see* Crohn's and Colitis UK
natalizumab   130
National Association for Colitis and
    Crohn's Disease *see* Crohn's and
    Colitis UK
networking   333–4
NOD2 gene   16
non-steroidal anti-inflammatory drugs   21,
    35–6
nuclear medicine   70
Nurse Consultant   375, 378

nurse-led clinics   326–327, 406
Nurses European Crohn's and Colitis
    network   391
nursing assessment   81–93
Nursing Process   83–4
nursing roles   376–7
nutrient malabsorption   142
nutrition   128–9
  growth failure   262
  parenteral   237
nutritional problems   141–5
nutritional therapy   211–12
nuts   148

obesity   141
obsessional behaviour   303–4
omeprazole   231
organisation of IBD care   359–73
osteopenia   142
  children   264
osteoporosis   55, 142, 144–5, 388
ostomates
  clothing   211
  cultural and religious issues   211
  exercise   210–11
  pregnancy   212
  quality of life   211
  sexual issues   212
  travel   210
  work and hobbies   210
outcomes, improving   431–3

paediatric services   273–4, 281–2
pain management   342–3
parallel clinic   284
pathogenesis   21–5
pathology   71–3
pathophysiology   3–25
patient advocacy   286–90
patient education   333–52, 388
  nursing role   335–44
patient education groups   351
Patient Group Directions   406
Patient Opinion   370
patients
  access to services   350–1
  putting first   426–9
  needs   365–6, 400–1
Patient-Specific Directions   406

pelvic sepsis   188–90
perianal disease   122
personal and family relationships   299
Porto criteria   266, 268
pouchitis   187–90
pouchoscopy   188
prebiotics   149, 151
pregnancy   191–2, 212, 241–54, 263–4
  delivery   252–3
  investigations during   74, 252
  medication   247–52
  remission and   246
  surgery   252
primary care   368
primary sclerosing cholangitis   182
probiotics   149, 151
proctitis   48, 105–6
proctocolectomy
  restorative *see* ileoanal pouch
  total   166–7
psychological problems   301–4
psychological support   369
psychosocial issues   295–309, 339
pubertal delay   263
PubMed   416
pyoderma gangrenosum   52–3

QOL *see* quality of life
quality of life   192–3, 296–8

radiology   65–70
rapid access clinics   385–6
Rating Form for Inflammatory Bowel
    Disease Patients' Concerns   297
rectal bleeding   47
rectal mucus   204
rectal stump blow out   163
remission   126
  Crohn's disease   147
renal calculi   54
research   415–23
  barriers to   418–21
  conducting   418
  funding   421–2
  lack of skills   419–20
  literature   416–17
  multidisciplinary   420–1
  nurse-led   421
  publishing   422–3

reviews   416–17
review of patients   385
RFIPC *see* Rating Form for Inflammatory
      Bowel Disease Patients' Concerns
rifabutin   130
RPC *see* ileoanal pouch

scoring systems   33–4
secretions   226
seeds   148
self-management   347–51, 366–7, 388
   programmes   305
sepsis   232–5
serology tests   73
service development   332–3
setons   218
sexual function   184–5
shared care   366–7, 349–50
short bowel syndrome   151, 227
   adaptation   232
small bowel
   enteroscopy   64–5
   length   225–6
   resection   149, 151
smoking   19, 32–4
   cessation   387
   passive   33–4
social function   298–9
socioeconomic class   32
specialist nurses   359, 367–8, 375–95
specialist nursing services   397–411
   annual reports   410
   collaboration   403
   core services   405
   education   409
   income generation   409
   organisational needs   402–3
   promotion of   408–9
   protocols, policies and guidelines   403–4
   purpose of   401–3
   team vision   402
staff education   389
stoma
   accessories   206
   appliances   205–6
      leakage   212–13
   bathing and showering   209
   blockage   150
   care   201–19

complications   212–13
diet and   149, 150
discharge from hospital   209
follow-up care   209
high-output   203, 28
lifestyle adjustment   208–9
management   205–7
post-operative care   208–9
pre-operative care   204
role of nurse   204
siting of   204
sore skin   213
surgery   205
types of   202
stool tests   72–3
stress   24, 299–301
stricturing, Crohn's disease   147
stricturoplasty   174
sugar   18
sulphasalazine   318, 321
sulphides   141
support groups   185, 220, 290–1, 325–32,
      352
surgery
   children   273
   complications   163–4, 170–1, 175
   counselling   183–4
   Crohn's disease   171–7
   during pregnancy   252
   laparoscopic   161, 173, 181
   post-operative care   164–5, 171, 175
   pre-operative preparation   161, 170, 172
   rate of recovery   164
   risks   172–3
   stoma   205
   ulcerative colitis   159–71
surgical management   159–77

tacrolimus   125, 251
tagged white blood cell scan   70
telephone advice line   405–6
thalidomide   250
therapeutic goals   120
therapeutic relationship   307
therapy
   optimising   64–71
   top-down versus step-up   126–7
thioguanine   125–6
thiopurines   249

toxic megacolon   160
transition clinic   284
transition from paediatric to adult
   care   281–91
   autonomy   286–9
   education   289
   models   284
   RCN clinical pathway   287
   setting up service   285–6
   timing   289–90
Truelove and Witt's criteria   48

UC *see* ulcerative colitis
UK IBD Audit Project   303–7
ulcerative colitis   8–9
   clinical course   49–50
   clinical features in children   267
   clinical presentation   47–8
   elective surgery   165–71
   emergency surgery   159–65
   histopathology   11
   immunosuppression   131
   Montreal classification   48

non-response to medical therapy   160
   pathology   11
   pattern of   8
   remission   49
   severity   48
   surgical management   159–71
   time trends   30
ultrasound   65–6
urostomy   203

vascular factors   24–5
vegetables   148
viral infections   127

Wadhwani, Sneha   317–23
WCE *see* wireless capsule endoscopy
weight loss   84–5
wireless capsule endoscopy   64–5
World IBD Day   372

X-rays   65

zinc deficiency   143